GUIDELINES FOR WOMEN'S HEALTH CARE

SECOND EDITION

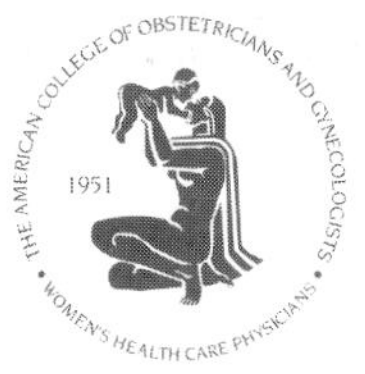

The American College of
Obstetricians and
Gynecologists
Women's Health Care Physicians
409 12th Street, SW
Washington, DC 20024–2188

Guidelines for Women's Health Care was developed under the direction of the Editorial Committee for *Guidelines for Women's Health Care* (1996–2002):

The information in *Guidelines for Women's Health Care* should not be viewed as a body of rigid rules. The guidelines are general and intended to be adapted to many different situations, taking into account the needs and resources particular to the locality, the institution, or the type of practice. Variations and innovations that improve the quality of patient care are to be encouraged rather than restricted. The purpose of these guidelines will be well served if they provide a firm basis on which local norms may be built.

Library of Congress Cataloging-in-Publication Data

Guidelines for women's health care.-- 2nd ed.
p. ; cm.
Includes bibliographical references and index.
ISBN 0-915473-76-3 (alk. paper)
1. Women's hospitals--Standards--United States. 2. Hospitals--Maternity services--Standards--United States. I. American College of Obstetricians and Gynecologists.
[DNLM: 1. Obstetrics and Gynecology Department, Hospital--standards--United States. 2. Ambulatory Care Facilities--standards--United States. 3. Gynecology--standards--United States. 4. Obstetrics--standards--United States. WP 27 AA1 G9 2002]
RG14.U6 A6 2002
362.1'98'021873--dc21

2001053863

12345/65432

CONTENTS

Preface VII

PART 1 Governance and Administration 1

Governance 3

Human Resources 13

Evaluating Credentials and Granting Privileges 31

Quality Assessment and Continuous Quality Improvement 40

Compliance with Government Regulations 50

Liability 57

Ethical Issues 62

PART 2 Organization of Services 77

Facilities and Equipment 79

Infection Control 86

Supporting Services 95

Information Management 99

Practice Management 105

PART 3 Patient Care 117

Primary and Preventive Care 121

Continuum of Women's Health Care 144

Routine Detection and Prevention of Disease **192**

Ambulatory Gynecologic Surgery **240**

PART 4 SELECTED ISSUES IN THE DELIVERY OF WOMEN'S HEALTH CARE **255**

Abnormal Genital Bleeding **257**

Abnormal Cervical Cytology **261**

Behavior Modification **266**

Breast Disorders **269**

Cholesterol **272**

Chronic Pelvic Pain **274**

Crisis Intervention **277**

Depression **279**

Domestic or Intimate Partner Violence **283**

Early Pregnancy Complications: Spontaneous Abortion and Ectopic Pregnancy **287**

Eating Disorders **291**

Endocrine Disorders **297**

Endometriosis **299**

Female Circumcision/Female Genital Mutilation **305**

Genetics **309**

Gynecologic Ultrasonography **312**

Hormone Replacement Therapy **314**

Human Immunodeficiency Virus **319**

Hypertension **321**

Immunizations **325**

Infertility **330**

Latex Allergy **336**

Neoplasms **339**

Osteoporosis and Bone Densitometry **350**

Pain Management **354**

Pediatric Gynecology 358

Pelvic Floor Dysfunction 360

Premenstrual Syndrome 362

Recurrent Pregnancy Loss 364

Sexual Assault or Rape 367

Sexual Dysfunction 370

Sexually Transmitted Diseases 372

Substance Use and Abuse: Tobacco, Alcohol, and Illegal Drugs 375

Termination of Pregnancy 382

Urinary Incontinence 386

Uterine Leiomyomata 388

Women with Disabilities 391

Appendixes

A. Code of Professional Ethics of the American College of Obstetricians and Gynecologists 397

B. Occupational Safety and Health Administration Regulations on Occupational Exposure to Bloodborne Pathogens 405

C. Clinical Laboratory Improvement Amendments of 1988 418

D. Federal Requirements for Patient Screening and Transfer 422

E. The Americans with Disabilities Act 428

F. Statement on Scope of Practice of Obstetrics and Gynecology 433

G. ACOG Woman's Health Record 434

H. Guide to Preventive Cardiology for Women 453

I. U.S. Organizations Concerned with Gynecology and Women's Health Care 469

Index 479

PREFACE

This second edition of *Guidelines for Women's Health Care* is a synopsis of policy and management issues relating to the health care of women. It was developed under the direction of the ACOG Editorial Committee for *Guidelines for Women's Health Care*, a diverse group of health professionals with representation from multiple areas: academic and private practice, nursing, and general and subspecialty medicine.

Over the past several years, the committee has reviewed information from a wide variety of sources (eg, ACOG and other nationally recognized organizations) to assemble a single volume that defines principles of health care management for diverse types of delivery systems to promote optimal health care for women. Guidelines is not intended to replace these other resources, but rather to serve as a cross-reference to them. Similarly, Guidelines does not aim to be a textbook. Many fine medical textbooks exist for the study of women's health; duplicating that information here is neither practical nor possible. The goal of Guidelines is to gather in one place administrative information and clinical pearls relevant to the practice of ambulatory and inpatient women's health care and to outline the role of obstetrician–gynecologists and other women's health care professionals. An emphasis is placed on important information that is not readily accessible in standard medical textbooks.

Guidelines is designed to serve as a resource to a wide variety of health care professionals involved in both policy making and patient care. Although some information relates specifically to obstetrician–gynecologists, most of it is relevant to all health care professionals who offer women's health care. The language of Guidelines is accordingly inclusive. *Guidelines for Women's Health Care* also will be a valuable aid to other professionals in the health care system who are not directly involved in providing patient care but who are instrumental in determining the quality and scope of that care. As an example, the information would be helpful to hospital administrators in determining hospital policy and defining the content of health care, to third-party payers in determining coverage, and to those involved in peer review and improvement activities.

Guidelines for Women's Health Care is published as a companion volume to *Guidelines for Perinatal Care*, published jointly with the American Academy of Pediatrics and now approaching its fifth edition. Although each book is developed with the aid of a separate committee, their contents are coordinated to provide a comprehensive reference to all aspects of women's health care—gynecologic, obstetric, and neonatal—with minimal duplication. The Editorial Committee for *Guidelines for Women's Health Care* notes that portions of the sections on patient transfer and patient care were originally published in *Guidelines for Perinatal Care*. The work of the Editorial Committee for *Guidelines for Perinatal Care* is gratefully acknowledged.

The content of the second edition of *Guidelines for Women's Health Care* has been extensively revised since the first edition. It is divided into four major segments: 1) Governance and Administration, 2) Organization of Services, 3) Patient Care, and 4) Selected Issues in the Delivery of Women's Health Care. In the first edition, information on health care organization and administration was covered in only one section. Recognizing the value of this information to health care professionals and administrators, the committee has greatly expanded these sections, which are now covered in Parts 1 and 2.

Part 1, Governance and Administration, focuses on the people who provide women's health care and the organizational structures through which they provide services. New to this edition is information on professional behavior, ethical issues, liability, and risk management, as well as information on patient transfer that also appears in *Guidelines for Perinatal Care*.

Part 2, Organization of Services, focuses on establishment and maintenance of the physical environment in which women's health care is delivered—both ambulatory and inpatient. This part aims to provide useful information for physicians and other health care professionals charged with establishing and maintaining a health care service, including important advice on safety considerations. New to this edition are expanded sections on safety measures, facility design, supporting services, information management, and practice management.

Part 3, Patient Care, incorporates information on patient care issues commonly faced by the generalist. Key knowledge needed to provide high-quality primary and preventive care and gynecologic surgical care is included. The section on primary and preventive care reviews recommended care throughout a woman's life span, including routine assessments. Included are screening, prevention, and counseling on gynecologic and selected other medical conditions—the information needed to provide a complete, high-quality "well-woman" examination. The section on gynecologic surgery does not aim to offer all the information found in a surgical textbook, but instead outlines key management principles for a surgical unit.

Part 4, Selected Issues in the Delivery of Women's Health Care, represents a new approach for Guidelines. This section addresses topics that may go beyond the well-woman examination or the generalist's knowledge. Policy and management issues are addressed for conditions that have a major impact on women's health such as depression, endometriosis, and abnormal genital bleeding. This part also includes information for health care professionals who wish to focus on special needs patients, for example, women with disabilities. Although this is not a comprehensive collection of health topics or a guide to day-to-day care, included are conditions and special needs that the Editorial Committee for *Guidelines for Women's Health Care* deemed to be of great concern to clinicians providing women's health care. The Editorial Committee welcomes suggestions for future topics to be included in this section.

Each part of Guidelines includes a detailed reading list for additional information. Part 4 also provides names and contact information—

including Internet addresses—for organizations that can be useful to professionals seeking to further expand their knowledge. To aid the reader, Guidelines also is extensively indexed.

Guidelines for Women's Health Care is the result of the efforts of many individuals who contributed their time and expertise. The committee wishes to extend its thanks to the following individuals:

Fredric D. Frigoletto, Jr, MD, chair of the development committee for the first edition, who shared his thoughts on new directions

Philip B. Mead, MD, for his review of the section "Infection Control" in Part 2

Peter A. Schwartz, MD, expert reviewer of the sections "Professional Behavior" and "Ethical Issues" in Part 1

Catherine Sewell, MD, contributor to the section on "Female Circumcision/Female Genital Mutilation" in Part 4

Henry A. Thiede, MD, member of this committee in the early development stages of this resource

Robert A. Wild, MD, member of this committee in the early development stages of this resource

Sandra Welner, MD, contributor to the information on women with disabilities in Parts 3 and 4

PART 1

Governance and Administration

The delivery of high-quality women's health care requires efficient systems of governance and administration that provide an organizational framework for the effective management of staff and patient care. This part provides guidance for the establishment of systems of governance, human resources, credentialing, quality improvement, regulatory compliance, liability, and ethics that offer a blueprint for quality women's health care services regardless of setting.

GOVERNANCE

In order to provide effective and efficient women's health care, a well-defined organizational structure must be in place. The structure will facilitate the organization's compliance with operational, regulatory, risk management, and ethical guidelines. This part will provide a framework for addressing these issues. Although organizational structure tends to be thought of as only applying to hospitals, all facilities providing women's health care need a clearly delineated structure. In many cases, the structure of the department of obstetrics and gynecology may serve as a model for other facilities, such as ambulatory surgical centers and offices.

The Department of Obstetrics and Gynecology

Open communication and a collegial approach to problem solving facilitate the growth and development of obstetric and gynecologic services within an institution—enabling it to better meet the needs of the community. Institutional administration and departmental leadership should strive to maintain such an approach in the management of these services.

The departmental organization should fulfill the following functions:

- Clarify issues of accountability
- Provide departmental representation in institutional policy-making decisions
- Provide a system of governance for clinicians providing obstetric and gynecologic services within an institution
- Provide a forum that fosters collaborative practice with other disciplines engaged in the care of women (eg, certified nurse–midwives [CNMs], nurses, technicians, therapists, clergy and others providing spiritual support, support personnel, clerical workers, and administrators)

The ultimate goal of the organization of a department of obstetrics and gynecology is to provide a mechanism that ensures the best possible patient care and treatment outcome. Each aspect of the department's structure and function should be directed toward that goal.

A department of obstetrics and gynecology should be organized as an independent department. In addition to the provision of quality patient care, the organization of the department should encompass concerns about cost, liability, fair treatment of departmental members, and the department's responsibilities to the institution as a whole. It should take into consideration educational and research responsibilities, including teaching services where applicable, as well as regulatory and cost-containment mechanisms and the need to maintain a relationship with the community. A sound organizational plan encourages both the prevention of problems and continuous quality improvement. It should include processes for the early identification of problems and fair and legally defensible mechanisms to address them. A department's structure should be evaluated in terms of improving the outcome of patient care.

The responsibilities of the department of obstetrics and gynecology are delegated by the institution's governing bodies. The responsibilities of each member of the department and the authority to carry out those responsibilities should be clearly delineated. All those who receive privileges in a department should be subject to the policies and procedures of that department and should respect them.

The size and type of institution, together with the bylaws of the medical staff, determine the type of organization appropriate for the department of obstetrics and gynecology. The organizational needs of a department in an institution devoted exclusively to patient care may differ in many details from those of a department in another institution with teaching and research responsibilities. Regardless, there are some basic components and key alliances that provide an organizational approach to quality patient care.

Officers

Each department should have a designated head or chair who may be either elected or appointed. That individual should be chosen on the basis of professional ability, experience, and commitment to continued improvement of patient care. Because not all members of a department are likely to have these attributes, it is not recommended that the position be rotated among all attending staff members. Also to be discouraged are short terms of office (eg, 1 year). Rotations of 3–5 years allow the department head adequate time to establish and implement plans for departmental improvement. If a term of office for department chair exceeds 5 years, it is recommended that an independent committee, which may include members of the medical staff and governing board, periodically review the appointment to ensure that administrative performance is optimal.

The responsibilities and the authority of the department head should be defined in writing by the medical staff and institution administration. They should be consistent with the general structure of the medical staff bylaws and other accepted external standards established for such facilities. Responsibilities of the department head generally include the following:

- Make recommendations on the appointment, reappointment, promotion, or suspension of staff who have been granted clinical privileges
- Make recommendations on the granting or withdrawal of privileges in the department as required in the bylaws
- Periodically evaluate in writing the professional performance of each member of the department and retain the documents in a confidential manner
- Provide a system whereby substandard performance of any departmental member can be identified and corrected
- Develop, institute, and oversee the quality assessment and quality improvement programs for the department
- Integrate the department's quality assessment and improvement activities with those of the institution
- Establish committees with clear charges regarding purpose, tenure, and reporting responsibilities; appoint members of the department to departmental committees; and either appoint the committee chairs or provide a mechanism for their election

- Recommend/approve members of the department for appointment to institutional committees
- Provide a continuing education program for departmental members and maintain records of attendance
- Establish and monitor policies, procedures, and protocols for patient care in collaboration with other professional health care practitioners, when appropriate
- Serve as a consultant or arbitrator for unresolved differences of opinion regarding patient care or questions of policy
- Make recommendations regarding policies for any obstetric or gynecologic care needed by patients admitted to other services for other diseases
- Establish responsibilities of all health care practitioners for teaching and patient care and prepare a schedule of assignments
- When responsible for medical student or resident education, ensure that standards for content, quality, and needs for supervision are met in accordance with the Liaison Committee for Medical Education and the Accreditation Council for Graduate Medical Education
- Serve as a voting representative of the department on the medical staff executive committee
- Participate in any institutional planning for further development or changes that may affect the department

The department head should have a strong influence on the development of policies and procedures within the department. Members of the department should be involved in the formulation of these policies to strengthen their commitment to quality patient care. A consensus should be achieved on these policies, and they should apply to all members of the department. Mechanisms by which these policies are formally adopted and reported should be established. When decisions made within the department of obstetrics and gynecology have an effect on other departments, on patients of other departments, or on the institution as a whole, those departments should be consulted and their concurrence obtained.

If there is a department staff fund, it is necessary to maintain accurate records of the use of that fund and to obtain an external audit at least annually. If the fund's size justifies it, a treasurer may be elected or a departmental advisory committee can be made responsible for overseeing it. Access to and management and disbursement of department funds must conform to the standards set by the department, the institution, and generally accepted accounting principles.

Committees

The purpose of committees is to address specific issues relating to patient care. The extent to which a department will have committees for certain functions will depend on the size and complexity of the institution and the department. In some instances, the institution's organizational structure may fill some of those needs and require only departmental participation. When an institution-wide committee performs any of these functions, the department of obstetrics and gynecology should have active membership on that committee.

The department head should be familiar with the institution's committee structure. The department of obstetrics and gynecology should be represented on committees making decisions that have substantial effects on patient care within the department. Other institutional committees are vitally important to issues of quality of care (see box). The department of obstetrics and gynecology should participate in these committee activities. Representatives to these committees should report on their activities and interpret their importance to the other members of the department.

All the department members should be strongly encouraged to participate in the responsibilities of the department, including serving on committees. Such involvement encourages interest and a better understanding among the members. Assignments are usually made by the department head and should be specific in terms of responsibility, authority, tenure, expectations, and reporting requirements. Committee activities should focus on assessment of the quality of both gynecologic and obstetric patient care through a variety of mechanisms: maternal, perinatal, and gynecologic morbidity and mortality review, tissue review, clinical indica-

Items for Quality Assessment

The institutional governance structure should ensure at a minimum the ongoing function of at least the following activities:

- Medical staff credentials review
- Reappraisal and reappointment
- Medical records review
- Bylaws/rules and regulations review
- Quality improvement
- Infection and environmental control evaluation
- Pharmacy and therapeutics control
- Laser safety control
- Risk management review
- Hospital admission/complications review
- Continuing education and performance standards review of all members of the health care team
- Operating room/tissue review
- Ethics review

tors, medical review criteria, or other measurable standards. These reviews should be directed toward identifying and correcting problems as well as seeking opportunities for implementing continued improvement in the quality of care.

Committees may be ad hoc or standing. Ad hoc committees are established for a limited purpose and a limited duration. Standing committees are required to carry out basic departmental functions. The department head should appoint members of ad hoc committees. These committees should have the broadest representation possible to include those who might be affected and those who can contribute. An ad hoc committee should have a specific charge and should be given specific time requirements for reporting. When the committee has achieved its goal and submitted its report, it should be formally discontinued unless there is a compelling reason to continue its function or to convert it to a standing committee.

In departments with large numbers of staff members, an executive or advisory committee is desirable to expedite the decision-making process and to provide for staff representation. When the staff is made up of full-time, part-time, and volunteer personnel, each component may be represented on the committee as deemed appropriate.

Meetings

Regular meetings and conferences of the department should be held, and a level of acceptable attendance for continued maintenance of privileges should be established. The number and complexity of these meetings will vary with the size and intricacy of the department. They should include administrative meetings so that needs, changes, or problems within the department can be discussed either for information or for advice. Reports from the various committees should be made on a regular basis and minutes maintained, including summations of quality assessment and risk management. Written minutes of department meetings are essential, both to provide continuity in the activities of the department and to keep the medical staff administration informed. Meetings or activities relating to quality assessment may have legal protection under state or federal laws and should conform to those requirements. Legal counsel should be sought in establishing and maintaining such committees. Records of such activities should be kept confidential and separate from the business minutes of the department. An agenda should be established before each meeting, and a summary of the minutes should be sent to all members. Certain issues, such as those relating to quality assessment, risk management, or personnel matters, should be handled in a sensitive and confidential manner.

In addition to regular meetings of the department, conferences should be held. These should include continuing educational activities provided either by the members of the institution or by visiting lecturers. Such activities create an opportunity to address issues identified in the quality assessment process. Educational conferences can provide an open forum for discussion of patient management that is thought to be suboptimal. These conferences also are opportunities for members of the administration or other clinical disciplines to share information with the attending staff of the department of obstetrics and gynecology.

Education and Research

Education is of key importance in all institutions. The medical staff and other health care practitioners achieved their degrees, certifications, and licensure through formal education processes. Maintaining and updating these skills and knowledge also require education. It is a responsibility of the institution and each department to have an organized educational program appropriate to its needs. The medical and nursing staff providing gynecologic care at any level should become knowledgeable about current gynecologic care through joint in-service sessions. Such educational programs should be sensitive and responsive to any deficiencies identified by either the institutional or departmental quality assessment and improvement programs. They also should consider the needs created by the introduction of new technology or treatment methods.

An educational program provides the opportunity to exchange useful information with others, including clinical departments, risk management programs, the ethics committee, or guest speakers. The sponsorship of guest speakers should be reviewed to avoid any actual or implied impropriety by linking program financing to sales of drugs or equipment (see the discussion of conflict of interest in "Human Resources" in Part 1).

Only certain institutions have active research programs. Most of these are teaching hospitals, which also offer residency programs for specialty training. Research experience is a special requirement for residents as defined by the Residency Review Committee for Obstetrics–Gynecology. When research is clinical in nature and affects patients, institutional rules should be in place to protect the welfare of each patient. In general, this function is best served by an institutional review board (IRB), which reviews research proposals and has the authority to approve or reject them based on their implications for patients' rights and safety. The IRB should have written policies that are consistent with federal guidelines. Its members should be selected to reflect expertise in science, ethics, and the sensitivities of the community. Research that affects patients must not be done without such review and written approval. Further information about IRBs is found in "Ethical Issues" in Part 1.

Ambulatory Surgical Facilities

A freestanding ambulatory care surgical facility should have a governing body, similar to a hospital's board of trustees, that has final authority and responsibility for patient care, facilities, services, appointment of the medical staff, and delineation of clinical privileges. A mechanism similar to that used in a hospital must be established for granting privileges. A hospital-based facility usually functions under the hospital's governing body, and hospital regulations determine the staff privileges granted in such a facility. If obstetric–gynecologic services are provided, obstetrician–gynecologists should be included in the process of developing policies related to overall operations, quality assessment activities, and patient care. Physicians should check state and federal laws and regulations on self-referral prohibitions before referring a patient for health care services in which the physician or a member of the physician's immediate family has a financial interest. These laws and regulations continue to evolve, and current requirements should be reviewed (see also "Human Resources" in Part 1).

Offices

Regular office staff meetings should be held for all office staff. These meetings can be useful in improving staff communication and in exploring ways to enhance patient relations and communications. The office staff meeting is the ideal setting to discuss quality assessment issues and risk management and to provide continuing medical education for both clinical and nonclinical staff members. Staff should be encouraged to make suggestions for improving office procedures.

Office staff should be reminded periodically of the need for maintaining strict confidentiality of all patient contacts, treatment, and records. A written personnel policy should exist that states that any violation of patient confidentiality is grounds for employee dismissal. Offices also should establish policies on sexual harassment and make all personnel aware of them (see "Human Resources" in Part 1). There should be a discussion with staff on the importance of considering chaperons when either male or female health care practitioners perform pelvic or breast examinations (see "Human Resources" in Part 1).

SUGGESTED READING

1999 Accreditation handbook for ambulatory health care. Skokie, Illinois: Accreditation Association for Ambulatory Health Care, Inc, 1999

American College of Obstetricians and Gynecologists. Code of professional ethics of the American College of Obstetricians and Gynecologists. Washington, DC: ACOG, 2002

American College of Obstetricians and Gynecologists. Guidelines for relationships with industry. In: Ethics in obstetrics and gynecology. Washington, DC: ACOG, 2002:40–42

American College of Obstetricians and Gynecologists. Quality improvement in women's health care. Rev. ed. Washington, DC: ACOG, 2000

Joint Commission on Accreditation of Health Care Organizations. Comprehensive accreditation manual for hospitals: the official handbook. Oakbrook Terrace, Illinois: JCAHO, 2000

Joint Commission on Accreditation of Healthcare Organizations. 2000–2001 comprehensive accreditation manual for ambulatory care. Oakbrook Terrace, Illinois: JCAHO, 1999

Human Resources

The successful delivery of women's health care depends on the people directly and indirectly involved with providing that care. For this reason, issues of human resources management must be addressed at all levels of health care delivery, including health systems, hospitals, surgical centers, and offices.

Human resources encompasses practical matters of hiring, managing and evaluating, and—when necessary—terminating staff. Equally important, however, is an understanding of the principles that drive these personnel management decisions and an understanding of what constitutes professional and unprofessional behavior. Human resources issues vary depending on the type of institution, scope of practice, union regulations, and staff needs.

Personnel

Regardless of the setting of delivery of health care services, certain elements constitute effective personnel management. Written job descriptions should exist for each staff position, and these descriptions should be reviewed periodically to be certain that staff members are not performing tasks beyond their licensing or training. Written policies indicating specific responsibilities and outlining a plan for continuing education of personnel should be prepared, approved by the medical staff, and reviewed periodically. Previous employment references should be checked for all new employees. Current licensure verification is mandatory for all licensed personnel. A system for accreditation of personnel should be in place and reviewed at least biennially (see "Evaluating Credentials and Granting Privileges" in Part 1).

The human resources operations in health care institutions are governed by the policies and procedures of that institution. The leadership of the women's health component should have extensive knowledge of and, ideally, a collegial working relationship with the overarching institutional human resources unit.

At the office practice level, human resource needs also must be addressed. An office-based medical practice or clinic should have an office manager or other key staff person assigned to personnel management. A personnel manual should be established for the entire office staff. Issues of preemployment screening, benefits, employee assistance programs, and performance reviews should be considered for inclusion in the manual.

Professional Behavior

It is vitally important in providing health care services that all staff be aware of what constitutes professional and unprofessional behavior. Such behavior can be outlined in codes of ethics, such as those developed by the American Medical Association (AMA) and the American College of Obstetricians and Gynecologists (ACOG). Institutions also may summarize the behavior expected of their staff in a personnel manual or similar guide.

Certain situations in the practice of women's health care merit special attention from an ethical perspective and are addressed here. Institutional ethics committees, when available, are valuable resources in determining the appropriate resolution of these and other situations (see "Ethical Issues" in Part 1).

Code of Professional Ethics of the American College of Obstetricians and Gynecologists

Obstetrician–gynecologists (and other clinicians caring for women) have ethical responsibilities to patients, society, and other health care professionals. The American College of Obstetricians and Gynecologists has developed a "Code of Professional Ethics" to provide guidance to its obstetrician–gynecologist Fellows (see Appendix A). Many of the ethical considerations described also apply to other health care professionals providing care to women.

This code of ethics describes the ethical foundations for professional activities in women's health care and summarizes the rules of ethical conduct built on these foundations. Noncompliance with this code may affect an individual's initial or continuing Fellowship in ACOG.

Confidentiality

Clinicians providing women's health care should respect the rights of patients, colleagues, and others and safeguard patient information and confidences within the limits of the law. Patient information ordinarily may not be revealed to others without the patient's express consent. Maintaining confidentiality is intrinsic to respect for patient autonomy and promotes the free exchange of information between patient and physician relevant to medical decision making (see "Ethical Issues" in Part 1 for a more detailed discussion of the ethical principle of autonomy and the ethical concept of confidentiality). Additionally, in certain situations, maintaining confidentiality is critical to ensuring a woman's safety from retaliatory actions by an abusive family member or partner. Institutions should have policies in place to safeguard patient information from inadvertent or inappropriate deliberate breaches of confidentiality. In addition, jurisdictions vary in their laws and regulations regarding reporting, disclosure, and breach of confidence. For example, the results of human immunodeficiency virus (HIV) testing may need to be recorded and stored in a certain way. Clinicians should become familiar with the legal requirements that exist in their communities.

In the past decade, there has been exponential growth in the variety of methods of communication. Patient information may be stored not only on a paper record but also electronically. It is exchanged over the telephone (including wireless cellular telephones), facsimile machines, and e-mail. Regardless of how a patient's health information is stored or exchanged, the same ethical principles of confidentiality apply.

Tests which may have multiple medical or psychosocial ramifications require comprehensive explanation of the process, goals, and implications. When such a test is recommended, the patient should be informed of pertinent policies regarding the use of information resulting from the test and the legal requirements relating to the release of information before she grants her consent. She should be aware of what information might be communicated and to whom and the potential implications of reporting the information.

Situations may arise in which a clinician has competing obligations: on the one hand to protect the patient's confidentiality and on the other to disclose test results to prevent harm to a third party. In these situations, the clinician should first explore every avenue of communication in discussions with the patient about rights and responsibilities. Consultation with an institutional ethics committee or a medical ethics specialist may be helpful in deciding whether or not to disclose the information. It may be prudent to seek legal advice.

In some situations, a violation of confidentiality may be appropriate. This may be justifiable only when it is required by law or when 1) there is a high probability of harm to a third party, 2) the potential harm is a serious one, 3) the information communicated can be used to prevent harm, and 4) greater good will result from breaking confidentiality than from maintaining it.

When a breach of confidence is contemplated, practitioners should be aware of other detrimental effects on the patient and on society at large if confidentiality is breached. In the case of breaching confidentiality about HIV seropositive status, for example, two other significant factors should be considered:

- There are personal risks to the individual whose confidence is breached. These include serious implications for the person's relationship with family and friends, the threat of discrimination in employment and housing, and the impact on family members.
- Loss of patient trust may reduce the physician's ability to help the individual patient and may deter other women at risk who are considering being tested. This latter result would have a serious negative impact on the educational efforts that lie at the heart of attempts to reduce the spread of disease.

If, on balance, a breach of confidence is deemed appropriate, practitioners should consider whether the goal of maintaining patient privacy would be better served by personal communication with the individual at risk or by notification of local public health authorities. In some areas, anonymous notification of contacts is possible.

A major obstacle to the delivery of health care to adolescents is concern about confidentiality. Although ensuring confidentiality is relatively simple when providing services to adults, providing the same degree of confidentiality to adolescents can be less straightforward. The legal status of a minor, requirements for parental consent before the provision of medical services, and economic considerations often encumber the physician–patient relationship.

Clinicians who care for adolescents should be familiar with current state statutes on the rights of minors to consent to health care services, as well as those laws that affect confidentiality. All states require consent for the treatment of a minor from a person legally entitled to authorize such care. Exceptions to this requirement for consent exist, however, and in these cases adolescents generally have the right to prevent clinicians from disclosing information about the care they receive. Examples of such exceptions include the following:

- Emergencies, when immediate treatment is needed to safeguard the life or health of the adolescent
- Treatment of "emancipated minors," including those who are married, those who are members of the armed forces, those who live apart from their parents and are self-supporting, and those who are themselves parents
- Statutes allowing minors to consent to at least some specific health care services, such as contraceptive services, prenatal care and delivery, sexually transmissible infection services, HIV testing and treatment, treatment of drug and alcohol abuse, and mental health treatment. These laws exist in all states and may specify the age at which a minor can begin to consent to such care.

Courts have increasingly recognized the growing independence of minors and the seriousness of their health care needs. Case law in some jurisdictions has established the right of a "mature minor" to consent to some forms of health care without prior parental consent. A mature minor is generally defined as an adolescent younger than the age of majority—set at 18 years in most states—who, although living at home as a dependent, demonstrates the cognitive maturity to give informed consent. When deciding whether to accept a mature minor as a patient, clinicians should evaluate their personal views. If their own views on confidentiality would restrict the provision of services to a minor, the patient should be referred to another caregiver whose personal views do not conflict with the provision of such services.

Adolescent confidentiality also may be compromised by economic considerations, because few adolescents have the ability to pay for health care services without the aid of a parent or other adult. Moreover, explanation of benefits forms issued by insurers are sent to parent policyholders, which also could compromise the confidentiality of care received by adolescents.

Clinicians should discuss confidentiality with the adolescent and, where appropriate, with her parent(s) or guardian(s). They should be informed that they each have a private and privileged relationship with the clinician and should be informed of any restrictions on confidentiality. For example, it should be explained that if the adolescent discloses any risk of significant bodily harm to herself or others, the clinician will breach confidentiality. In addition, state laws mandate the reporting of physical or sexual abuse of minors. The goal is to encourage and facilitate family communication; maintaining confidentiality need not preclude working toward this goal.

Chaperons

Local practices and expectations differ with regard to the use of chaperons, but the presence of a third person in the room during the physical examination can confer benefits for both the patient and the clinician, regardless of the gender of the chaperon. Chaperons can provide reassurance to the patient about the professional context and content of the examination and the intention of the clinician and offer witness to the actual events taking place should there be any misunderstanding. The request by either a patient or a health care practitioner to have a chaperon present during a physical examination should be accommodated irrespective of the health care practitioner's gender.

The presence of a third party in the room may, however, cause some embarrassment to the patient and limit her willingness to talk openly with the clinician. If a chaperon is present, the clinician should provide a separate opportunity for private conversation. If the chaperon is an employee of the practice, the clinician must establish clear rules about respect for privacy and confidentiality. In addition, some patients (especially, but not limited to, adolescents) may consider the presence of a family member as an intrusion. Family members should not be used as chaperons unless specifically requested by the patient.

Referral

Relationships with other health care professionals should reflect fairness, honesty, and integrity, sharing a mutual respect and concern for the patient. Clinicians often may best fulfill their obligations to patients through referral to other professionals who have the appropriate skills and expertise to address the situation. Therefore, they should consult, refer, or cooperate with other health care professionals and institutions to the extent necessary to serve the best interests of their patients.

With respect to referrals, the role of the referring clinician is to identify the most appropriate resources. Referrals—whether medical, psychologic, or social—carry with them the ethical obligation to investigate the skills and credentials of the consultant. As with other potential conflicts of interest, physicians should be aware of how their referring relationships could be construed as being inappropriate or might be prohibited by state and federal law.

In the current health care climate, however, clinicians may find barriers to making the referrals they deem appropriate. Managed care plans may, for example, prohibit obstetrician–gynecologists or other clinicians from making referrals for such services as surgical consultation following abnormal mammography or dermatology consultation for skin disorders. In other cases, referrals must be made to a narrowly defined panel of specialists. Women who have relied on their obstetrician–gynecologists for referrals may find their access to specialized services impeded. Clinicians who believe that a patient's health is jeopardized by these policies are obligated to appeal to the plan or medical director (see "Conflict of Interest" in this section).

It is in everyone's best interest—practitioners with primary clinical responsibility, consultants, patients, and health care plans—that the criteria for consultation be mutually agreed on in advance and stated clearly in writing. Open communication and established professional relationships facilitate effective consultation and referral. However, at times a consultant may be called on unexpectedly, inconveniently, and sometimes inappropriately to be involved in or to assume the care of a patient. In these situations, a physician is only obligated to provide consultation or assume the care of the patient if there is a contractual agreement or a preexisting patient–physician relationship or if there is a severe medical emergency in which there is no reasonably available alternative caregiver. Hospital or departmental guidelines for consultation and referral may prevent such confrontations.

Expert Witnesses

Clinicians have a continuing responsibility to society as a whole and should support and participate in activities that enhance the community. As professionals and members of medical or nursing societies, they are required to uphold the dignity and honor of their professions. One way health care professionals can do this is through serving as expert witnesses on behalf of defendants, the government, or plaintiffs.

The moral and legal duty of health care professionals who testify before a court of law is to do so in accordance with their expertise. This duty implies adherence to the strictest personal and professional ethics. Truthfulness is essential. Misrepresentation of one's personal clinical opinion as an absolute right or wrong may be harmful to individual parties and to the profession at large.

Health care professionals who serve as expert witnesses should have experience and knowledge in the areas of clinical medicine that enable them to testify about the standards of care that applied at the time of the occurrence that is the subject of the legal action. Their review of the facts should be thorough, fair, and impartial and should not exclude any relevant information. It should not be biased in favor of the defendant, the plaintiff, or the government. The role of an expert witness should be to provide testimony that is complete, objective, and helpful to a just resolution of the proceeding.

Testimony should evaluate performance in light of generally accepted standards, neither condemning performance that falls within generally accepted standards nor endorsing or condoning performance that falls below these standards. The expert witness should clearly distinguish between medical malpractice and medical maloccurrence and should make every effort to assess the relationship of the alleged substandard practice to the outcome. Deviation from a practice standard is not always substandard care or causally related to a bad outcome. Expert witnesses should be prepared to have testimony they have given in any judicial proceeding subjected to peer review by an institution or professional organization to which they belong.

The acceptance of fees for testifying that are greatly disproportionate to those customary for professional services can be construed as influencing the testimony given by the witness. It is clearly unethical for health care professionals to accept compensation that is contingent on the outcome of litigation.

Impaired Clinicians

Physicians and advanced practice health care clinicians are considered "impaired" when their ability to practice is impaired by chemical dependency or inappropriate personal conduct. Many states have laws requiring health care practitioners to report to the state medical or nursing licensing board a physician or advanced practice health care clinician who is reasonably believed to be guilty of prohibited conduct. Those actions to be reported include but are not limited to impairment by alcohol, drugs, physical disability, or mental instability as well as practice misconduct or practicing medicine fraudulently or with gross incompetence or gross negligence. The institution's legal counsel should have information on the individual state's "duty to report" laws, and departmental members should be aware of the content of these laws.

Signs of impairment include behavior changes such as decreasing quality of record keeping, frequent absences, unexplained isolation from the staff, and suspicious prescribing habits. The failure of a colleague to take action or any action taken to shield the impaired clinician from disclosure can result in serious consequences for those who should have recognized the situation. The reluctance of a colleague to become involved is understandable. It is necessary, however, to obtain as much specific and well-documented evidence of the impairment as is reasonable. Rather than having a single individual confront the impaired practitioner, it is better that a group of respected peers accept this responsibility. A representative of the county or state medical society impaired physician program, when such a program is available, and a family member, if practical, should be included in the process. The impaired practitioner should be approached in a nonjudgmental manner. These techniques are more likely to result in an admission of impairment by the health care clinician. Less direct efforts are more likely to result in denial. When facing an impaired health care practitioner, one should address the following questions:

- Is there evidence of impaired ability to practice?
- Is there imminent danger to patients?
- Is there a history of previous treatment for impairment?
- Is the practitioner motivated to enter a treatment program for impairment?

An impaired health care practitioner should be obligated to enter a treatment program, taking into account state legal requirements, the requirements of the state licensure board, and the preferences of the impaired practitioner. State and local medical societies are valuable sources of information regarding both the evaluation and the treatment of impaired health care practitioners. In many states, the health care practitioner is provided protection from disciplinary action and confidentiality is assured. Such protection usually is withdrawn if the practitioner refuses to cooperate or does not follow treatment plans. Obviously there is considerable advantage to the impaired practitioner, the practitioner's family, the department, the medical staff, the institution, and the public when a colleague's suspicion leads to early identification and successful rehabilitation. Guidelines on what should be covered in an institutional policy on reporting and investigating suspected impairment have been published by the AMA.

The voluntary entrance of an impaired practitioner into a rehabilitation program is not reportable to the National Practitioner Data Bank (NPDB) if no professional review action was taken and the practitioner did not relinquish clinical privileges. Furthermore, when a health care practitioner takes a leave of absence and clinical privileges have not been taken away, no report to the NPDB is required. However, if a professional review action requires an impaired physician to enter a rehabilitation program involuntarily, that review action is reportable to the NPDB if it is based on the physician's competence or professional conduct and adversely affects the physician's clinical privileges for more than 30 days.

Most state medical societies have a committee on physicians' health serving as an advocate and referral resource for physicians at risk for alcohol and drug dependence. For example, in one such program administered by a medical society, the committee on physicians' health enters into a contract with the physician in need of rehabilitation to guide treatment resources and provide documentation of recovery and freedom from substance abuse. The contract is for a 3-year period and can be extended. Two health care practitioners serve as a team to monitor the progress of therapy. Under the terms of the contract, the physician must fulfill the following obligations:

- Be in regular contact with the team
- Identify his or her primary care physician
- Identify the person or facility chosen for the evaluation and supervision of treatment
- Identify the continuing after-care activities or support group, including meetings to be attended and the frequency of attendance
- Submit to regular urine screens for chemical abuse or identify a monitor who will attest daily to sobriety

- Agree to make the department head or other responsible person aware of the problem and to provide reports to the committee on physicians' health

Practitioners who have developed a degree of chemical dependency or inappropriate behavior that causes stress within their families and in their personal lives but has not impaired their medical practice are considered to be "troubled." A colleague's ability to identify a health care practitioner in this state carries with it the responsibility to make an effort to be of help personally or to guide the individual to competent help. Ignoring the issue is a disservice to the affected practitioner and is a dereliction of duty by the practitioner.

Other personal, medical, or family problems may negatively affect a practitioner's professional function. Such problems are not ordinarily included under the term "impaired practitioner;" nevertheless, they cannot be ignored. The department head or other responsible person should be informed and should consult personally with the health care practitioner involved.

Communicable Diseases

Another factor that may impair a clinician's ability to practice is the presence of a communicable disease. The welfare of the patient is central to all considerations in the patient–clinician relationship. Chief among the clinician's responsibilities is to "first, do no harm."

For this reason, health care professionals should seek to avoid contracting infectious diseases by availing themselves of recommended immunizations (see the recommendations in "Primary and Preventive Care" in Part 3) and following standard precautions for patient care. Although it appears that surgeons who follow recommended infection-control procedures are at little risk of acquiring HIV while caring for HIV-infected patients, surgeons readily can acquire hepatitis B virus (HBV) from infected patients. The risk of acquiring hepatitis C virus (HCV) appears to be lower than the risk of acquiring HBV and higher than the risk of acquiring HIV.

Health care professionals who have reason to believe that they are infected with HIV or other serious infectious agents that might be communicated to patients should be tested voluntarily for the protection of their patients. Surgeons who perform invasive procedures and who do not have evidence of immunity to HBV should know their hepatitis B surface antigen status and, if it is positive, they also should know their hepatitis B e antigen status. Surgeons who perform exposure-prone procedures should consider being tested for the anti-HCV antibody and, if positive, should confirm seropositivity status by documenting HCV RNA in the serum with reverse transcription polymerase chain reaction testing. Institutional and local health department rules usually are available to guide health care workers who test positive for bloodborne viruses.

Each HIV-positive physician must make a decision as to which procedures he or she can continue to perform safely. This decision will depend on the physician's level of expertise, the particular surgical techniques involved, and the physician's medical condition, including mental status. There are aspects of obstetrics and gynecology that do not involve measurable risk of transmission of infection. Some patient care activities, however, such as surgery and obstetric deliveries, may involve some potential exchange of bodily fluids. The decision should be made in conjunction with such responsible individuals as his or her personal physician, the chief of the department, the hospital's director of infectious diseases, the chief of the medical staff, or with a specialized advisory panel.

Physicians who are infected with HIV should follow standard precautions. They also should comply with current guidelines for disinfection and sterilization of reusable devices used in invasive procedures.

Conflict of Interest

Potential conflicts of interest are inherent to the practice of medicine. Clinicians are expected to recognize these and resolve them according to the patient's best interest, respecting her autonomy. If there is concern about a possibly significant conflict of interest, the clinician should disclose his or her concerns to the patient. To aid in resolving these concerns, consultation with colleagues or an institutional ethics committee may be sought. If a conflict of interest cannot be resolved, the clinician should take steps to withdraw from the care of the patient.

Today, clinicians find themselves caught between the health care industry—which urges the use of its procedures and products—and managed care organizations—which may seek to limit the care that is provided. Both can present conflicts of interest.

Clinicians should choose diagnostic procedures and treatments on the basis of medical considerations and patient needs, regardless of any direct or indirect interest that they may have in the health care industry or any benefits they receive from industry. Advertising or product marketing must not influence a clinician's accuracy, completeness, or balanced presentation of medical advice to patients. Clinicians have an obligation to go beyond the information provided through such promotional strategies in selecting the most appropriate care for the patient. When any product promotion leads to inappropriate or unbalanced medical advice or recommendations to patients, an ethical problem exists.

Promotions that involve the provision of gifts, parties, trips, or services must be assumed to aim to create both a sense of obligation and attitudes or practices that favor the donor. This may result in a real or perceived conflict of interest for the recipient, whether it is an individual clinician or an institution. Such ethical conflicts can interfere with patient care and are not in keeping with standards of professional behavior. In certain situations, however, the acceptance of gifts is ethical—for example, gifts that primarily entail a benefit to patients and are not of substantial value (eg, textbooks, modest meals). Gifts should not be accepted if conditions or obligations are attached (eg, gifts given in relation to prescribing practices), and no cash payments should be accepted.

The American Medical Association and the Accreditation Council for Continuing Medical Education have developed guidelines for relationships with industry as they pertain to the support of educational programs. Industry subsidies to underwrite the costs of continuing medical education conferences or professional meetings can contribute to the improvement of patient care and are permissible. However, control over the selection of content, faculty, educational methods, and materials should belong to the organizers of the conference. Presentations must give a balanced view of all therapeutic options. Use of generic names will contribute to this impartiality. If trade names are used, those of several companies should be used rather than only those of a single company. Subsidies may not be used to pay for the costs of travel, lodging, or other personal expenses of clinicians who are attending the conferences, nor should subsidies be accepted to compensate for the clinician's time.

An area of contemporary and growing concern is the patenting of medical procedures. In addition to raising problems of efficacy and safety, the patenting of medical procedures may jeopardize patients' interests by delaying the rapid transmission of new scientific knowledge and adding costs to a procedure that might put it out of reach of patients. Academic health care professionals should be aware of the powerful incentives placed on them by their universities to maximize extramural revenues and should urge that such policies not encourage the patenting of procedures.

The shift to managed care also has created potential conflicts of interest for women's health care professionals. Clinicians have an obligation to serve as patient advocates to ensure that patients receive appropriate medical care. As noted previously in this section, those who believe, based on clinical evidence, that a patient's health is jeopardized by the policies, coverage limits, or utilization restrictions of a plan are obligated in their role as patient advocates to appeal to the plan or medical director. To ensure that a health plan's policies do not endanger patient welfare, health care professionals should become actively involved with the policy-making boards of managed care plans in which they participate and should contribute to the quality improvement processes that result in plan guidelines. They should refuse to participate in managed care arrangements with unethical policies.

Billing Fraud

To avoid problems with billing, practitioners should thoroughly understand billing and coding requirements or have staff on whom they can rely for this expertise (see "Practice Management" in Part 2). Even honest mistakes have caused clinicians difficulties in this area. Dishonest billing is illegal under most circumstances and is an abdication of the clinician's responsibilities to society. This is true even when deceptive practices are meant to benefit the patient. For example, clinicians may be tempted to add a covered diagnostic category to patient information so that the patient may receive treatment that is believed to be necessary but is not covered. However well intentioned such strategies may be, they introduce dishonesty into the practitioner–patient relationship.

Sexual Harassment

Sexual harassment is a form of sex discrimination prohibited under Title VII of the Civil Rights Act of 1964. Unwelcome sexual advances, requests for sexual favors, and other verbal or physical conduct of a sexual nature constitutes sexual harassment. In one of its publications, the AMA states that the following conditions apply to sexual harassment:

- Submission to such conduct is made either explicitly or implicitly a term or condition of an individual's employment or academic success.
- Submission to or rejection of such conduct by an individual is used as the basis for employment or academic decisions affecting such individuals.
- Such conduct has the purpose or effect of unreasonably interfering with an individual's work or academic performance or creating an intimidating, hostile, or offensive working environment.

Both men and women can be victims of sexual harassment. Institutions and other facilities should have policies on sexual harassment that are known to all personnel and should offer guidance for employees and supervisors on reporting and following up complaints.

Sexual Misconduct

The practice of obstetrics and gynecology includes interaction at times of intense emotion and vulnerability for the patient and involves both sensitive physical examinations and medically necessary disclosure of especially private information about symptoms and experiences. Children and adolescents are particularly vulnerable to emotional conflict and damage to their developing sense of identity and sexuality when roles and role boundaries with trusted adults are confused. It is essential to ensure privacy, particularly the young person's privacy, and to prevent subtly coercive violations from occurring (see "Confidentiality" in this section).

Sexual misconduct is not a new issue in the practice of medicine. It has been reevaluated in terms of current medical ethics to give additional consideration to respect for the rights of individuals, the unusual power relationship between a professional and a patient, and the potential for abuse of that power.

The American College of Obstetricians and Gynecologists' Committee on Ethics agrees with the AMA's Council on Ethical and Judicial Affairs statement on this issue:

> *Sexual contact that occurs concurrent with the physician–patient relationship constitutes sexual misconduct. Sexual or romantic interactions between physicians and patients detract from the goals of the physician–patient relationship, may exploit the vulnerability of the patient, may obscure the physician's objective judgment concerning the patient's health care, and ultimately may be detrimental to the patient's well-being.*

The AMA council provided the following guidelines, and ACOG's Committee on Ethics first affirmed these principles in 1994:

- Mere mutual consent is rejected as a justification for sexual relations with patients since the disparity in power, status, vulnerability, and need make it difficult for a patient to give meaningful consent to sexual contact or sexual relations.
- Sexual contact or a romantic relationship concurrent with the physician–patient relationship is unethical.
- Sexual contact or a romantic relationship with a former patient may be unethical under certain circumstances. The relevant standard is the potential for misuse of physician power and exploitation of patient emotions derived from the former relationship.
- Education on ethical issues involved in sexual misconduct should be included throughout all levels of medical training.
- Physicians have a responsibility to report offending colleagues to disciplinary boards.

Although the AMA and ACOG statements were developed specifically in reference to physicians, sexual misconduct by any health care practitioner is an abuse of professional power and a violation of patient trust. Regardless of societal changes, rigid conformance to ethical principles in this regard is considered essential.

SUGGESTED READING

American College of Obstetricians and Gynecologists. Code of professional ethics of the American College of Obstetricians and Gynecologists. Washington, DC: ACOG, 2002

American College of Obstetricians and Gynecologists. Coding responsibility. ACOG Committee Opinion 249. Washington, DC: ACOG, 2001

American College of Obstetricians and Gynecologists. Confidentiality in adolescent health care. ACOG Educational Bulletin 249. Washington, DC: ACOG, 1998

American College of Obstetricians and Gynecologists. Ethical dimensions of seeking and giving consultation. In: Ethics in obstetrics and gynecology. Washington, DC: ACOG, 2002:28–31

American College of Obstetricians and Gynecologists. Ethical guidance for patient testing. In: Ethics in obstetrics and gynecology. Washington, DC: ACOG, 2002:32–34

American College of Obstetricians and Gynecologists. Ethical issues related to expert testimony by obstetricians and gynecologists. In: Ethics in obstetrics and gynecology. Washington, DC: ACOG, 2002:38–39

American College of Obstetricians and Gynecologists. Guidelines for relationships with industry. In: Ethics in obstetrics and gynecology. Washington, DC: ACOG, 2002:40–42

American College of Obstetricians and Gynecologists. Sexual misconduct in the practice of obstetrics and gynecology: ethical considerations. In: Ethics in obstetrics and gynecology. Washington, DC: ACOG, 2002:89–91

American College of Surgeons. The impaired surgeon: diagnosis, treatment, and reentry. Chicago: ACS, 1995

American Medical Association. Council on Ethical and Judicial Affairs reports on managed care. Chicago: AMA, 1998

American Medical Association. Guidelines for establishing sexual harassment prevention and grievance procedures. Chicago: AMA, 1990

American Medical Association Council on Ethical and Judicial Affairs. Code of medical ethics: current opinions and annotations. Chicago: AMA, 2000

Kane B, Sands DZ. Guidelines for the clinical use of electronic mail with patients. The AMIA Internet Working Group, Task Force on Guidelines for the Use of Clinic-Patient Electronic Mail. J Am Med Inform Assoc 1998;5:104–111

Sexual misconduct in the practice of medicine. Council on Ethical and Judicial Affairs, American Medical Association. JAMA 1991;266:2741–2745

SOGC resolution on sexual abuse by physicians. Society of Obstetricians and Gynaecologists of Canada. J SOGC 1992;14(9):96

Evaluating Credentials and Granting Privileges

Evaluating credentials and granting privileges are essential parts of ensuring the provision of quality care. During the initial application for staff membership at a hospital or other institution, the applicant is responsible for demonstrating his or her qualifications. Once an applicant is accepted on staff, it becomes the institution's responsibility to determine which privileges should be granted. Standards for granting privileges should be established by the institution's governing board and applied uniformly. The standard of training should allow any practitioner, regardless of specialty, to meet the criteria for privileges in a specific area of practice as long as training criteria and experience are documented. Therefore, the credentialing and granting of privileges are local activities that should be based on training, experience, and demonstrated competence.

Medical Staff Appointments

The institution is responsible for verifying the information in the applicant's credentials from the primary source, whenever feasible. It is important to review individual state laws and regulations as well as the requirements of accrediting agencies when systems for evaluating credentials and granting privileges are designed. These documents should include, but may not be limited to, the following information:

- Education
- Residency and subspecialty training

- Status of American Board of Obstetrics and Gynecology certification or equivalent
- Technical experience and verification of competence
- State licensure
- Medical liability experience
- Letters of recommendation assessing professional judgment and behavioral characteristics

Information should be obtained directly from the practitioner's liability insurance company and, as required by law, the NPDB (see box). Hospitals must query the data bank when screening applicants for a medical staff position (courtesy or otherwise) or when granting, adding to, or expanding clinical privileges. The data bank also must be queried every 2 years as to health care practitioners on the medical staff and those who have clinical privileges. There are no requirements to query the data bank about interns and residents because they are trainees in a graduate medical education program; however, hospitals are required to check the data bank when residents or interns are appointed to the medical staff or are granted clinical privileges beyond the aegis of the residency program, such as "moonlighting" in the emergency room. Inquiries regarding the extent of privileges and any negative actions also should be directed to any other institution where the health care clinician practiced.

Many institutions require medical specialty board certification for membership and often accept certification from other countries, such as Canada. Such institutions may grant medical staff membership to physicians and advanced practice health care clinicians in the certification process for a limited period with the understanding that at the end of that period privileges may be withdrawn or reduced. For physicians, the term *board-eligible* has been replaced with the term *active candidate*, which indicates that the individual has passed the written examination and has not exceeded the limitations of eligibility for the oral examination. The education and experience of noncertified physicians should be reviewed carefully to determine that institutional standards for awarding privileges are met.

The National Practitioner Data Bank

National Practitioner Data Bank
PO Box 10832
Chantilly, VA 20153-0832
800-767-6732
(703) 802-4869
www.npdb-hipdb.com

The National Practitioner Data Bank (NPDB) was established by the Health Care Quality Improvement Act of 1986. The NPDB is an information repository that includes reports of medical malpractice payments and disciplinary actions against physicians, dentists, and, in some cases, other licensed health care practitioners in regard to licensure, clinical privileges, and professional society standing.

Practitioners can query the NPDB regarding information about themselves. All queries require payment of a fee. Hospitals are required by law to query the NPDB; other entities that may be eligible to query the NPDB include state boards of medical examiners or state licensing boards, professional societies that follow a formal peer review process, and entities that provide health care services and follow a formal peer review process. Practitioners who are the subject of a report receive notification when a report is submitted. Subjects may contact the reporting entity to make corrections to a report, may add a statement to a report, or may dispute the report.

The Help Line number listed above provides recorded information 7 days a week, 24 hours a day. Information specialists are available at the same number weekdays from 8:30 AM to 6:00 PM (5:30 PM on Fridays) eastern standard time. The web site also provides detailed information.

Although usually licensed, residents do not ordinarily have independent admitting privileges. Fellows (eg, those in subspecialty training who usually have completed basic specialty requirements) may have admitting privileges if allowed by the institution's bylaws; however, their privileges and appointments should be regarded as time limited for the term of training. Under these circumstances, the discontinuation of the appointment at the completion of the program need not be reported to the NPDB. Institutions should develop specific policies governing dual employment (moonlighting) for residents that adhere to state requirements. The institution's policy regarding dual employment should be clearly articulated in residents' contracts. Dual employment should not interfere with residents' obligations to their institutions or with the effectiveness of their educational program.

Incorporating CNMs, nurse practitioners (NPs), and physician assistants (PAs) into the same credentialing process used by physicians is increasing. This process will allow these individuals to function to the full extent of their educational preparation and legal scope of practice. Such advanced practice health care clinicians may work in association with a specific physician or may be employed by an institution. They must be properly licensed and certified by their state, and they should have adequate professional liability insurance, either through an individual policy or through the physician's or institution's policy.

Delineation of Privileges

The authority for granting privileges, including special or temporary certification or other special appointment, is established by the governing body of an institution and should be delineated in the institution and medical staff bylaws. Granting privileges should be based on the individual's training, experience, and demonstrated competence. The department head, after a careful review of all available data, should make recommendations for the initial awarding of privileges, the renewal of privileges, and the addition or denial of new privileges. The recommendations of the department head regarding appointments and privileges often are reviewed and acted on by institution committees, which forward their recommendations to the institution's board. The ultimate responsibility for the quality of medical care rests with the governing board, with the medical staff being responsible for effective self-governance.

After an applicant's credentials have been verified, the specific privileges that have been requested should be considered carefully. The granting of privileges should be based on training, experience, and demonstrated competence. Physicians who are appropriately trained in a technique, have sufficient experience performing it, and have demonstrated current competence should be granted privileges accordingly.

Assessment for granting privileges may vary according to the risk of the procedure or illness and the newness of technology. For example, the review for dilation and curettage will be less rigorous than the review for hysterectomy. Also basic to this review is the capacity of the institution to meet the requirements for the privileges granted. Privileges should not be granted for treating illnesses or for performing procedures that cannot be supported properly by the facilities and the staff.

Blanket approval for all aspects of patient care under the designation "obstetric and gynecologic privileges" fails to recognize the reality of tertiary care issues and variations in training in technical procedures. The institution should have in place a policy that allows for differentiation of privileges, even within one department. This policy may be in the form of a list of specific procedures for which privileges may be granted, which is applicable to surgical specialties, or categorical privileges, which are more applicable to medical specialties. Although the criteria and process by which clinical privileges are granted should be outlined in the medical staff bylaws, the actual privileges that may be granted should be stated in the medical staff rules and regulations, where they can be amended more easily. For advanced practice health care clinicians, the privilege list also should delineate the level of physician involvement required for each privilege requested.

Advanced practice health care clinicians may have delineated clinical privileges or may function under a job description. In either case, specific guidelines established by the Joint Commission on Accreditation of Healthcare Organizations (JCAHO) and state regulatory authorities govern the scope and independence of their practice. Physician assistants are regarded as supervised clinical practitioners, while the requirements for CNM and NP collaboration with physicians vary by state. Both CNMs and NPs generally operate under guidelines, developed collaboratively and subject to institutional approval, that define their role in the institution and protocols that govern their practice. These documents should define conditions that require referral and include guidelines for physician collaboration.

Temporary Privileges

On occasion there is a need to provide access to the facilities for a practitioner who, although fully qualified, is not a member of the institution's medical staff. The reasons for providing temporary access should be reviewed for appropriateness and to ensure that they serve the best interests of patients. The practitioner's qualifications and the adequacy of the practitioner's medical liability insurance should be verified before privileges are granted. The institution's bylaws should specify who has authority to award such privileges and should limit their duration. Generally, temporary privileges should not exceed 30 days.

Provisional Status

An individual's initial appointment to the medical staff should be based on a thorough review of the individual's credentials. The classification of privileges should be designated and a provisional period specified (usually 6–12 months). Medical staff bylaws may provide for an extension of the provisional period if the volume of work or the opportunity for observation has not been sufficient to satisfy the requirements for regular staff eligibility.

At the end of the provisional period an appointee found to be professionally competent and ethical should be granted regular staff membership with an appropriate classification of privileges. If, however, at the end of or during the provisional period there is objective and documented evidence that the individual is not professionally competent or ethical, the department head should recommend to the privileging committee and, thereby, to the institution's governing body that privileges should be restricted or denied. Any such action is subject to the provisions of applicable medical staff bylaws.

Added Skills or Qualifications

Special credentials and privileges may be necessary for areas of new technology when the technology is introduced subsequent to an individual's residency training, involves areas requiring special competence, or both. Examples include operative laparoscopy, radical surgery for cancer, and assisted reproductive techniques. Gynecologic surgeons should restrict their activities to equipment they are qualified to use and procedures for which they have credentials. Privileges can be extended to perform specific operative procedures based on the applicant's documented education, personal experience, and supervision by a qualified physician.

Outreach Surgeons

Surgeons who occasionally commute as needed to perform surgery (for example, to rural areas) often are referred to as outreach surgeons. Outreach surgeons sometimes can provide a community with services it would not otherwise have. When outreach surgery is an appropriate option for the community and the patient, hospital standards should impose the following requirements:

- A written, complete preoperative workup
- A written plan for postoperative care
- Regular review of the records and outcomes

Evaluation for Continuing Competence

The performance of each staff member and documentation of continuing competence should be reviewed periodically. Institutions should establish objective standards of evaluation that can be applied to procedures or services rendered by clinicians of different specialties or backgrounds. Similarly, women's health care should be judged by the established criteria, regardless of whether it is provided by a nurse–midwife, an NP, a PA, a family physician, or an obstetrician–gynecologist. Standards of evaluation may include such matters as additional medical education for new skills, continuing education, professional recognition, results of departmental assessment of quality of care, and consideration of any untoward actions taken at that or any other institution. Recertification requirements for board-certified specialists should be considered when establishing criteria for continuation of privileges.

The quality assessment and improvement process should be designed to detect variations from the established norms for clinical practice in areas that are considered important aspects of care. The process should determine, in each instance, whether a variation is acceptable or unacceptable. Unacceptable variations are considered deficiencies. Deficiencies found through this process should be entered in the file on each practitioner. Remedial action and its outcome also should be recorded. This information forms an important basis for the recommendations made for the renewal of privileges.

It is preferable that privileges be reappraised annually, but it should be done at least biennially. The law requires that hospitals query the NPDB every 2 years to determine whether any negative actions have been taken or malpractice payment made against any practitioner who is on the medical staff or who has privileges. A decision should be made as to whether privileges are to be continued in full, restricted, or terminated. Expansion of privileges should come through formal application and appropriate review.

Established policies and procedures should be followed, in consultation with legal counsel, whenever privileges are to be restricted or terminated. When a negative action is recommended, all applicable bylaw procedures must be followed. The final authority for such action resides with the institution's governing body. Professional review actions that restrict the clinical privileges of a physician for more than 30 days for reasons relating to professional competence or conduct must be reported to the state licensing board and the NPDB. If a physician voluntarily surrenders or restricts his or her own privileges while under investigation (or to avoid it), this information also must be reported. These actions may be reported, but are not required to be reported, when taken against practitioners who are not physicians.

Suggested Reading

Accreditation Council for Graduate Medical Education. Manual of policies and procedures for graduate medical education review committees. Chicago: ACGME, 1999

American Academy of Family Physicians, American College of Obstetricians and Gynecologists. Maternity and gynecologic care—recommended core educational guidelines for family practice residents. ACOG Statement of Policy 73. Leawood, Kansas: AAFP; Washington, DC: ACOG, 1998

American College of Obstetricians and Gynecologists. Guidelines for implementing collaborative practice. Washington, DC: ACOG, 1995

American Medical Association. Licensing and credentialing: what every physician needs to know. Chicago: AMA, 1999

Joint Commission on Accreditation of Health Care Organizations. Comprehensive accreditation manual for hospitals: the official handbook. Oakbrook Terrace, Illinois: JCAHO, 2000

Joint Commission on Accreditation of Health Care Organizations. 2000–2001 comprehensive accreditation manual for ambulatory care. Oakbrook Terrace, Illinois: JCAHO, 1999

QUALITY ASSESSMENT AND CONTINUOUS QUALITY IMPROVEMENT

The concept of quality in the assessment of hospitals and other health care organizations has been promoted by JCAHO and others for many years (see box on page 41). Continuous quality improvement (CQI) has evolved from the traditional, problem-focused process of quality assurance. The quality assessment process can be used to establish clinical indicators, measurable dimensions of care (eg, a medical event, diagnosis, or outcome) that reflect aspects of care whose importance is gauged by frequency, severity, or cost (see box on page 42). Clinical indicators alone do not measure quality, but they can be quantified and compared with predetermined goals. When the care given to patients by a health care practitioner (such as a physician, CNM, or NP) who has privileges at the institution deviates from established goals, clinical indicators can identify the need for additional peer reviews.

One of the most important first steps in developing a departmental CQI program is to establish leadership. Regardless of the structure within a given hospital, the need for responsive leadership among general medical staff and the department of obstetrics and gynecology is key to an effective CQI program and to the overall operation of the department.

The American College of Obstetricians and Gynecologists' quality assessment screening tools, formerly known as criteria sets, have been developed to assist in retrospective chart review to evaluate the quality of patient care. They are derivative documents based primarily on ACOG publications and consensus opinions. These screening tools do not necessarily mention all clinical approaches and may be modified to reflect local practice.

The screening tools are primarily intended for use by medical record screeners to aid in identifying practice variations that might indicate the need for further review, documentation, or justification. Charts that fail these screens should go through peer review by a committee of practitioners who have sufficient knowledge, experience, and judgment to make

The American College of Obstetricians and Gynecologists' Voluntary Review of Quality of Care

The Voluntary Review of Quality of Care program, conducted under the auspices of the Committee on Quality Improvement and Patient Safety of ACOG, is available to assist hospitals and physicians in assessing the quality of care provided in their departments of obstetrics and gynecology. The evaluation may assess the department as a whole, the obstetrics or gynecology service, an individual procedure, or the quality assessment process within the department. When a quality-of-care issue has been identified by a hospital regarding an individual physician, a tailored review of the physician's records may be conducted. The program concerns itself only with quality of care and provides no consultation in legal, architectural, marketing, or other issues. For more information about the Voluntary Review of Quality of Care program, call ACOG at (202) 638-5577 or visit the ACOG web site at www.acog.org.

a determination as to whether the variations are appropriate. The use of these screening tools alone for utilization review or as the basis for denying reimbursement for health care services is inappropriate. The American College of Obstetricians and Gynecologists' screening tools are not intended to establish standards of care.

The quality of a practitioner's care cannot always be determined on the basis of an individual case because differences of opinion may exist regarding management. Therefore, the ability of the practitioner may need to be assessed by reviewing more than one case. When a single questionable case is identified that involves a health care practitioner who has demonstrated exemplary skills in the management of all other patients, the department head might conclude that no further action is necessary. However, continued monitoring over time, referred to as trending, may demonstrate that this physician has a higher rate of variation than the department as a whole. Trending data may suggest a concern that an individual case review may not identify. If a questionable case is one of many questionable cases managed by the same practitioner, this pattern might indicate the need for corrective action. Continuous quality improvement focuses on the premise that although most medical care is good, there can always be improvement.

Gynecologic Quality Indicators

- Unplanned readmission within 14 days
- Admission after a return visit to the emergency room for the same problem
- Cardiopulmonary arrest, resuscitated
- Occurrence of an infection not present on admission
- Unplanned admission to special (intensive) care unit
- Unplanned return to the operating room for surgery during the same admission
- Ambulatory surgery patient admitted or retained for complication of surgery or anesthesia
- Gynecologic surgery, except radical hysterectomy or exenteration, using 2 or more units of blood, or postoperative hematocrit of less than 24% or hemoglobin of less than 8 g
- Unplanned removal, injury, or repair of organ during operative procedure
- Initiation of antibiotics more than 24 hours after surgery
- Discrepancy between preoperative diagnosis and postoperative tissue report
- Removal of uterus weighing less than 280 g for leiomyomata
- Removal of follicular cyst or corpus luteum of ovary
- Hysterectomy performed on a woman younger than 30 years of age except for malignancy
- Gynecologic death

American College of Obstetricians and Gynecologists. Quality improvement in women's health care. Rev. ed. Washington, DC: ACOG, 2000

Collecting and Analyzing Data

The concurrent or retrospective collection of data is critical to the quality improvement process. Concurrent data are most commonly used for purposes of risk management and utilization review. Retrospective data retrieval is more commonly used for quality assessment. For inpatient care, analysis soon after discharge is considered the most accurate method. This can be accomplished by the use of a trained data abstractor using preestablished practice norms, such as clinical indicators and screening tools, to identify records for practitioner review. The data obtained by this process also can be used for educational purposes to make all staff members aware of the performance of the unit as a whole. Data collected for quality measurement should focus either on the processes used to deliver care or the outcomes of the care provided.

An institutional CQI program gathers data that will be used to evaluate the systems and processes that affect patient care. The data also should permit assessment of the effectiveness of changes that are made. These findings can be a major mechanism for future quality improvement.

To encourage self-policing by physicians, both federal and state laws provide some protection for physician peer review. The Health Care Quality Improvement Act, passed by Congress in October 1986, grants immunity from damages under federal and state laws (including antitrust provisions) to health care practitioners engaged in good faith peer review. Most states also have adopted laws to encourage and protect physician peer review, although the type of immunity offered and the class of persons protected from personal liability for participating in peer review varies from state to state.

Most states safeguard the confidentiality of records used in peer review actions. Again, the extent of the protection varies from jurisdiction to jurisdiction, and anyone engaged in peer review should know the laws of his or her state. For example, some states recognize confidentiality only for the peer review records of a hospital review committee, while others protect all information reported to the committee. In some states, the information is not admissible as evidence in a trial but may be discoverable in pretrial proceedings. To ensure the maximum protection of records, those individuals formulating a hospital's quality review program should seek legal advice.

Corrective Action

When the quality assessment process or other mechanisms have identified a variation, a specific problem, or an opportunity to improve care or performance, a plan should be formulated to address it. A record should be maintained of all of the actions taken. The fact that a problem was identified, that it was addressed, and that action was instituted to correct the problem should be documented. This documentation should include a statement of the expectations for change and the means by which change will be measured. Most corrective actions can be handled under the authority of the department head or other responsible person. When the recommended action requires the involvement of a higher authority, procedures should be in place to facilitate necessary decision making. When the action required involves a reduction in privileges, it is critical to have legal consultation beforehand.

Any negative actions must be taken in accordance with the institution's bylaws and applicable legal requirements. Careful documentation is of critical importance. Due process procedures must be in place in the medical staff bylaws prior to the institution of reviews that could result in disciplinary action.

A follow-up evaluation of the problem practitioner's quality of care is necessary to document the effectiveness of the actions. The findings, actions, and outcome of the quality assessment process should be reported in a timely manner to the institution-wide quality assessment committee.

Remedial education may be necessary because of an identified deficiency in care. When this occurs, a remedial program for that individual may be provided or obtained elsewhere. When a deficiency involves several staff members, it is more appropriate to direct the education toward the unit as a whole. The concept of CQI involves the entire hospital.

Whereas the quality assessment process for remedial action or improvement often can be done within a single department, which would report its process and findings to an institutional quality assessment committee, the CQI process tends to be interdepartmental and incorporate not only all clinical services but also laboratory services and other clinical support functions. For example, in a review of repeated delays in the treatment of patients with ectopic pregnancy, the department would evaluate not only the actions of the health care practitioner but also other services, including the emergency room, admissions office, laboratory, transportation, and any other services which may have contributed to the delay.

Continuous quality improvement requires a data system that will provide information that can be analyzed and reported statistically. Quality assessment and CQI, although related, have independent purposes and both are necessary at present. The current direction of JCAHO and other such bodies is to promote the CQI philosophy in health care facilities throughout the nation.

When a quality assessment process identifies deficiencies in the quality of care provided by a specific individual, the department head or other responsible person has the responsibility and should have the authority to take steps to correct the deficiency. Discussion and counseling with the practitioner should always be the first step in the process. In certain circumstances it may be all that is required. Other possible actions that may be instituted include:

- Observation of the practitioner's skills—either by the department head or by a designated staff member who may have the skills required to assess a particular procedure or treatment
- Proctoring—which requires the direct observation of an individual's practice by a peer or by a review of the charts of current or recently treated patients to ensure that the standards are being met
- External peer review—which may be used when there is interpersonal conflict, disagreement as to the appropriate action, or a lack of comparable skill within the department
- Remedial education—which may take the form of special programs focused on needs

When the initial remedial action does not result in the anticipated improvement, the problem must be reassessed. A second effort should be made to provide a solution, and the result of this effort must be evaluated. Results should be recorded in the department's quality assessment file and reported to the institution's quality assessment committee. Failure may occur, however, and further steps may be necessary. The department head and the quality assessment committee may need to take disciplinary action against a physician who fails to comply or improve. Because such action has important legal ramifications, it is critical that legal counsel, usually supplied by the institution, be consulted in advance.

A period of observation may be instituted during which the practitioner is allowed to continue to practice but under conditions that have been established for the protection of the public. A decision on whether privileges should be continued is dependent on the assessment of the practitioner's skills. It is imperative that the institution's due process provisions in the medical bylaws be reviewed and strictly followed.

When the deficiency is considered more serious, privileges may be reduced. Reducing privileges requires formal proceedings, which should be prescribed in the medical staff bylaws and may be subject to reporting to the NPDB.

Revoking privileges, including summary suspension, is an extreme step ordinarily not taken unless all other measures have failed or the behavior of the health care practitioner is so egregious that the safety of patients is jeopardized. The legal implications of such action require that the processes identified in the institution's administrative documents be reviewed carefully by legal counsel and followed with precision.

Quality Improvement in the Office

The medical office or clinic is well suited to modern methods of quality improvement, and programs and resources addressing quality improvement in the office continue to evolve. Ideally, a written quality management plan should be established. The office staff should meet periodically as a quality management team to discuss methods of measuring and improving the quality of the care administered by the office. As a means of assessing and improving the quality of care, consideration should be given to monitoring medical records, appointments and scheduling, patient relations and communication, telephone communication, personnel management, equipment and drugs, and complications and adverse outcomes of medical activities and procedures (see box).

Quality management activities within the medical office should concentrate on assessing and improving function in one specific system at a

Suggested Items to Monitor for Quality Improvement in the Office

Medical Records/Information Systems

- Legibility
- Organization
- Documentation—general (including the problem list)
- Documentation of drug allergy
- Lost medical records
- Misfiled medical records
- Breach of confidentiality
- List of current medications

Appointments and Scheduling—Patient Flow

- Acceptable waiting time for appointments
- Appropriate waiting time in office to see clinician
- Follow-up on missed or canceled appointments, tests, and procedures

Patient Relations

- Periodic patient survey on perceived quality
- Patient exit evaluation forms
- Evaluation of patient complaints
- Periodic assessment of waiting room reading materials and patient information material for timeliness and appropriateness

Patient Communications

- Compliance with established protocol for informing patient of the results of laboratory studies and procedures
- Method of informing patients of a delayed or rescheduled appointment
- Monitoring appropriateness of method of terminating practitioner–patient relationship

Telephone Communications

- Excessive busy signals (data are available from the telephone company)
- Excessive holding time

(continued)

Suggested Items to Monitor for Quality Improvement in the Office
(continued)

- Documentation of telephone contact in medical records, with disposition documented
- Monitoring of telephone prescription refills for doctor approval
- Monitoring amount of "dropped" or lost calls

PERSONNEL MANAGEMENT

- Employee morale
- Absenteeism
- Periodic employee performance assessment
- Maintenance of patient confidentiality

EQUIPMENT AND DRUGS

- Periodic equipment check for proper function
- Maintenance logs of equipment repair
- Security system for controlled drugs
- Security system for syringes and needles
- Method of monitoring drugs for expiration dates (including samples)

COMPLICATIONS AND ADVERSE OUTCOMES OF MEDICAL ACTIVITIES AND PROCEDURES

- Drug reactions
- Wound infections
- Delayed complications from hospitalized patients (eg, episiotomy infections, postpartum endometritis)
- Equipment failure

time. Once the function has improved to a level of quality acceptable to the practice, the quality management team would then move to another system for review. Several systems may be optimally monitored by monthly tracking (eg, patient complaints, complications of office procedures). Medical offices also may wish to measure the quality of care administered by their practitioners in the hospital setting separate from the hospital's quality management program.

Risk management activities in the office setting will generally overlap with quality improvement activities. The two programs may be done in tandem. The risk management emphasis should be on patient safety and reduction of liability (see "Liability" in Part 1).

Suggested Reading

American College of Obstetricians and Gynecologists. Institutional responsibility to provide legal representation. In: Ethics in obstetrics and gynecology. Washington, DC: ACOG, 2002:48

American College of Obstetricians and Gynecologists. Quality improvement in women's health care. Rev. ed. Washington, DC: ACOG, 2000

Berwick DM. Continuous improvement as an ideal in health care. N Engl J Med 1989;320: 53–56

Gaucher EJ, Coffey RJ. Total quality in healthcare: from theory to practice. San Francisco: Jossey-Bass Publishers, 1993

Lohr KN, ed. Medicare: a strategy for quality assurance. Washington, DC: National Academy Press, 1990

Parsons MC, Murdaugh CL, Purdon TF, Jarrell BE. Guide to clinical resource management. Gaithersburg, Maryland: Aspen Publishers, 1997

Schoenbaum SC, Sundwall DN, Bergman D, Buckle JM, Chernov A, George J, et al. Using clinical practice guidelines to evaluate quality of care. Rockville, Maryland: Agency for Health Care Policy and Research, U.S. Department of Health and Human Services, Public Health Service, 1995 March; AHCPR publication no. 95-0045

COMPLIANCE WITH GOVERNMENT REGULATIONS

In recent years an increasing number of government regulations, both state and federal, have had a significant impact on the health care workplace. Practitioners and managers of medical offices and clinics should recognize the regulations that affect the office and clinic setting and properly implement those procedures required by law. Among those that have the most significant impact are the Occupational Safety and Health Administration's (OSHA) Occupational Exposure to Bloodborne Pathogens Standard (Appendix B), regulations imposed by the Clinical Laboratory Improvement Amendments of 1988 (CLIA) (Appendix C), legal requirements regarding patient screening and transfer (Appendix D), U.S. Food and Drug Administration (FDA) regulations governing mammography, and the Americans with Disabilities Act (Appendix E).

In addition, the Health Insurance Portability and Accountability Act of 1996 expanded the federal government's ability to enforce measures against health care fraud. Physicians should be aware of their potential liability in the event they inappropriately submit a claim. To reduce liability exposure, individual physicians should implement and maintain a compliance plan to ensure required standards are met.

Occupational Exposure to Bloodborne Pathogens Standard

In 1991, OSHA issued regulations designed to minimize the transmission of HIV, HBV, and other potentially infectious materials in the workplace. The regulations, which went into effect March 6, 1992, and were revised in 2001, cover all employees in clinician offices, hospitals, medical laboratories, and other health care facilities where workers could be "reasonably anticipated" to come into contact with blood and other potentially infectious material. The OSHA regulations require employers to implement an exposure control plan to minimize employees' exposure to bloodborne pathogens. The plan must contain the following components: personal protective equipment for employees exposed to blood and other body fluids, adoption of certain work practice controls (eg, hand-washing facilities, disposal of contaminated needles, handling and storage of specimens), housekeeping requirements, provision of hepatitis B vaccination to employees, postexposure evaluation and follow-up procedures, employee training, use of warning labels, and record-keeping requirements. These requirements are enforced by OSHA or, in the case of states having OSHA-approved comparable job safety and health plans, by state agencies. Violations are punishable by fines.

In 1999, OSHA issued a revised compliance directive for the bloodborne pathogens standard. This directive clarifies the standard and emphasizes that employers must use readily available technology in their safety and health programs. For example, employers must ensure that their exposure review plans are reviewed annually and reflect consideration and use of commercially available safer medical devices, such as shielded needles. The directive also includes the U.S. Centers for Disease Control and Prevention guidelines on vaccinations against HBV and on postexposure evaluation and follow-up for HIV and Hepatitis C. It requires employee training on implementation of the new and safer medical devices. The directive can be obtained from the OSHA home page at www.osha.gov under the "Directives" link or by calling (202) 693-1888.

As mandated by the Needlestick Safety and Prevention Act in 2001, OSHA revised its bloodborne pathogens standard to clarify the need for employers to select safer needle devices as they become available, to involve employees in identifying and choosing the devices, and to incorporate other mandates of the new statute. Several states have enacted needlestick laws and many more are considering such legislation. Practitioners can expect this standard to continue to evolve.

Clinical Laboratory Improvement Amendments of 1988

In 1988, Congress enacted CLIA in response to growing public concerns regarding the quality and accuracy of laboratory testing. In September

1992, regulations promulgated by the Health Care Financing Administration (currently known as the Centers for Medicare and Medicaid Services [CMS]), the federal agency charged with implementation and enforcement of CLIA, took effect. Since 1992, regulations revising CLIA have been issued periodically.

Under CLIA, federal oversight is required for all laboratories, including physician offices, that perform tests that examine human specimens for the diagnosis, prevention, or treatment of any disease, impairment of health, or health assessment. All physician offices that conduct any such tests must register with CMS and obtain a certificate. Even if the office is performing minimal testing (eg, urine pregnancy tests) or not charging fees for testing, the laboratory still must obtain the appropriate certificate.

Categories of Testing

There are three levels of test categories based on the complexity of the testing: 1) waived tests; 2) tests of moderate complexity, including provider-performed microscopy procedures; and 3) tests of high complexity. These test categories determine the type of certificate a laboratory is issued. Each category of testing has different regulatory requirements; the more complex the category of testing, the more stringent the regulations. Most obstetrician–gynecologists' offices do only waived tests or provider-performed microscopy procedures. Appendix C provides some basic information on these categories of tests and CLIA regulations governing these procedures.

Clinical Laboratory Improvement Amendments Certificates

A "registration certificate" is the initial certificate obtained by laboratories conducting tests of moderate and high complexity. It authorizes the laboratory to conduct moderate- or high-complexity testing for up to 2 years or until the laboratory is inspected and an appropriate certificate is issued. After CMS or its agent inspects the laboratory and finds it to be in compliance with CLIA, the laboratory is issued a certificate of compliance authorizing performance of designated tests. Two other types of certificates, based on the complexity of the testing performed, are "certificates of waiver" and "certificates for provider-performed microscopy procedures." Laboratories can choose to obtain a "certificate of accreditation" from a CMS-approved accreditation organization to fulfill compliance with CLIA.

Patient Screening and Transfer

Specific federal legal requirements apply to patient screening in emergency rooms and the transfer of patients by Medicare-participating hospitals. It is essential that institutions and health care practitioners understand their obligations under the law. Even hospitals that are not capable of handling high-risk deliveries or high-risk infants and have written transfer agreements must meet all the screening, treatment, and transfer requirements before transferring a patient. For detailed information about the federal requirements for patient screening and transfer, see Appendix D.

Interhospital Care and Transfer

Federal law mandates that all Medicare-participating hospitals provide an appropriate medical screening examination for any individual who seeks medical treatment at an emergency department and places strict requirements on the transfer of these patients. Both the facilities and the professionals providing care must understand their obligations under the laws regarding patient transfer.

Interhospital transport is appropriate and recommended if services and staff are not available at the referring facility to care for the patient. Prior to transport, the hospital must still meet the screening, treatment, and transfer requirements. Many legal details of transport are not well defined, but all involved parties assume a number of responsibilities. Some of these include:

- Each transport system must comply with the standards and regulations established by local, state, and federal agencies

- Informed consent for transfer, transport, and admission at the receiving hospital should be obtained before the transport team moves the patient
- Formal agreements between hospitals should be developed to outline procedures and responsibilities for patient care
- Relevant patient identification should be provided for the patient to wear during transport
- Patient care guidelines, orders, and verbal communication are to be used to care for the patient during transport

Referring Hospital

The referring hospital and physician are responsible for the care of patients until they arrive at the receiving hospital. The referring physician is responsible for evaluating and stabilizing the patient before transfer. Both the referring physician and the hospital should understand the transport system, including how to gain access to and appropriately use its services. When transferred, each patient should be accompanied by a form that includes general information about the patient, reason for transfer, transport mode, and medical information that may enhance the understanding of the patient's needs or problems.

Receiving Hospital

The receiving hospital is responsible for the overall coordination of the transport program. It should ensure that the interhospital transport system is organized to provide appropriate care for the transported patient. Contingency plans should be established to avoid a shortage of beds for patients requiring transport. The receiving center is responsible for providing consultant physicians with the following abilities:

- Communication capability 24 hours per day
- Reports that describe the patient's condition and planned therapy
- Summary of the hospital course and recommendations for ongoing care after discharge

Transport Team

The transport team should have the necessary expertise to provide supportive care for a wide variety of emergency conditions that can arise during transport. The composition of the team should be consistent with the expected level of medical needs of the patient being transported. The transport unit should:

- Provide rapidly available vehicles and staff
- Provide communication between the transport team and the receiving hospital
- Coordinate all levels of transfer (air and ground)
- Maintain sufficient patient care equipment for safe transport, the most necessary of which will include:
  —Physiologic function monitors (eg, heart rate, blood pressure, temperature, respiratory rate, transcutaneous oxygen assessments)
  —Resuscitation and support equipment (eg, intravenous pumps, suction apparatus, ventilators)
  —Medical gas tanks
  —Functional capabilities to support electrical equipment

Air Transport

Hospital-based equipment may develop flaws in flight and affect the safety of the patient. All equipment should be tested regularly to ensure accuracy and safety during air transport. The following agencies can offer assistance in choosing or testing medical equipment used during air transport:

- The U.S. Army Aeromedical Research Laboratory, Fort Rucker, AL
- Armstrong Laboratory, Brooks Air Force Base, TX
- Association of Air Medical Services, Pasadena, CA
- Emergency Care Research Institute, Plymouth Meeting, PA
- Federal Aviation Administration, Washington, DC

Education

An education program that informs users and the public about the capabilities of the interhospital transfer service is fundamental to the success of the operation. Outreach education should reinforce cooperation between all referring hospitals, and the practitioners in the system should know about the clinical capabilities and special resources of each institution. A mechanism should exist to rapidly inform all participants in the transport program about new changes or procedures.

Mammography Quality Standards Act

In 1992, Congress enacted the Mammography Quality Standards Act in response to concerns about breast cancer and the quality of mammography services in the United States (see box). To operate lawfully after October 1, 1994, all mammography facilities, including physician offices, must be certified by the FDA as providing quality mammography services. This is true even if an office has only one mammography unit and the film is processed and interpreted elsewhere. If films are interpreted and processed or record-keeping services are provided for mammography performed elsewhere and the physician is only a "partial clinician" of mammography services, that physician still must be part of a certified system (ie, certified under the primary facility). For a facility to be certified,

The Mammography Quality Standards Act

For more information on the Mammography Quality Standards Act, go to the Mammography Quality Standards Act home page on the Internet (www.fda.gov/cdrh/mammography). For details about compliance, see *Small Entity Compliance Guide: An Overview of the Final Regulations Implementing the Mammography Quality Standards Act of 1992*, published by the U.S. Department of Health and Human Services in October 1997.

Physicians also can call the Facility Hotline (800-838-7715) or "Facts on Demand," a 24-hour automated fax system (800-899-0381). To find a mammography facility certified by the U.S. Food and Drug Administration, call the National Cancer Institute at 800-422-6237.

it must be accredited by a federally approved private nonprofit or state accreditation body. In addition, a facility's clinical images must be periodically reviewed, and the facility must be inspected annually and meet federally developed standards. Comprehensive regulations governing the requirements for mammography personnel, quality control, record keeping, and medical audits became effective April 28, 1999.

In October 1998, the Mammography Quality Standards Reauthorization Act, which extends the program through September 2002, was signed into law. In part, this act requires that all women be sent a lay summary of their mammography results directly from the facility. Physicians referring patients to mammography facilities will still receive the examination report.

LIABILITY

Risk management is an approach to practice that minimizes the risk of lawsuits by 1) practicing in a manner that reduces the possibility of actual error, 2) ensuring the best chance of obtaining desired results in patient care, and 3) presenting the most defensible treatment history. Risk management cannot always prevent a lawsuit; however, it often can protect a clinician against nonmeritorious claims and help improve the outcome of medical malpractice litigation.

The goal of risk management is quality medical practice. Risk management is a team effort, and all participants must understand that the acts of one can easily lead to liability for others. Staff members should be knowledgeable about professional liability risk management.

Risk Reduction

A program of risk management should be developed and maintained, with an emphasis on patient safety and a reduction of practitioner liability. This program should have the following elements:

- A person responsible for the risk management program and, if applicable, the risk management committee

- Periodic review of clinical records and clinical care policies
- Education in risk management activities for all staff within the institution or office
- Methods to identify incidents and adverse occurrences arising in the practice setting

The risk management program should address important clinical care issues, which may include, but are not limited to:

- Periodic review for legal and medical accuracy of any forms used for informed consent
- Procedures by which a patient may be dismissed from care or refused care
- Procedures for transfer of medical information at the patient's request to other health care practitioners
- Periodic performance reviews of employees and allied health personnel
- Review of all incidents and complaints reported by employees, visitors, and patients
- Periodic review of patient office records
- Review of all deaths, trauma, or adverse outcome events
- Review of obligations under any managed care contracts; ensure proper procedures are followed
- Procedures for how and when to communicate with the professional liability insurance carrier
- Procedures for dealing with inquiries from governmental agencies, attorneys, consumer advocate groups, and the media
- Procedures for addressing relationships with competing health care organizations so as to avoid antitrust and restraint of trade concerns
- Procedures for managing situations in which a physician becomes acutely incapacitated during a medical or surgical procedure

- Identification and management of the impaired health care practitioner
- Procedures for complying with applicable state and federal laws and regulations
- Procedures for complying with contractual agreements
- Procedures for the prevention of unauthorized prescribing and the use of drugs
- Procedures for communicating with laboratories to ensure efficient handling and follow-up of clinical information
- Procedures for communicating with patients: confidentiality issues and follow-up of abnormal tests or other results, as well as missed appointments
- Methods for maintaining a realistic patient schedule and allowing for emergencies
- Protocols for introducing the use of new technologies, devices, or medications

Practice Coverage and Referrals

Physicians are urged to coordinate patient care among partners, covering physicians, and consultants. Practice coverage outside of normal business hours should be established and documented. When possible, covering physicians should have the same privileges as the treating/attending physician. Any coverage arrangements will need to comply with the managed care plan requirements that apply to a given patient. It must be determined whether the covering physician has professional liability insurance coverage and to what extent.

Patients should be advised if their physician will be absent from practice, and the physician should recommend or make available a qualified substitute. This discussion should be documented as to the scope of the physician's absence, the substitute, and patient acceptance. The hospital and answering service need to be advised of the treating physician's absence and of the name and contact information of the covering physician.

Physicians can be subject to professional liability allegations involving referrals of patients to other physicians and acceptance of patients for consultations. Common elements of claims involve criticism for failure to refer for a second opinion or failure to recognize one's personal or professional limitations.

In some instances, a physician's reluctance to refer patients to another physician is based on an unrealistic sense of his or her own abilities. Often it is the physician's sincere effort to personally provide answers and services to the patient that prevents him or her from referring the patient to another physician. No physician should expect to have complete and superior knowledge in all instances. There also are those physicians who are reluctant to refer because they wish to save the patient the costs of extra professional care or they fear they will lose a patient to the referred physician. Physicians also might be reluctant to refer patients because of pressures from their managed care contracts. Courts have little sympathy when a collective approach to treatment might have resulted in better patient care.

Sometimes the patient is reluctant to see another physician. If consultation is recommended and the patient refuses or fails to comply with the recommendation, it should be clearly documented in the patient's record.

Once a physician is aware that the patient's medical needs may fall outside of the realm of his or her expertise, appropriate care should be arranged. It is the duty of the physician to alert the patient to the situation and arrange for a consultation with a competent specialist. Other responsibilities of referring and consulting clinicians are outlined in "Human Resources" in Part 1. Communicating to the patient the urgency as well as the scope of the consultation is imperative. In addition, the attending physician should be attentive to the feelings of the patient. Problems may arise if the patient feels slighted or abandoned by the delegation of care. The patient and her primary physician should be kept informed by the consultant during the entire treatment process.

If feasible, all active patients should be given adequate notice that a medical practice is closing and that they must find another physician. What constitutes adequate notice may vary. For gynecologic patients, 30–60 days' notice should be sufficient. Obstetric patients may need more time to find another physician. Physicians should assist their patients in finding other care and provide the name and telephone number of the local medical society so that patients can find other obstetrician–gynecologists in the area or provide the names of other obstetrician–gynecologists. For convenience, the notification should include an authorization form to transfer copies of the patient's records to the physician of her choice. Physicians should retain copies of all correspondence and any authorization forms returned by patients. Only copies of records should be sent, not originals.

Billing

A billing system should be established to ensure that visits and procedures are coded accurately and payment and reimbursement requests comply with all federal requirements. Physicians should develop a program of checks and balances to maintain the system properly. Methods of collection of unpaid accounts should be reviewed before referral to a collection agency.

Heightened federal scrutiny of Medicare billing entities has brought a need for physicians to develop fraud and abuse compliance plans. Compliance plans are not currently required for physician practices by the U.S. Department of Health and Human Services. However, establishing and following a compliance plan could potentially reduce the severity of a federal audit.

Suggested Reading

Accreditation Association for Ambulatory Health Care, Inc. Accreditation handbook for ambulatory health care. Skokie, Illinois: AAAHC, 1999

American College of Obstetricians and Gynecologists. The assistant: information for improved risk management. Washington, DC: ACOG, 2001

American College of Obstetricians and Gynecologists. Ethical dimensions of informed consent. In: Ethics in obstetrics and gynecology. Washington, DC: ACOG, 2002:19–27

American College of Obstetricians and Gynecologists. Ethical dimensions of seeking and giving consultation. In: Ethics in obstetrics and gynecology. Washington, DC: ACOG, 2002:28–31

American College of Obstetricians and Gynecologists. Informed refusal. ACOG Committee Opinion 237. Washington, DC: ACOG, 2000

American College of Obstetricians and Gynecologists. Litigation assistant: a guide for the defendant physician. 2nd ed. Washington, DC: ACOG, 1998

American Medical Association. Risk management principles and commentaries for the medical office. 2nd ed. Chicago: AMA, 1995

The Office of the Inspector General's compliance program guidance for hospitals. Plymouth Meeting. Pennsylvania: ECRI, 1998

Publication of the OIG's provider self-disclosure protocol—Office of Inspector General (OIG), HHS. Notice. Fed Regist 1998;63:58399–58403

ETHICAL ISSUES

Recent growth in scientific technology has expanded medicine's ability to affect the processes of human birth, life, and death. In no specialty is this more apparent than in the field of obstetrics and gynecology. Assisted reproductive technologies, fetal surgery, and interventions at the end of life raise questions that cannot be addressed with medical knowledge alone. Good decisions in these areas depend on a thoughtful consideration of the values, desires, and goals of those involved. Before an ethical approach to confronting difficult problems can be achieved, however, certain fundamental issues must be addressed:

- The clinician should have an understanding of the structure of his or her own value system and of the ways in which personal judgments about right and wrong, and good and bad, influence decisions in various areas of life.
- The clinician should have a general background of knowledge in the discipline of ethics.
- The process by which a clinician makes and implements ethical decisions should be systematic and logically consistent.

Ethics is the formal study of moral behavior in which moral obligations are analyzed in terms of recognized ethical principles. After critical reflection, an attempt is made to determine which of a number of commonly held moral assumptions are justifiable. In applying moral rules and principles to human action, the discipline of ethics does not identify any particular moral view as the correct one. It serves instead as a framework for systematically analyzing different moral points of view and rationally justifying one course of action over another, based on consideration of recognized principles and accepted values.

Ethical principles and concepts encompass a variety of actions. They are the foundation of professional behavior (see "Human Resources" in Part 1) and serve to underpin actions taken to protect the interests of patients. A basic understanding of ethical principles and concepts will aid in ethical decision making. Institutions and individuals should be ethically guided in policy making, and institutional ethics committees may be helpful in determining ethically appropriate courses of action.

Ethical Principles and Concepts

Ethical principles include autonomy, beneficence, and justice. These principles, when put into practice, lead to the common ethical concepts of informed consent, honesty, and confidentiality.

Ethical Principles

Autonomy. Autonomy refers to respect for person or self-rule. A person is free to establish personal norms of conduct and to voluntarily choose a course of action based on her own values and principles. This freedom imposes on others an obligation not to interfere with the right to exercise autonomy. Autonomy is considered by some to be almost absolute unless it infringes on the personal freedom of others. Other views impose narrower limits on individual autonomy. Respect for autonomy plays an important role in many areas of medical practice. Although a clinician may consider a particular course of treatment to be best for a patient, the clinician may agree to a somewhat different therapy at the patient's request.

Beneficence. Beneficence is the obligation to promote the well-being of others. The related principle of nonmaleficence obliges one to avoid doing harm. With roots in the Hippocratic tradition, beneficence and nonmaleficence are fundamental to the ethic of medicine. The application of these principles consists of balancing benefits and harms. The concept of "harms" in this context includes intentional harms as well as those harms that can be anticipated to arise despite the best intentions (eg, unwanted side effects of medication or complications of surgical treatment). These principles, therefore, are the source of a clinician's obligation to act with due care. In balancing beneficence with autonomy, the patient's "best interests" should be defined as objectively as possible. Attempting to override patient autonomy to promote what the clinician perceives as a patient's best interests is called "paternalism."

Justice. Justice is the right of individuals to claim what is due them. Some theories of justice determine distribution of benefits and burdens based on criteria such as need, effort, contribution, or merit. Other theories specify that all benefits and burdens are distributed equally (distributive justice). It is important that the criteria to be used are determined in advance and selected in a manner consistent with accepted moral rules and principles and that they are relevant to the benefits and burdens being assigned. In this society, for example, race, sex, and religion are not considered to be morally legitimate criteria for the distribution of benefits such as employment and housing. Justice generates an obligation to treat equally those who are alike according to whatever criteria are selected. Patients with identical needs should receive equal treatment unless it is demonstrated that they differ from others in a way that is relevant to the treatment in question.

At times, constraints such as a scarcity of resources force moral judgments about competing claims made to appear equal based on previously used criteria. Different criteria must then be chosen, and selection of these criteria is in itself a moral decision.

Ethical Concepts

Several ethical norms can be derived from the fundamental ethical principles of autonomy, beneficence, and justice. These norms or concepts are important because they influence many of the decisions made in obstetrics and gynecology. An understanding of these concepts will facilitate ethical decision making.

Informed Consent. Informed consent is the willing and uncoerced acceptance of a medical intervention by a patient after appropriate disclosure by the clinician of the nature of the intervention and its risks and benefits, as well as the risks and benefits of alternatives. The primary purpose of the consent process is the exercise of patient autonomy. A patient's right to make her own decisions about medical issues extends to the right of informed refusal—the right to refuse recommended medical treatment. By encouraging ongoing and open communication about relevant information, the health care professional enables the patient to exercise personal choice. This sort of communication is central to the clinician–patient relationship.

At times, a patient's capacity to comprehend and process the medical information presented to her may be in doubt. This capacity may wax and wane, and as a first step in such cases, the health care professional should, through consultation and further discussion with the patient, attempt to clarify and improve the patient's ability to provide consent. For example, medication may be appropriate. The decision as to competence to consent, however, is a legal one. If a patient is unable to provide consent, a substitute decision maker should be sought.

It is important to emphasize that informed consent is a process. In some minds, it has become synonymous with the informed consent forms used to document that the informed consent process has taken place. Documenting the informed consent process is important from a medical–legal perspective (see "Information Management" in Part 2).

Specific requirements for informed consent of U.S. research subjects have been codified in the Code of Federal Regulations. They are addressed later in this section in "Institutional Review Boards."

Honesty. Beneficence or autonomy is the principle honesty serves. The principle of autonomy requires that a patient be given complete and truthful information about her medical condition and about any proposed treatment. Only with such information is she able to exercise her right to make choices about health care. If complete information is not available, existing uncertainty should be shared with the patient. The perception that a health care professional has concealed the truth or has engaged in deception will weaken patient trust and undermine the clinician–patient relationship. This is true regardless of the intent of the clinician; for example, improper diagnostic coding to allow insurance coverage of a service the clinician judges to be medically indicated is nonetheless deception.

Confidentiality. A patient's right to make decisions about health care includes a right to decide how and to whom personal medical information will be communicated. The principle of autonomy underlies a health care professional's duty to respect patient privacy. As is the case with dishonesty, breaches of confidentiality threaten the patient's trust and may destroy the clinician–patient relationship. How the health care professional's responsibility to respect confidentiality plays out in daily practice and guidance on setting up systems to maintain confidentiality are detailed elsewhere (see "Human Resources" in Part 1 and "Information Management" in Part 2, respectively).

Situations may arise in which maintaining patient confidentiality results in harm to a third party. The clinician then faces an ethical dilemma: the obligation to respect the patient's autonomy comes into conflict with the obligation to avoid harm to others who are at risk. An examination of the competing principles and of the claims arising from them will aid the health care professional in reaching a decision. In general, the duty to maintain confidentiality takes precedence over other obligations.

Patient Protection

A variety of mechanisms have been put in place to help ensure that patients' rights are respected and that patients are protected from harm. Patients' bills of rights outline the rights and, sometimes, responsibilities of patients receiving care at a health care facility. Patients who are receiving experimental care through a research protocol have the same rights as other patients. In addition, special policies provide for protection of research subjects, and these policies are overseen by IRBs.

Patient Bill of Rights

The intent of a patient's bill of rights is to outline the rights and responsibilities of a patient within the health care system. Various versions of these bills of rights exist. Among the primary examples are those developed by the American Hospital Association (first adopted in 1973), AMA, and JCAHO.

Regardless of origin, patients' bills of rights tend to agree on certain core rights of patients:

- The right to considerate and respectful care
- The right to relevant, current, and understandable information concerning their condition
- The right to be involved in all aspects of their care and to provide informed consent or refusal of care
- The right to know the identity of their caregivers
- The right to be informed of institutional policies, including those that could affect patient choice
- The right to make an advance directive (see also "Continuum of Women's Health Care" in Part 3)
- The right to privacy and confidentiality except when otherwise mandated by law
- The right to review their own medical records
- The right to know about the institution's charges and payment methods
- The right to know about potential conflicts of interest, including business relationships among institutions and health care professionals that may affect patient care
- The right to consent or decline participation in research studies; participants have the right to a full explanation of potential risks and benefits, procedures to be followed, and alternative services available; those who decline participation have the right to the most effective care the institution can otherwise provide

- The right to reasonable continuity of care, when appropriate
- The right to know about resources available for resolving conflicts and grievances
- The right to have available adequate health care

In addition, JCAHO states in its *Hospital Accreditation Standards* that patients should receive a written statement of their rights, appropriate to their age, understanding, and language, on admission to a health care facility. This statement should be available to them throughout their stay and can be posted in public areas accessible to patients and their visitors. Patients' rights should be described to them if written communication is not effective. Clinicians should be aware of the availability of their institution's patient's bill of rights and its content.

The idea that every American has a right to some level of health care has developed since the end of World War II. Both the United Nations and the World Health Organization support this right. The issue of access to care has engendered much discussion in recent years. Recently, the President's Advisory Commission on Consumer Protection and Quality in the Health Care Industry has echoed this call in its "Patients' Bill of Rights."

The American College of Obstetricians and Gynecologists has called for quality health care appropriate to every woman's needs throughout her life and for ensuring that a full array of clinical services are available to women without costly delays or the imposition of geographic, financial, attitudinal, or legal barriers. When health care institutions have policies based on religious beliefs that limit patient options, patients should be advised of these policies openly and as early as possible.

Fellows of the College should exercise their responsibility to improve the health status of women. They can do this both in the traditional patient–physician relationships and by working within their community and at the state and national levels to ensure access to high-quality programs meeting the health needs of all women.

Patients rightfully share responsibility for their care. The American Hospital Association identifies core patient responsibilities as follows:

- The responsibility to provide personal medical information

- The responsibility to request additional information if they do not fully understand information or instructions
- The responsibility to ensure that institutions have copies of their advance directives, if they exist
- The responsibility to inform their health care professional if they anticipate problems in complying with treatment
- The responsibility to make reasonable accommodations to the needs of health care institutions and their employees, other patients, and health care professionals
- The responsibility to provide information for insurance claims and to work with the institution to make payment arrangements, when necessary
- The responsibility to recognize the impact of their lifestyle on their personal health

Institutional Review Boards

The role of an IRB is to review and monitor biomedical research involving human subjects, with the goal of ensuring the protection of the rights and the welfare of the subjects. Although institutions sponsoring research usually will form their own IRBs, an institution that does not have its own IRB is permitted to use "outside" IRBs for approval and review of research.

General regulations affecting the protection of human subjects are contained in Title 21 of the Code of Federal Regulations, Part 50. The general standards for the composition, operation, and responsibility of an IRB that reviews research regulated by the FDA are contained in Title 21 of the Code of Federal Regulations, Part 56. In addition, the FDA has developed information sheets that offer guidance for IRBs and clinical investigators. The information presented here is excerpted from these sources.

Each IRB should have at least five members, with varying backgrounds, to promote complete and adequate review of research activities commonly conducted by the institution. Selection of IRB members should be based on experience and expertise and should aim for diversity of gender, race, and cultural background. At least one member should represent the scientific area, at least one should represent nonscientific areas, and at least one should not be otherwise affiliated with the organization. Individuals such as lawyers, clergy, and ethicists are commonly chosen to represent nonscientific areas.

The IRB should document that informed consent has been obtained. In some cases, the IRB may waive the requirement that the subject or her representative sign the consent form. The informed consent provided to the subject should include the eight basic elements of informed consent:

- A statement that the study involves research, an explanation of the purposes of the research and the expected duration of the subject's participation, a description of the procedures to be followed, and identification of any procedures that are experimental
- A description of any reasonably foreseeable risks or discomforts to the subject
- A description of any benefits to the subject or to others that may reasonably be expected from the research
- A disclosure of appropriate alternative procedures or courses of treatment, if any, that might be advantageous to the subject
- A statement describing the extent, if any, to which confidentiality of records identifying the subject will be maintained and that notes the possibility that the FDA may inspect the records
- For research involving more than minimal risk, an explanation as to whether any compensation is available and an explanation as to whether any medical treatments are available if injury occurs and, if so, what they consist of or where further information may be obtained
- An explanation of whom to contact for answers to pertinent questions about the research and research subjects' rights, and whom to contact in the event of a research-related injury to the subject
- A statement that participation is voluntary, that refusal to participate will involve no penalty or loss of benefits to which the subject is otherwise entitled, and that the subject may discontinue participa-

tion at any time without penalty or loss of benefits to which the subject is otherwise entitled

Other elements of informed consent may be required when appropriate.

An IRB should notify investigators and the institution of its decision to approve or disapprove proposed research or of modifications required to secure IRB approval. Disapprovals should include the reason and give the investigator an opportunity to respond. Continuing review of research performed at the institution should be conducted at intervals appropriate to the degree of risk, but not less than once per year. For certain categories of research, expedited reviews are possible. These categories are updated from time to time and are published in the *Federal Register.*

All IRB activities should be documented. These records should be kept for at least 3 years after the completion of research, and the records should be accessible for inspection and duplication by the FDA. The FDA has developed a checklist, included in its information sheets, that may be helpful in ensuring appropriate functioning and documentation of IRB activities.

Ethical Decision Making

In most cases, there is no conflict among patient, family, health care professional, and health care facility in selecting the most appropriate health care option even though more than one course of action may be morally and ethically justifiable. Sometimes there may be disagreements among parties as to the most appropriate choice. If the risk–benefit relationship is not optimal, no course of action will seem acceptable. Rarely, research goals might appear to conflict with the patient's best interests. Attempts to resolve such difficulties can be aided by a rational analysis of the various factors involved.

Although the key to ethical decision making is the patient–clinician dyad, the involvement of individuals with a variety of backgrounds and perspectives can be useful, especially if the dyad has reached an impasse. Through establishment of IRBs and institutional ethics committees, health care facilities can support the protection of patient rights and assist in ethical decision making in difficult situations. Institutions also have obligations to support their officers, employees, and health care professionals who are seeking to fulfill their ethical obligations.

Institutional Ethics Committees

Changes in medical technology and social structure have moved the site of much medical decision making from the home to health care facilities. Decisions once made privately and confidentially now are made publicly, with wide social, economic, and ethical consequences. Accordingly, patients, practitioners, and health care administrative personnel need a forum for discussion and education. Moreover, more and more often nonmedical institutional decision making (eg, third-party contracts, institutional purchasing, cancellation of financially negative services) is having a greater influence on patient care. An institutional ethics committee can provide such a forum. Ethics committees typically have the following functions:

- To foster awareness of ethical issues and create an environment of ethical concern
- To establish educational programs regarding ethical principles, biomedical ethics literature, and relevant legal decisions
- To act as an informational resource concerning medical ethics in the institutional setting
- To offer counsel on ethical issues and problems in individual cases
- To help create, promote, and audit a code of ethical behavior for the entire institution

Institutional ethics committees should represent disciplines from the health care facility and the community. Membership should be broad to minimize the possibility that the committee will be limited to those holding a specific point of view. Although religious attitudes and viewpoints may be valuable and welcome for decision makers, members holding such viewpoints should avoid advancing a particular religious or philosophical view without identifying it as such or misrepresenting it as medical advice.

The American Society for Bioethics and Humanities strongly opposes certification of ethics consultants and accreditation of educational programs to train individuals or groups to conduct ethics consultations. Interaction between the committee and the medical and nursing staff should be determined by the institution.

Most committees serve in advisory, rather than decision-making, capacities. However, authority exists within health care institutions to enforce institution policies and standards and to assume appropriate legal responsibility for practices within the institution. Specific duties for the committee may be mandated by law. In general, the committee may aid the patient, health care professional, and institution by serving as a resource for education, support, and institutional quality improvement.

An institutional ethics committee should first educate itself, using consultants, attending seminars, reviewing the literature, and using other resources to rigorously study the discipline of biomedical ethics. This information should then be disseminated to the hospital community. For example, the committee can educate staff about state laws (such as those defining death) and federal legislation (such as the law regarding informing patients about advance directives). The committee also can educate itself about varying cultural, religious, or professional perspectives (eg, religious attitudes toward autopsy, blood transfusion, and donation and reception of transplanted organs). Such education will help to anticipate conflicts and to accommodate or tolerate different points of view. The committee also can serve as a forum for the discussion of unresolved biomedical issues, such as the application of new reproductive technologies.

One of the primary functions of the committee is to advise and support primary decision makers (patients, families, and health care professionals) when difficult decisions must be made. As a part of this function, it can connect patients and families to social support and advocacy groups, which may increase their options.

Institutional ethics committees can assist in ensuring that the process of informed consent is followed with patients or their proxies. Consent for acceptance or refusal of treatment should be based on accurate and current medical information that presents all reasonable options. The committee should establish programs to promote this goal. The committee also should determine that the institution has systems to ensure that 1) the patient has the capacity to choose and 2) appropriate decision makers are identified when the patient does not have this capacity.

The committee also can assist in institutional quality assessment and improvement functions. For example, it can review the facility's experience for the purpose of identifying problems that are recurrent, in order to devise useful guidelines, and continually evaluate the guidelines for effectiveness.

The use of institutional ethics committees is an evolving technique for helping with difficult decisions. Continuing appraisal of their form and function is important. They are not meant to supplant other good techniques that have been found effective in the institution.

Institutional Responsibility

The *Code of Professional Ethics of the American College of Obstetricians and Gynecologists* states, "The obstetrician–gynecologist should strive to address through the appropriate procedures the status of those physicians who demonstrate questionable competence, impairment, or unethical or illegal behavior. In addition, the obstetrician–gynecologist should cooperate with appropriate authorities to prevent the continuation of such behavior." Institutions share in the responsibility to address unprofessional behavior.

Academic institutions, professional corporations, and health care facilities should have policies and procedures by which alleged violations of professional behavior can be reported and investigated (see "Governance" in Part 1). These institutions also should have policies in place regarding legal representation and indemnification for their employees or others acting in an official capacity who, in discharging their obligations relative to unethical or illegal behavior of individuals, are exposed to potentially costly legal actions. The American College of Obstetricians and Gynecologists agrees with the position of the American Association of University Professors that institutions should ensure effective legal and other necessary representation and full indemnification for any faculty member named or included in lawsuits or other legal proceedings arising from an act or omission in the discharge of institutional or professional duties.

Suggested Reading

American College of Obstetricians and Gynecologists. Code of professional ethics of the American College of Obstetricians and Gynecologists. Washington, DC: ACOG, 2002

American College of Obstetricians and Gynecologists. Ethical dimensions of informed consent. In: Ethics in obstetrics and gynecology. Washington, DC: ACOG, 2002:19–27

American College of Obstetricians and Gynecologists. Ethics in obstetrics and gynecology. Washington, DC: ACOG, 2002

American College of Obstetricians and Gynecologists. Informed refusal. ACOG Committee Opinion 237. Washington, DC: ACOG, 2000

American College of Obstetricians and Gynecologists. Institutional responsibility to provide legal representation. In: Ethics in obstetrics and gynecology. Washington, DC: ACOG, 2002:48

American Hospital Association. A patient's bill of rights. Chicago: AHA, 2001. Available at http://www.aha.org/resource/pbillofrights.ospj. Retrieved September 28, 2001

American Medical Association. Fundamental elements of the patient-physician relationship. In: Code of medical ethics: current opinions with annotations. Chicago: AMA, 2000:xv–xvi

American Society for Bioethics and Humanities. Core competencies for health care ethics consultation. Glenview, Illinois: ASBH, 1998

Information sheets: guidance for institutional review boards and clinical investigators. Rockville, Maryland: Food and Drug Administration, 1998

Institutional responsibility for legal demands on faculty. American Association of University Professors. Academe 1999;85(1):52

Institutional review boards, 21 C.F.R. § 56.101–56.124 (2000)

Joint Commission on Accreditation of Healthcare Organizations. Comprehensive accreditation manual for hospitals: the official handbook. Oakbrook Terrace, Illinois: JCAHO, 2000

Quality first: better health care for all Americans. Washington, DC: President's Advisory Commission on Consumer Protection and Quality in the Health Care Industry, 1998

Protection of human subjects, 21 C.F.R. § 50.1–50.27 (2000)

PART 2

Organization of Services

The delivery of high-quality obstetric and gynecologic care requires the establishment of efficient systems that can fulfill certain functions regardless of whether the care is provided in a hospital or an ambulatory setting. Such systems should support health care practitioners with essential human and material resources and foster interdisciplinary collaboration. Facilities should be organized in a manner that provides high-quality, efficient services. How practitioners define their scope of practice will affect how their office is organized and managed.

Common to all medical practices are certain principles and processes necessary to maintain an efficient and safe atmosphere in which to practice. The following principles of management for the organization of facilities and equipment, infection control procedures, supporting services, and information and practice management systems are recommended as guidelines that may be applied regardless of the size of the office or clinic or the scope of women's health care to be administered.

Facilities and Equipment

The facilities in which gynecologic care is provided should be conducive to the efficient and compassionate delivery of health care to all women, regardless of whether it is an office setting, an outpatient surgical facility, or an inpatient hospital setting. The following section describes many of the characteristics necessary for all facilities delivering gynecologic care as well as some of the most important specific requirements for individual settings.

General Requirements

Whether the facility in question is an office, an ambulatory surgical facility, or an inpatient hospital area, there are certain requirements for optimum delivery of gynecologic care. Building codes are city, county, and state specific. Facilities should adhere to all applicable codes.

Specific plans and procedures should be established for the health and safety of patients and personnel. Such plans and procedures should encompass the following items:

- Mechanisms to minimize the risk of the hazards of electrical and mechanical failure, explosion, and fire
- Comprehensive emergency plans, including but not limited to patient evacuation and the proper use of safety, emergency, and fire-extinguishing equipment
- Management of reasonably foreseeable medical emergencies arising from services rendered
- Transfer of patients to a nearby backup hospital in the event of an unanticipated emergency
- Training of personnel in cardiopulmonary resuscitation

- Control and disposal of needles, syringes, glass, knife blades, and contaminated material
- Proper storage, preparation, and administration of drugs
- Facilities that are accessible, free of barriers, and safe for all, including the physically disabled
- Adequate maintenance and cleanliness of facilities

Because one of the primary concerns is the safety of the patient and any accompanying individuals such as children, attention should be given to childproofing all reception areas as well as clinical areas. This should include moving any dangerous instruments or solutions out of lower cabinets or installing childproof locks on cabinet doors. Sharps containers should be placed back from the edge of countertops, and waste containers should be covered. There should be proper lighting and flooring to minimize any accidents, and at least some areas, including examination rooms and restrooms, should be wheelchair accessible.

Electrical, lighting, air quality, and temperature systems must function appropriately and safely, and a program for regular maintenance should be in place. An environmental engineer's assistance may be necessary to ensure proper functioning and maintenance. The safety and reliability of medical and other equipment must be established and maintained; this may require the assistance of mechanical engineers and biomedical technicians. Standards for electrical outlets and electrical equipment have been developed by the Joint Commission on Accreditation of Healthcare Organizations (JCAHO).

Emergency equipment and supplies should be readily available and maintained. Personnel should be instructed periodically in the proper use of safety, emergency, and fire-extinguishing equipment. Plans should be developed for emergency situations, including assisting individuals who have difficulty walking. Drills should be regularly conducted to ensure preparedness. Alternate sources of power should be adequate for staff to manage patients in the event of an emergency.

Medical equipment, such as ultrasonography equipment, should be operated only by properly trained personnel. Equipment should be well maintained and inspected at regular intervals for proper functioning and safety as specified by the manufacturer's operations manual. A log should be maintained of routine checks as well as repairs and service calls on medical equipment.

Policies and assessments to avoid potential hazards should be established. Smoking on the premises should be prohibited. Hazards that might result in accidents, electrical shock, or trauma should be minimized or eliminated. Sources of infections also should be minimized, and the adequacy of the infection control program should be periodically assessed (see "Infection Control" in Part 2). A system must be in place for the identification, safe handling, and disposition of hazardous materials and waste (see "Practice Management" in Part 2). Radiation exposure should be minimized.

Violence against physicians and other health care workers has raised concerns about personal safety in health care settings. The following are suggestions to enhance the safety of physicians, staff, and patients:

- Establish a relationship with the local police force and other security personnel
- Obtain a security audit of the office or institution
- Review emergency plans periodically
- Restrict after-hours access
- Improve lighting at entrances and in parking areas
- Install security cameras, mirrors, and panic buzzers
- Install deadbolt or electronic locks
- Lock all doors except the main entrance
- Preprogram 911 (emergency phone number) into all phones
- Enclose and secure reception areas
- Develop an emergency notification system

Office and Other Ambulatory Settings

The office or clinic, no matter how small or how large, should be well organized and clean. The reception area should be pleasantly decorated and comfortable and should have adequate seating capacity to accommodate patients. Current general interest reading material and patient education materials should be available. The reception area should be separate from yet visible to the receptionist. Ideally, patients in the reception area should not be able to overhear telephone conversations or business conducted by the receptionist. A telephone should be available for patients to make outgoing calls. Restrooms and a patient changing area that is adequate in space for undressing and dressing should be available. Accessories, such as mirrors and hangers for a patient's personal belongings, should be provided in the changing area.

There should be a comfortable, private area for discussing confidential information and for interviewing and counseling the patient and her family. There should be a utility area, separate from the examination rooms, equipped with work counters, closed cabinets for storage, locked medicine cabinets, a refrigerator, and facilities for sterilization and hand-washing.

The physician's office may serve as a consultation room; however, separate rooms, other than the physician's office and examining rooms, are desirable for use by nurses, social workers, health educators, or other members of the health care team. The number of examining rooms will depend on the patient profile and the size of the practice. A minimum of two examination rooms per practitioner is recommended.

Some obstetrician–gynecologists provide mammography screening in their offices. Mammography equipment is now subject to regulation by the U.S. Food and Drug Administration (FDA). For further details, refer to "Compliance with Government Regulations" in Part 1.

Surgical Facilities

A freestanding surgical facility should be organized and equipped for a variety of uses. These uses are to provide preoperative and postoperative care; to assess the quality of that care, including regular periodic review of practice procedures, governance, and outcome; and to arrange for the transfer of a patient if an emergency arises.

The American College of Surgeons has classified ambulatory facilities providing surgical services as follows:

- Class A—Provides minor surgical procedures performed under topical, local, or regional anesthesia without preoperative sedation
- Class B—Provides minor or major surgical procedures performed in conjunction with oral, parenteral, or intravenous sedation or under analgesic or dissociative drugs
- Class C—Provides major surgical procedures that require general or regional block anesthesia and support of vital bodily functions

Various requirements have been defined by the American College of Surgeons for each of these classes of units. For example, for all classes of facilities, there is a requirement that space and equipment be adequate to provide safe delivery of surgical and anesthesia services, appropriate monitoring and resuscitation equipment must be available and suited for each level of facility, and acceptable standards of cleanliness and sterility must be maintained. Specifically, for all classes of facilities, blood pressure monitoring apparatus is required. For Class B and C facilities, an electrocardiographic oscilloscope, a defibrillator, and a pulse oximeter with an alarm also are required. Class B and C facilities also require appropriate intravenous fluids and administration equipment, appropriate stretchers and wheelchairs, and dressing and lounge areas for surgical personnel that do not adversely affect the care of patients. Class C facilities require all of the above as well as an oxygen analyzer with an alarm and a CO_2 monitor.

The appropriate physical design for an ambulatory surgical facility depends on the number and types of surgical procedures to be performed. The facility should provide a comfortable, safe environment with minimal architectural barriers. The requirements of the Occupational Safety and Health Administration (OSHA) should be met as well as state and local requirements (see box). Traffic flow should be convenient and efficient. A multilevel facility should have elevators that can accommodate gurneys.

Occupational Safety and Health Administration Compliance Consultation

A free, confidential consultation service is available to evaluate a facility's safety and ability to comply with Occupational Safety and Health Administration (OSHA) standards. Consultation is performed by state government professionals; it is completely independent of OSHA inspection, and no citations or penalties are given. For more information, visit the OSHA web site at www.osha.gov.

The facility also should include adequate space for the following functions:

- Reception and waiting
- Administrative activities such as patient admission, record storage, and business affairs
- Patient dressing and locker storage
- Preoperative evaluation, including physical examination, laboratory testing, and preparation for anesthesia
- Performance of surgical procedures
- Preparation and sterilization of instruments
- X-ray capability (eg, to check for items missing from the equipment count at the end of the procedure)
- Storage of equipment, drugs, and fluids
- Postanesthetic recovery
- Staff activities
- Janitorial and utility support

Inpatient Facilities

Within inpatient hospital settings, as well as emergency and urgent care settings, a private, secure examination room appropriate for gynecologic examinations should be available. The room should be of adequate size, with a door that locks from the inside or a curtain to pull across the doorway. It should be equipped with a sink and adequate counter space or a tray stand to hold the supplies needed for the examination. This room should be equipped with an examination table with stirrups or footrests and adequate lighting to perform a pelvic examination. Basic equipment, including patient drapes, a sharps disposal container, vaginal specula of various sizes, and supplies to perform cervical cytology tests, wet preps and cultures (subject to certification), and biopsies of the endometrium, cervix, and vulva also should be readily available. Equipment needed for minor surgical procedures should be accessible. In essence, this room should be of similar size and layout and equipped like an examination room in an outpatient office.

High-quality care is more easily attained in a specialty service. When hospital size permits, the gynecologic inpatient service should be consolidated in one designated area. In smaller hospitals where the number of patients may not justify the establishment of a separate area, gynecologic patients may be treated in either a medical or surgical area. Gynecologic patients who do not have transmissible infections may be treated in the obstetric area when hospital policy permits and when their care does not interfere with the operation of the obstetric unit.

Suggested Reading

American College of Surgeons. Guidelines for optimal ambulatory surgical care and office-based surgery. 3rd ed. Chicago: ACS, 2000

American Institute of Architects Academy of Architecture for Health. Guidelines for design and construction of hospital and health care facilities, 1996–97. Washington, DC: The American Institute of Architects Press, 1996

Joint Commission on Accreditation of Healthcare Organizations. A crosswalk between the American College of Surgeons' guidelines for optimal office-based surgery and the Joint Commission's ambulatory care standards. Oakbrook Terrace, Illinois: JCAHO, 1998

Recommended practices for sterilization in perioperative practice settings. AORN: Association of periOperative Registered Nurses. AORN J 1999;70:283–293

Sibbald B. Physician, protect thyself. CMAJ 1998;159:987–989

INFECTION CONTROL

All women's health care facilities need effective infection control procedures to protect patients and staff. The following recommendations for the cleaning, disinfecting, and sterilizing of patient care equipment, bloodborne pathogen contamination, and isolation and standard precautions provide an infection control framework for all health care facilities.

Cleaning, Disinfecting, and Sterilizing Patient Care Equipment

To reduce the risk of disease transmission in the health care environment, it is imperative that all facilities follow established infection control practices in cleaning, disinfecting, and sterilizing patient care equipment (Table 2–1). The risk of disease transmission from patient to health care worker, from health care worker to patient, and from patient to patient can be reduced significantly if proper preventive procedures are established and followed rigorously.

Health care workers should be aware that practices regarding the selection and use of sterilization methods and disinfectants continue to evolve, with new recommendations coming forth as new products and information become available. In each facility, one person should be charged with the responsibility for infection control. This employee should be guided by current information published in the scientific literature. Facilities must be in compliance with OSHA requirements (see "Compliance with Government Regulations" in Part 1 and Appendix B). Periodic publications and guidelines issued by the Centers for Disease Control and Prevention (CDC) and by the Association for Professionals in Infection Control and Epidemiology, Inc, are valuable sources for such information. Hospital infection control professionals also are excellent resources.

Cleaning

Before sterilization or high-level disinfection, instruments should be cleaned thoroughly to remove debris. All methods of sterilization and disinfection are ineffective if equipment is not cleaned thoroughly. Cleaning may be accomplished by a thorough scrubbing with soap and water, a detergent or enzymatic/detergent solution, or with a mechanical device such as an ultrasonic cleaner. Special cleaning brushes are made available by instrument companies for more difficult to clean items. Ideally, mechanical devices should be used for sharp objects to lessen the possibility of injury to personnel during cleaning. Heavy-duty gloves lessen the risk of hand injuries if such items are cleaned by hand. If an instrument is not cleaned immediately after use, it should be placed into a container of water or disinfectant–detergent to prevent drying of material on the instrument before it is cleaned.

Disinfecting and Sterilizing

For purposes of infection control, all medical and surgical instruments are generally classified into three categories—critical, semicritical, or noncritical—depending on the risk that they might transmit infection and the need to sterilize or disinfect them between uses. All health care facilities should evaluate each item used and classify it accordingly.

Critical Items. Critical items are defined as surgical or other instruments that penetrate sterile tissue or the vascular system (eg, scalpels, biopsy forceps, endometrial biopsy instruments, urinary catheters, needles). Many of these items are available in sterile disposable form.

The only completely reliable methods for sterilizing reusable instruments in the office setting are steam under pressure (autoclaving), gaseous ethylene oxide, and dry heat. Ethylene oxide is not commonly used; it is not practical in the office setting. Autoclaving devices are practical, relatively inexpensive, and safe to use. They are the method of choice for instruments that can tolerate moist heat. Steam sterilization requires appropriate preparation, packaging, monitoring (biological, chemical, and mechanical), and storage of items. Continuous dry heat at 170°C for 1 hour sterilizes articles that cannot tolerate moist heat. Superheated gas bead sterilizers are useful and effective for rapid sterilization of the distal end of the metal instruments frequently used in the office setting (eg, biopsy forceps).

Table 2–1. Methods of Sterilization and Disinfection

	Sterilization		Disinfection		
	Critical Items (will enter tissue or vascular system or blood will flow through them)		**High Level (semicritical items [except dental[*]] will come in contact with mucous membrane or nonintact skin)**	**Intermediate Level (some semicritical tems[†] and noncritical items)**	**Low Level (noncritical items; will come in contact with intact skin)**
Object	*Procedure*	*Exposure Time (h)*	*Procedure (exposure time ≥20 min)* [‡,§]	*Procedure (exposure time ≤10 min)*	*Procedure (exposure time ≤10 min)*
Smooth, hard surface[†]	A	MR	C	G[‖]	H
	B	MR	D	H	I
	C	MR	E	J	J
	D	6	F[¶]	K	K
	E	MR	G		L
Rubber tubing and catheters[§]	A	MR	C		
	B	MR	D		
	C	MR	E		
	D	6	F[¶]		
	E	MR			
Polyethylene tubing and catheters[§,#]	A	MR	C		
	B	MR	D		
	C	MR	E		
	D	6	F[¶]		
	E	MR			
Lensed instruments	B	MR	C		
	C	MR	D		
	D	6	E		
	E	MR			

Thermometers (oral and rectal)**				H**
Hinged instruments	A	MR	C	
	B	MR	D	
	C	MR	E	
	D	6		
	E	MR		

*Semicritical dental items (eg, handpieces, amalgam condensers) should be heat sterilized; refer to Am J Infect Control 1996;24:313–342.

†See Am J Infect Control 1996;24:313–342 for discussion of hydrotherapy.

‡The longer the exposure to a disinfectant, the more likely it is that all microorganisms will be eliminated. Ten minutes' exposure is not adequate to disinfect many objects, especially those that are difficult to clean because they have narrow channels or other areas that can harbor organic material and bacteria. Twenty minutes' exposure is the minimum time needed to reliably kill *M. tuberculosis* and nontuberculous mycobacteria with glutaraldehyde.

§Tubing must be completely filled for chemical disinfection; care must be taken to avoid entrapment of air bubbles during immersion.

||Used in laboratory where cultures or concentrated preparations or microorganisms have spilled. This solution may destroy some surfaces.

¶Pasteurization (washer disinfector) of respiratory therapy and anesthesia equipment is a recognized alternative to high-level disinfection. Some data challenge the efficacy of some pasteurization units (J Hosp Infect 1983;4:199–208).

#Thermostability should be investigated when appropriate.

**Do not mix rectal and oral thermometers at any stage of handling or processing.

Key
- A. Heat sterilization, including steam or hot air (see manufacturer's recommendations)
- B. Ethylene oxide gas (see manufacturer's recommendations)
- C. Glutaraldehyde-based formulations (2%) (Caution should be exercised with all glutaraldehyde formulations when further in-use dilution is anticipated)
- D. Stabilized hydrogen peroxide 6% (will corrode copper, zinc, and brass)
- E. Peracetic acid, concentration variable but ≤1% is sporicidal
- F. Wet pasteurization at 70°C for 30 minutes after detergent cleaning
- G. Sodium hypochlorite (5.2% household bleach) 1:50 dilution (1,000 ppm free chlorine)
- H. Ethyl or isopropyl alcohol (70–90%)
- I. Sodium hypochlorite (5.2% household bleach) 1:500 dilution (100 ppm free chlorine)
- J. Phenolic germicidal detergent solution (follow product label for use-dilution)
- K. Iodophor germicidal detergent solution (follow product label for use-dilution)
- L. Quaternary ammonium germicidal detergent solution (follow product label for use-dilution)
- MR. Manufacturer's recommendations

Adapted from Rutala WA. APIC guideline for selection and use of disinfectants. 1994, 1995, and 1996 APIC Guideline Committee. Association for Professionals in Infection Control and Epidemiology. Am J Infect Control 1996;24:313–342

Liquid chemical germicides (cold sterilization) may be used to sterilize instruments that may be damaged by heat; however, complete sterilization may take up to 10 hours of exposure time, so this method is used more commonly for semicritical items. Several commercial germicides are registered with the U.S. Environmental Protection Agency as sterilant–disinfectants and are identified as such by the U.S. Environmental Protection Agency label on the container. They may be used for both critical and semicritical items. It is imperative that the user follow the manufacturer's recommendations for activation, shelf life, temperature requirements, monitoring, concentration of active ingredients, and exposure time. Exposure time varies greatly depending on whether the instruments require sterilization or high-level disinfection.

The following agents are used for cold sterilization or high-level disinfection:

- Glutaraldehyde-based formulations
- Stabilized hydrogen peroxide (6%)
- Orthophalaldehyde solutions
- Peracetic acid
- Peracetic acid—hydrogen peroxide

The glutaraldehyde-based formulations have gained widespread acceptance because of several advantages, including excellent biocidal properties, activity in the presence of organic matter, and noncorrosive action on endoscopic equipment. Rubber and plastic equipment generally are not damaged by this solution.

Semicritical Items. Semicritical items are defined as instruments that come in contact with mucous membranes or with skin that is not intact (eg, metal vaginal speculums and diaphragm fitting rings). Semicritical items may be sterilized as discussed previously but can be disinfected with wet pasteurization at 75°C for 30 minutes after detergent cleaning or by the use of chemical germicides as listed in the previous section.

Ideally, instruments that enter sterile tissue should be sterilized; however, high-level disinfection is frequently used. Endoscopic equipment often is difficult to clean and disinfect because of narrow channels and joints. Extended exposure to a chemical germicide makes it more likely that all contaminating microorganisms will be deactivated; however, extended exposure to these agents may damage delicate and lensed instruments. Users of these instruments should ask the manufacturers about the proper method of cleaning, sterilizing, and disinfecting. In general, such instruments should be exposed to a high-level chemical disinfectant for at least 20 minutes at room temperature after thorough cleaning. Disinfection must be followed by a sterile water rinse, then drying with a 70% ethyl or isopropyl alcohol rinse, followed by purging with air. Key points for disinfecting endoscopes are: meticulous cleaning, leak testing, following manufacturer's recommendations, training of personnel, use of standard procedures, and monitoring of concentrations. Nonimmersible scopes should be phased out.

Some semicritical items, such as oral or rectal thermometers or objects with smooth hard surfaces, may be disinfected with intermediate-level disinfectants, such as ethyl or isopropyl alcohol. Phenolic germicidal detergent solution or iodophor germicidal detergent solution also may be used for intermediate-level equipment items.

Noncritical Items. Noncritical items are those that come into contact with the skin but not with mucous membranes. Examples of commonly used noncritical items are bedpans, blood pressure cuffs, patient furniture, instrument stands, and countertops. A chemical germicide registered with the U.S. Environmental Protection Agency as a "hospital disinfectant" and labeled for "hepatitis B" or "tuberculocidal activity" is recommended for disinfection of surfaces that have been soiled by patient contact. These disinfectants include phenolics, iodophors, and chloride-containing compounds. Sodium hypochlorite (household bleach), prepared daily, is an inexpensive and effective intermediate-level germicide. A 1:100 dilution of bleach in tap water, or 1/4 cup of bleach in 1 gallon of water, is effective on surfaces that have been cleaned of visible contamination. Gross spills of blood or other body fluids should first be cleaned mechanically, then disinfected with a hospital-grade disinfectant with tuberculocidal activity or a 1:10 to 1:100 dilution of bleach. Convenient spray bottles of this concentration of household bleach and water allow for effective and inexpensive application. They should be freshly prepared.

Low-level disinfectants that are registered with the U.S. Environmental Protection Agency as hospital disinfectants, but not labeled for tuberculocidal activity, are appropriate for general housekeeping purposes such as cleaning floors and walls. Quaternary ammonium compounds are ideal and inexpensive for this purpose.

Bloodborne Pathogen Contamination. Possible contamination of instruments by bloodborne pathogens such as human immunodeficiency virus, hepatitis B virus, and hepatitis C virus is of increasing concern. Standard sterilization and disinfection procedures, if carried out as recommended, are adequate to sterilize or disinfect equipment and protect against these viruses.

Isolation Precautions

In 1996, the Hospital Infection Control Practices Advisory Committee of the CDC revised its "Guideline for Isolation Precautions in Hospitals." These recommendations for reducing transmission of microorganisms also can apply to the office setting. All personnel should be educated about the use of precautions and their responsibility for adhering to them.

The Centers for Disease Control and Prevention recommends that blood and body fluid standard precautions should be used consistently for all patients. Because medical history and examination cannot reliably identify all patients infected with human immunodeficiency virus or other bloodborne pathogens, the CDC recommends standard precautions for all patients to protect health care workers from infectious body fluids.

These recommendations incorporate the prior concept of universal precautions to prevent transmission of bloodborne pathogens and recognize the importance of all body fluids, secretions, and excretions in the transmission of nosocomial pathogens. These precautions apply to 1) blood; 2) all body fluids, secretions, and excretions except sweat, regardless of whether they contain visible blood; 3) nonintact skin; and 4) mucous membranes. Standard precautions include some of the following techniques:

- *Hand-washing* after touching blood or body fluids and contaminated items, whether or not gloves are worn, and between patient contacts
  - —Use of a plain soap for routine hand-washing
  - —Use of an antimicrobial agent after patients with known or suspected illnesses easily transmitted by direct patient contact (eg, wound infection or respiratory infections)
- Wear *gloves* when touching blood, body fluids, and contaminated items and remove them promptly after use, before touching noncontaminated surfaces
- Wear a *mask* and eye/face protection during activities that may generate a splash or spray of blood or body fluids to the face
- Wear a *gown* during activities that may generate a splash or spray of blood or body fluids to clothing or skin
- Handle used *patient care equipment* soiled with blood or body fluids so as to prevent contamination of skin, mucous membranes, clothing, and other surfaces. Single-use items should be discarded properly, and reusable equipment must be cleaned and reprocessed appropriately.
- Have written *procedures for routine cleaning*, care, and disinfection of frequently touched surfaces
- Have written procedures for handling soiled *linen* to prevent contamination of clean surfaces
- Take care to prevent injuries when using *sharp instruments.* Never recap used needles; place used disposable syringes, needles, scalpel blades, and other sharps in puncture-resistant, disposable containers located as close as practical to the area where the items are normally used.
- Have *mouthpieces* readily available to use as an alternative to mouth-to-mouth resuscitation

SUGGESTED READING

Alvarado CJ, Reichelderfer M. APIC guideline for infection prevention and control in flexible endoscopy. Association for Professionals in Infection Control. Am J Infect Control 2000;28:138–155

American Society for Anesthesiologists. Recommendations for infection control for the practice of anesthesiology. 2nd ed. Park Ridge, Illinois: ASA, 1998

Association for Professionals in Infection Control and Epidemiology, Inc. APIC text of infection control and epidemiology. Washington, DC: APIC, 2000

Garner JS. Guideline for isolation precautions in hospitals. The Hospital Infection Control Practices Advisory Committee [published erratum appears in Infect Control Hosp Epidemiol 1996 Apr;17(4):214]. Infect Control Hosp Epidemiol 1996;17:53–83

Updated U.S. Public Health Service Guidelines for the Management of Occupational Exposures to HBV, HCV, and HIV and Recommendations for Postexposure Prophylaxis. MMWR Morb Mortal Wkly Rep 2001;50(RR-11):1–52

Rutala WA. APIC guidelines for selection and use of disinfectants. 1994, 1995, and 1996 APIC Guidelines Committee. Association for Professionals in Infection Control and Epidemiology. Am J Infect Control 1996;24:313–342

Supporting Services

Ancillary services, including pharmacy, radiology, laboratory, and anesthesia, often are a component of patient care. The following recommendations for supporting services should be considered general guidelines and are not necessarily requirements or mandates. Such services, whether on-site or off-site, should be accredited, and their guidelines or policies should be acceptable to patients and clinicians. Physicians should check state and federal laws and regulations on self-referral prohibitions before referring a patient for health care services in which the physician or an immediate family member has a financial interest (see "Human Resources" in Part 1). These laws and regulations continue to evolve, and current requirements should be reviewed. All ancillary services must meet all applicable federal and state requirements.

Pharmacy Services

There should be an appropriate selection of medications available and means for obtaining medications not on-site. Prescribing, preparing, and dispensing medication should follow established procedures that are in compliance with legal regulations, licensure, and professional practice standards. Appropriate records and security must be kept to maintain the safe and controlled dispensing of medications and to allow patient notification in the event of a drug recall or newly reported complications. The pharmacy must be supervised by a licensed pharmacist or physician.

When medications are dispensed, patients should be given instructions and important medication information. The quality and appropriateness of medication usage should be monitored as part of the quality improvement program. Adverse medication effects should be monitored and addressed. The FDA has established MedWatch, which is the FDA Medical Products Reporting Program. The American College of Obstetricians and Gynecologists (a MedWatch Partner) encourages women's health care clinicians to participate in MedWatch. More information is available on the FDA web site, www.fda.gov. Reports also can be made online.

Laboratory and Pathology Services

All laboratory and pathology services must serve patient and clinician needs and meet professional practice standards and state and federal legal requirements. Procedures to control for quality should include validating test results through the use of standardized controls and appropriate documentation. A written report should be generated for all laboratory and pathology examinations performed. This report should be included in the patient's medical record, and there should be documentation of review by the clinician. A qualified physician should oversee the laboratory. Competent, appropriately trained personnel should conduct the laboratory work.

Radiology Services

Diagnostic imaging services including, but not limited to, radiographic, fluoroscopic, and ultrasonographic services must be available to meet patient and clinician needs. There should be adequate space and equipment to ensure the safe delivery of these services. This includes policies for handling, storing, and disposing of potentially hazardous materials and proper shielding where potentially hazardous energy sources are used. A radiologist or physician qualified and credentialed to interpret examinations must be available to authenticate reports. Written reports must be generated in a timely manner. Dated reports of service and diagnostic images must be maintained and available in the patient's file. Quality assurance must be maintained by periodic review. Imaging services should be performed only on the order of a qualified clinician.

Acceptable monitoring devices should be provided to personnel who might be exposed to harmful energy, and personnel exposure records should be maintained in accordance with relevant regulations. Proper warning signs must be posted to alert the public and office personnel to the presence of hazardous energy fields with particular attention to pregnant women and patients with pacemakers.

Anesthesia and Analgesia

A preanesthetic assessment should be conducted for any patient for whom anesthesia is planned (see "Ambulatory Gynecologic Surgery" in Part 3). Administration of any anesthetic must be performed or supervised by a qualified physician. Adequate space and equipment should be provided for safe delivery of anesthesia services. No explosive anesthetics should be used. General or spinal anesthesia must be administered by an anesthesiologist, a physician eligible to take the anesthesiology board examination, or a registered nurse–anesthetist under the direct supervision of an anesthesiologist. Local or regional block anesthesia with or without sedation should be administered by or under the supervision of a qualified physician. Clinicians administering intravenous conscious sedation must have sufficient training and experience related to the use, administration, side effects, and complications of all applicable medications. Knowledge of airway management, basic life supports, and emergency medical management is required. The patient must be closely monitored during the procedure and postprocedure until she is adequately recovered with particular attention to physiologic and mental status, pathologic findings, intravenous fluids and drugs administered, and any unusual events or complications (see "Ambulatory Gynecologic Surgery" in Part 3).

Follow-up Services

Discharge plans should attempt to address the patient's needs in all of the following areas: physical, emotional, housekeeping, transportation, and social. Follow-up services may include adult foster care, case management, home health services, hospice, long-term care facilities, ambulatory care, support groups, and rehabilitation services. Follow-up care practitioners should receive a summary of the care previously provided, the patient's progress toward goals, and information regarding instructions and referrals provided to the patient. The patient, her family, her primary health care practitioners, and her ancillary practitioners should communicate clearly with one another and understand the patient assessment and plan. The patient and her family should receive written and verbal education regarding their responsibilities for daily care and follow-up appointments, the safe use of prescribed medications, adverse reactions or complications that must be reported to the clinician, and a name and phone number to call in an emergency.

SUGGESTED READING

American Association of Blood Banks. Standards for blood banks and transfusion services. 19th ed. Bethesda, Maryland: AABB, 1999

American College of Radiology standards. Reston, Virginia: ACR, 1990

Glenn GC, Altshur CH, Gambino R, Henry JB, Hostetter A, Ohrt DK, et al. Practice parameter on laboratory panel testing for screening and case finding in asymptomatic adults. College of American Pathologists. Arch Pathol Lab Med 1996;120:929–941

Joint Commission on Accreditation of Healthcare Organizations. A crosswalk between the American College of Surgeons' guidelines for optimal office-based surgery and the Joint Commission's ambulatory care standards. Oakbrook Terrace, Illinois: JCAHO, 1998

Joint Commission on Accreditation of Healthcare Organizations. 2000–2001 standards for pathology and clinical laboratory services. Oakbrook Terrace, Illinois: JCAHO, 2000

Practice guidelines for sedation and analgesia by non-anesthesiologists. A report by the American Society of Anesthesiologists Task Force on Sedation and Analgesia by Non-Anesthesiologists. Anesthesiology 1996;84:459–471

INFORMATION MANAGEMENT

Because modern medical practice frequently involves several clinicians and other professionals, every health care facility needs information management systems in place to provide effective means of communication among all members of the health care team. This section provides guidelines for the maintenance of medical records and the documentation of all patient communication, including informed consent.

Medical Records

An accurate medical record should be maintained for each patient in a secure, confidential, and readily accessible way. The patient's name should appear on each page of the record, pertinent information should be firmly attached, and a problem list should be maintained. The record should be legible, concise, cogent, and complete. It should be completed promptly and signed by the qualified health care practitioner. Depending on the services provided to the patient, the medical record should contain the following information, when appropriate:

- Patient identification data
- History and physical findings
- Provisional diagnosis
- Prior medical procedures, including those provided at other facilities
- Diagnostic and therapeutic orders
- Surgeons' and nurses' notes
- Results of laboratory tests
- Signed, dated, and witnessed operative consent forms
- Operative report
- Anesthesia report
- Tissue report
- Medications record

- Progress notes
- Discharge notes and instructions

When surgery has been performed, the medical record should contain sufficient information to justify the preoperative diagnosis and the operative procedure and to document the postoperative course. Where feasible, medical records used in an ambulatory surgical facility should conform to a standard record used in the community or backup hospital. In addition, an ambulatory surgical facility should keep registers of admissions and discharges, operations, results of follow-up contacts, and controlled substances dispensed.

The medical record should allow an easy assessment of the care provided to determine whether the patient's health care needs have been identified, diagnosed, and managed effectively. Because modern medical practice frequently involves several physicians and professionals, the medical record should serve as a vehicle for communication among all members of the health care team. Entries by all health care workers should be signed or initialed and dated. Any abbreviations should be clear to all health care workers using the patient's medical record.

Medical records should be organized in a consistent manner. A system should be in place to avoid misplacing or misfiling medical records. Records should be protected against fire, theft, and other damage. Records may be kept in their original format or transferred to another media. When disposing of records, physicians should ensure the records are completely destroyed to protect confidentiality.

The medical staff should be made aware of the need for strict confidentiality of a patient's medical records (see "Human Resources" in Part 1). Patient information stored and transferred electronically requires safeguards to limit access and protect confidentiality.

There should be an established protocol for handling requests for records by the patient, her family, an attorney, an insurance company, or another third party. A signed authorization must be obtained from the patient prior to the release of any medical information contained in her medical record. Only copies should be transmitted; the original record should be retained in the office. When copies of the medical records are transferred to another institution, the institution must be expected to maintain the confidentiality of the patient's records.

Where feasible, patient financial records should be kept in a separate confidential file, apart from the patient's medical record. All correspondence or notation of conversations between physicians and professional liability insurance carriers or defense counsel pertaining to a patient should be kept in a confidential file, separate from the patient's medical record.

Medical and legal considerations determine the length of time records are retained. When records are no longer needed for medical purposes, state law determines how long medical records are kept. Some states have specific legal requirements for retaining medical records, specific requirements for retaining business records, or both; a medical record is considered a business record. Another determining factor regarding retaining medical records is the statute of limitations for filing medical malpractice actions. Most states have different statutes of limitations for adults and minors, and these statutes vary from state to state. Frequently, statutes of limitations for medical malpractice actions involving an adult provide for a 2- to 5-year period in which to bring a lawsuit. A minor usually has more time to file a malpractice suit, and in some states a minor may have 18 years or more to sue. Physicians should consult their state medical society or professional liability insurance carrier for information on retaining medical records. Records of Medicare or Medicaid patients must be retained for at least 5 years, and immunization records must be kept permanently. After ascertaining the applicable time frames for retaining records, physicians should keep records for the period that is the longest for the particular record.

Patient Communication

There is increasing use of technology for exchanging medical information between patients and health care practitioners. Cellular telephones, telephone answering machines, facsimile machines, and electronic mail all improve access among clinicians and patients but increase the possibility of a breach of patient confidentiality (see "Human Resources" in Part 1).

Third parties may have authorized or unauthorized access to the health care practitioner's or the patient's communication system. Prior to communicating with a patient using these technologies, the health care practitioner should discuss the security risks of these systems and obtain the patient's consent to this form of communication. A medical history may contain information so sensitive that the patient may judge that the risk of losing confidentiality outweighs the sought-after benefit. Reasonable precautions should be taken to achieve computer and telecommunication security, and patients must be educated to understand that no clinician or institution can guarantee complete security of electronically transmitted data.

Physicians should become familiar with their own state's regulations concerning telemedicine. Some states require that all physicians, wherever located, who provide medical advice to patients in that state have a medical license for that state. Practice web sites should carry clear disclaimers stating that the site is for informational purposes only and is not intended to give medical advice and that use of the site does not establish a physician–patient relationship.

All telephone contact regarding clinical matters should be documented in the patient's medical record. A method should be established to document or log such contacts both during and after office hours. An answering service for telephone calls or specific equipment to receive and transmit patient messages after normal office hours should be in place. The practitioner should be notified when a telephone message from a patient specifically requests that care be provided by that practitioner. Ideally, staff should inform the patient of an approximate time when the call would be returned by the practitioner. All telephone prescription renewals should be verified by the practitioner.

A protocol should exist for processing pertinent clinical information that may arrive by telephone, facsimile, or mail. A clear procedure should be in place to ensure that clinical information, such as laboratory, radiology, and pathology reports, and pertinent patient telephone messages are reviewed by the health care team. All such information should be initialed or signed and dated by the physician or qualified health care worker, then filed in the medical record.

Office tracking systems should be created for laboratory and imaging studies. These systems could include patient name; date of office visit; name of laboratory or imaging service; type of test or study; date the specimen is sent to the laboratory site or date the patient is referred to the imaging service; date the results are returned; the results; date the results are relayed to the patient, by whom, and in what way; and the date of the follow-up appointment. These systems could be either in the form of a paper medical record log or computerized.

A protocol should be established to ensure that patients are informed of all significant abnormal test results. This notification should be documented in the patient's medical record. A method should exist for monitoring patients' compliance with recommendations that are made based on abnormal test results. The patient or her family should be given individualized instructions for continuing care following office operative procedures, and this instruction should be documented in the patient's medical record. An established protocol also should exist for follow-up with any patient whose disease or condition may be life threatening or may have a serious effect on her life if she fails to keep appointments.

Missed appointments, noncompliance with medical advice, and refusal of a recommended test or procedure should be documented in the patient's medical record. Clinicians have the right to terminate practitioner–patient relationships. The clinician should be aware of legal and any managed care contractual requirements that apply to termination of the practitioner–patient relationship. Documentation of all steps undertaken to terminate the relationship should be present in the patient's medical record. Recommendations regarding the closing of a practice are found in "Liability" in Part 1.

Issues of cultural competency and barriers to effective communication must be examined and addressed when developing patient communication and documentation systems. Increased sensitivity to cultural issues can facilitate more positive interactions. In certain practices, consideration should be given to providing translated patient information. Patient communication procedures should allow for cultural differences in the role of the extended family in health care decision making. In addition, clinicians should be attuned to the possible intimidation of those with little exposure to the health care system. The volume of paperwork and the use of professional jargon often associated with women's health care information systems can be intimidating.

Informed Consent

The health care practitioner is responsible for securing the patient's informed consent. The risks and benefits of and alternatives to the proposed procedure, test, or treatment should be discussed with the patient (see "Ethical Issues" in Part 1). Patient education information, when available, should be provided to supplement informed consent and discussions relating to specific treatments, tests, operations, and procedures. The patient should be informed of the common adverse effects of prescribed drugs, as well as the importance of reading the patient package inserts for drugs or devices. All informed consent discussions and information material provided should be documented appropriately in the patient's medical record.

If a patient refuses a recommended test, treatment, or procedure, this refusal also should be documented. It should be noted that the physician recommended a particular test, treatment, or procedure to the patient, that the material risks and benefits were explained to her, and that the patient refused the treatment or procedure.

Practitioners also should comply with specific state and federal informed consent laws and regulations that apply to specific treatments or procedures. This may include informing patients of risks and benefits contained in the laws and having patients sign an approved consent form. Specific additional requirements may apply to patients younger than 21 years of age (see "Human Resources" in Part 1).

Suggested Reading

American College of Obstetricians and Gynecologists. The assistant: information for improved risk management. Washington, DC: ACOG, 2001

American College of Obstetricians and Gynecologists. Cultural competency in health care. ACOG Committee Opinion 201. Washington, DC: ACOG, 1998

Kane B, Sands DZ. Guidelines for the clinical use of electronic mail with patients. The AMIA Internet Working Group, Task Force on Guidelines for the Use of Clinic-Patient Electronic Mail. J Am Med Inform Assoc 1998;5:104–111

Practice Management

Staffing

Staffing Levels

Staffing requirements for an office or institution will vary. Factors in setting staffing levels and types include the anticipated need for chaperoning, population served, and scope of services to be provided. State regulations may be relevant depending on the health care practitioners needed and their scope of practice. In some cases, contractual arrangements may be required to assist patients with their health care needs (eg, nutrition, ultrasonography, social services).

The efficient operation of an ambulatory surgical facility requires that the assignment of administrative and professional personnel be based on the number of patients, the patient characteristics, the types of procedures performed, and the facility design. A sufficient number of staff members who possess the skills needed for optimal care for specific procedures should be available to prevent undue delays in the provision of care.

Departments in larger institutions will generally derive their staffing levels from guidelines established within the institution. Some professional organizations, such as the Association of Women's Health, Obstetrics, and Neonatal Nurses, have established staffing guidelines for patients in the labor and delivery suite and mother/baby nursing ratios (see box). Institutions may use these as guidelines to establish their own staffing levels. There are no established national staffing guidelines regarding gynecologic care for patients.

Types of Practitioners

A health care team may include many professionals. These professionals should be licensed and possess the credentials required by their respective professional organizations. More information about the health care professionals listed here is available from their respective associations (see box on page 106).

Obstetrician–Gynecologists. Obstetrician–gynecologists are physicians with additional education and experience in reproductive medicine and women's health care. They have completed a 4-year residency, and many go on to be board certified by the American Board of Obstetrics and

Associations Representing Women's Health Care Professionals

American Academy of Physician Assistants
950 N Washington Street
Alexandria, VA 22314-1552
(703) 836-2272
www.aapa.org

American College of Nurse–Midwives
818 Connecticut Avenue, NW, Suite 900
Washington, DC 20006
(202) 728-9860
www.acnm.org

American College of Obstetricians and Gynecologists
409 12th Street, SW
Washington, DC 20024
(202) 638-5577
www.acog.org

American College of Surgeons
633 N Saint Clair Street
Chicago, IL 60611-3211
(312) 202-5000
www.facs.org

American Nurses Association
600 Maryland Avenue, SW,
Suite 100 West
Washington, DC 20024
800-274-4262
www.ana.org

Association of Operating Room Nurses, Inc.
2170 S Parker Road, Suite 300
Denver, CO 80231-5711
800-755-2676
www.aorn.org

Association of Women's Health, Obstetric, and Neonatal Nurses
2000 L Street, NW, Suite 740
Washington, DC 20036
800-673-8499
www.awhonn.org

National Association of Inpatient Physicians
190 N Independence Mall
Philadelphia, PA 19106-1572
800-843-3360
www.naiponline.org

National League for Nursing
61 Broadway, 33rd Floor
New York, NY 10006
800-669-1656
www.nln.org

National Organization of Nurse Practitioner Faculties
1522 K Street, NW, #702
Washington, DC 20005
(202) 289-8044
www.nonpf.com

Gynecology. Those who received their initial board certification in or after November 1986 have time-limited certificates that must be renewed every 10 years. Obstetrician–gynecologists who are board certified or board eligible may become members of the American College of Obstetricians and Gynecologists. Some obstetrician–gynecologists seek additional training in a subspecialty area, such as reproductive endocrinology or infectious disease. At present, the American Board of Obstetrics and Gynecology offers subspecialty certification in three areas: 1) reproductive endocrinology and infertility, 2) maternal–fetal medicine, and 3) gynecologic oncology. In addition, fellowships are being offered in urogynecology/reconstructive pelvic surgery, although certification examinations in this area have not yet been offered.

Registered Nurses. Nursing personnel who care for gynecologic patients should be familiar with the special aspects of gynecologic conditions and the equipment needed to care for these patients. Delivery of safe and effective nursing care requires appropriately qualified registered nurses in adequate numbers to meet the needs of each patient in accordance with the care setting. The number of staff and level of skill required are influenced by the scope of nursing practice and the degree of nursing responsibilities within an institution. Nursing responsibilities in individual hospitals vary according to the level of care provided by the facility, practice procedures, number of professional registered nurses and ancillary staff, and professional nursing activities in continuing education and research.

Changing trends in medical management and technological advances influence and may increase the nursing workload. Each hospital should determine the scope of nursing practice for each nursing unit and specialty department. The scope of practice should be based on national nursing standards and guidelines for the specialty area of practice and should be in accordance with state law or regulations. A multidisciplinary committee comprising representatives from hospital, medical, and nursing administration should follow published professional standards and guidelines, consult state nurse practice acts and any accompanying regulations, identify the types and number of procedures performed in each unit, delineate direct and indirect nursing care activities performed, and identify activities to be performed by nonnursing personnel.

Hospitalists. The term *hospitalist* refers to a physician whose practice emphasizes providing care for hospitalized patients. Although some doctors have emphasized inpatient care for many years, there has been an explosive growth of such doctors since 1994. These doctors may or may not provide 24-hour inpatient coverage. Some hospitalists are in private practice and rotate to inpatient care days. Many more hospitals are putting hospitalists on their payroll and giving physicians the option to use hospitalists while their patients require inpatient care. Patient care is transferred back to the original clinician when the patient is discharged from the hospital.

Certified Nurse–Midwives. Certified nurse–midwives have been educated in both nursing and midwifery. The American College of Nurse–Midwives has established requirements for certification that are implemented by the American College of Nurse–Midwives Certification Council, Inc. Nurse–midwifery education includes training in the sciences and clinical preparation for the judgment and skills needed to manage the obstetric and, perhaps, the gynecologic care of women as well as the care for their patients' newborns.

Clinical Nurse Specialists. Clinical nurse specialists are registered nurses who have completed a formal educational program at the master's degree level. Clinical nurse specialists can handle a wide range of physical and mental health problems. They generally work in inpatient settings and are certified by the credentialing unit of the American Nurses Association.

Nurse Practitioners. Nurse practitioners are licensed registered nurses with advanced practice education, including supervised clinical instruction in health maintenance and diagnosis and treatment of illness. Completion of a nurse practitioner program may lead to a certificate or a master's degree.

Certification as a nurse practitioner is required in some jurisdictions and is voluntary in others. Certification is based on completing an approved educational program, passing a national certification examination, or both. Nurse practitioners who specialize in women's health are certified by the National Certification Corporation for Obstetric, Gynecologic, and Neonatal Nursing Specialties. Requirements for certification vary according to the specialty area and are determined by the certifying organization.

Nurse practitioners are qualified to provide a wide range of primary–preventive health care services, including obtaining medical, surgical, and psychosocial histories; performing physical examinations; and diagnosing and treating common illnesses and injuries. They generally work in primary care outpatient clinics, health maintenance organizations, specialty clinics, and schools. An increasing number of nurse practitioners are employed in inpatient settings.

Physician Assistants. Physician assistants enter training from a variety of backgrounds and are educated to provide medical care under the direction and supervision of a physician. The Commission of Accreditation of Allied Health Education Programs accredits physician assistant programs. Most of these programs have been established in, or with strong attachments to, medical schools. Applicants generally are required to have at least 2 years of college education and prior experience in health care. The educational program traditionally consists of a minimum of 2 years of classroom instruction and clinical rotation. Curriculum design for most physician assistant programs involves basic sciences, introduction to clinical sciences, and supervised clinical instruction. Completion of a physician assistant program may lead to a certificate or to an associate, baccalaureate, or master's degree.

Physician assistants practice in virtually all specialty areas, in outpatient and inpatient settings, as first or second assistants in surgery, and in providing preoperative and postoperative care. Most jurisdictions require physician assistants to pass a national certification examination. The examination is given only to graduates of accredited physician assistant programs and is developed by the National Board of Medical Examiners and administered by the National Commission on Certification of Physician Assistants. To maintain national certification and use the credential "Physician Assistant-Certified" an individual must complete 100 hours of continuing medical education every 2 years and take a recertification examination every 6 years.

Surgical Assistants. Competent surgical assistants should be available for all major obstetric and gynecologic operations. In many cases, the complexity of the surgery or the patient's condition will require the assistance of one or more physicians or other personnel with special surgical training to provide safe, quality patient care. Often, the complexity of a given surgical procedure cannot be determined prospectively. The judgment and prerogative of the primary surgeon to determine the number and qualifications of appropriately compensated assistants should not be overruled by public or private third-party payers. Registered nurses and other personnel assisting in the provision of surgical services should be appropriately trained, granted privileges to assist in specific procedures, and remain under the direct supervision of the surgeon.

Registered nurse first assistants are employed in hospital-based settings, ambulatory care settings, collaborative practice with physicians, and independent practice. The role of the registered nurse first assistant falls within the scope of nursing in all 50 state boards of nursing. Registered nurse first assistants must demonstrate:

- Competency in performing individualized surgical nursing care management before, during, and after surgery
- Competency in recognizing surgical anatomy and physiology and operative technique related to first assisting
- Competency in carrying out intraoperative nursing behaviors of handling tissue, providing exposure, using surgical instruments, suturing, and controlling blood loss
- Competency in recognizing surgical hazards and initiating appropriate corrective and preventive action including, but not limited to, recognizing abnormal laboratory values and diagnostic test results

- Achievement of Basic Cardiac Life support and Advanced Cardiac Life Support Certification or both
- Achievement of national Certification in Operating Room Nursing

Billing and Collections

The billing and collections process begins prior to the first visit. On scheduling an appointment, the office staff should discuss with the patient methods of payment, billing, third-party insurance procedures, requirements for copayments, practitioner participation, facility affiliation, and preauthorization or referrals that may be required at the visit. When the patient changes health care coverage, these issues may need to be addressed again. Verification of third-party coverage and compliance with continuing authorization requirements should be ensured at each visit. During the initial visit, the patient should be advised of the clinician's customary fees. An area of the office should be provided where these matters can be discussed in confidence.

Medical plan participation and identification of contractual requirements, including laboratory and imaging facility designations, should be discussed with the patient. A system should be in place to ensure proper participating laboratory and imaging service referrals. Appropriate referrals and approvals should be verified. Consideration of emergency medical conditions should be addressed and the practitioner informed prior to denial of care based on lack of required referral/approval documentation (see also "Human Resources" in Part 1).

Staff should be aware of third-party contractual requirements for service and billing and participate in ensuring compliance with payor contracts. Staff assigned to billing and coding should be aware of the service requirements for designated codes, and the clinician who must designate the billing code should ensure appropriate documentation in the record to justify the level of service billed. Information regarding the Medicare *Documentation Guidelines* for evaluation and management services appears in the "Primary and Preventive Care" section of Part 3. A system should be established to ensure that all preprocedure requirements (laboratory tests, consents, examination records, and third-party authorizations) are met in advance of the procedure.

The clinician is responsible for ensuring accuracy in the coding on bills. If a patient questions the customary fees, the clinician should be informed and should advise staff as to the appropriate method of addressing the patient's concerns. Ideally, a specific staff person should be assigned responsibility for handling the financial concerns or complaints of patients. If delinquent accounts are referred to an outside billing and collection service, the practitioner should be informed before an account is assigned to such an agency.

Appointments, Scheduling, and Patient Flow

Ambulatory Care

The most efficient method of managing patient flow in an office setting or clinic begins with appointment scheduling. Appointments should be booked realistically to maintain the clinician's schedules and allow sufficient time for emergency appointments. The personnel in each facility should establish a realistic goal for minimizing waiting time. The average time a practitioner spends with a patient for various procedures (new patient visit, yearly checkup, gynecologic procedure) can be analyzed easily to form a basis by which scheduling can be optimized. Such scheduling should be analyzed periodically to ensure minimal patient waiting. There should be established procedures for the following circumstances:

- Rescheduling missed or canceled appointments
- Informing patients when their appointments will be delayed significantly or when an emergency situation may prevent the clinician from keeping appointments
- Processing patients in a timely manner
- Guiding patients to specific areas of the facility (eg, laboratory, insurance office)

Operating Room Data and Data Tracking

Operating room data tracking is a basic function necessary for scheduling procedures and personnel, as well as billing. Data tracking provides a means to evaluate the operating room's utilization, efficiency, and productivity. Specific data points to be tracked depend on the needs of the institution. Data commonly collected include:

- Type of procedure
- Surgeon
- Length of procedure by surgeon
- Time of:
  - —Patient arrival in unit
  - —Patient in procedure room
  - —Anesthesia induction
  - —Incision
  - —Patient out of room
  - —Room clean up start and finish
  - —Case time (time from room set up to clean up)
  - —Turnover time (time from preceding patient out of room to next patient in room)

Practice Coverage

All obstetrician–gynecologists should have appropriate coverage agreements with practitioners within their own group practice or other practitioners to care for their patients in their absence. When possible, these clinicians should be obstetrician–gynecologists. Careful consideration should be given to managed care contractual agreements and participating physician coverage. Billing policies and procedures should be established in advance and consideration given to reimbursement agreements. The clinicians should be familiar with each other's practice style and capabilities, and practitioners should have privileges at the same hospital or other facilities. An established protocol should exist to introduce the covering practitioner to hospitalized patients and those with special problems. The institution and answering service should be advised of the dates of a clinician's absence or unavailability and the names, telephone numbers, and office addresses of the covering practitioner. The covering practitioner, when feasible, should have access to patients' medical records (see also "Liability" in Part 1).

Control and Disposal of Drugs and Other Sensitive Materials

A system must be in place for maintaining the security of all controlled drugs. Ideally, a secure system also should be in place for the control of syringes, needles, and prescription pads. An established procedure should exist for monitoring the expiration date of drugs, including sample drugs and laboratory reagents, and proper disposal techniques.

SUGGESTED READING

American College of Obstetricians and Gynecologists. The assistant: information for improved risk management. Washington, DC: ACOG, 2001

American College of Obstetricians and Gynecologists. CPT coding in obstetrics and gynecology—2000. Washington, DC: ACOG, 2000

American College of Obstetricians and Gynecologists. Guidelines for implementing collaborative practice. Washington, DC: ACOG, 1995

American College of Obstetricians and Gynecologists. ICD-9-CM diagnostic coding in obstetrics and gynecology—2000. Washington, DC: ACOG, 1999

American College of Obstetricians and Gynecologists. Statement on surgical assistants. ACOG Committee Opinion 240. Washington, DC: ACOG, 2000

American College of Surgeons. Physicians as assistants at surgery: 1999 study. Chicago: ACS, 1999

Donham RT. Defining measurable OR-PR scheduling, efficiency, and utilization data elements: the Association of Anesthesia Clinical Directors procedural times glossary. Int Anesthesiol Clin 1998;36:15–29

Health Care Financing Administration. Documentation guidelines for evaluation and management services. Baltimore, Maryland: HCFA, 1997

Joint Commission on Accreditation of Healthcare Organizations. Comprehensive accreditation manual for hospitals. Oakbrook Terrace, Illinois: JCAHO, 2000

PART 3

Patient Care

The practice of obstetrics and gynecology encompasses a broad spectrum of care directed to all aspects of a woman's health (see Appendix F). The obstetric–gynecologic practitioner often serves as a woman's point of entry into the health care system and as her main source of continuity in health care. A modern approach to obstetric–gynecologic practice requires an organized system that can administer to a broad range of women's health care needs—medical, surgical, and psychosocial. Awareness of and response to women with special concerns, such as women with disabilities, and issues of cultural competence play an important role in the delivery of women's health care. The scope of services provided by obstetric–gynecologic practitioners in the ambulatory setting will vary from practice to practice (see box). Similarly, the scope of services provided in inpatient settings varies. Credentialing for surgical services is a local issue that is determined based on an individual's training, experience, and demonstrated competence.

The American College of Obstetricians and Gynecologists (ACOG) calls for quality health care appropriate to every woman's needs throughout her life and for assuring that a full array of clinical ser-

Scope of Ambulatory Women's Health Care Services

Primary and Preventive Services

- Age-specific routine assessment (asymptomatic women)
- Health status evaluation and counseling
  - —Fitness
  - —Nutrition
  - —Exercise
- Routine detection and prevention of disease
  - —Cardiovascular disorders
  - —Diabetes
  - —Cancer
  - —Smoking
  - —Substance abuse
- Psychosocial issues: early detection and management
  - —Sexuality
  - —Domestic violence
  - —Child abuse
  - —Abuse/neglect of the elderly
- Family planning
- Preconceptional care
- Menopausal management

Obstetrics

- Obstetric care: high and low risk

Gynecologic Services

- Initial and periodic evaluation and treatment of gynecologic conditions (including breast conditions)
- Abortion-related services
- Evaluation and treatment of incontinence
- Gynecologic ultrasonography
- Evaluation and treatment of endocrine dysfunction and infertility

vices be available to women without costly delays or the imposition of geographic, financial, attitudinal, or legal barriers. The American College of Obstetricians and Gynecologists and its membership are committed to facilitating quality women's health care as well as access to it. To ensure access to high-quality programs meeting the health care needs of all women, ACOG Fellows should exercise their responsibility to improve the health status of women and their offspring both in the traditional patient–physician relationships and by working within their community and at the state and national levels.

In addition, it is critical that all Americans be provided with adequate and affordable health coverage. Despite economic prosperity and substantial job creation in recent years, there remains a considerable and increasing portion of the American population that does not have health insurance coverage. As a result, those individuals often defer obtaining preventive and medical services, jeopardizing the health and well-being of themselves and their families. Accordingly, ACOG supports universal coverage that is designed to improve the individual and collective health of society. Expanding health coverage to all Americans must become a high priority.

Primary and Preventive Care

Obstetrician–gynecologists have a tradition of providing primary and preventive care to women. Primary care emphasizes health maintenance, preventive services, early detection of disease, availability of services, and continuity of care. The obstetrician–gynecologist often serves as a primary medical resource and counselor to the patient and her family for a wide range of medical conditions. However, all clinicians, regardless of the extent of their training, have limitations to their knowledge and skills and should seek consultation at appropriate times for the benefit of their patients in providing both reproductive and nonreproductive care. This section focuses on primary and preventive care as it relates to routine assessments for asymptomatic women, special concerns for specific women based on their age and risk factors, and counseling that can help engage a woman in maintaining a healthy lifestyle and in minimizing health risks.

The following guidelines indicate routine assessments for women based on age groups and risk factors (Table 3–1; see boxes). These assessments, yearly or as appropriate, should include screening, evaluation, and counseling based on age and risk factors. Recommendations for screening have been considered within the context of accuracy, risks, and cost. Increasingly, managed care plans dictate the amount of time spent with patients during office visits. Unless flexibly applied, such an attempt to standardize caregiving threatens to overlook any nonstandard needs of an individual woman. Populations such as adolescents, the elderly, and the very sick may have needs that require more than the standard time allotted. If it is not possible to address all the patient's needs in one visit, additional visits may need to be scheduled. If a clinician believes, based on clinical evidence, that a patient's health interests are jeopardized by the policies of her plan, his or her role as the patient's advocate demands that an appeal be made to the plan or medical director.

Table 3–1. High-Risk Factors

Intervention	High-Risk Factor
Bacteriuria testing	Diabetes mellitus
Cholesterol testing	Familial lipid disorders; family history of premature coronary heart disease; history of coronary heart disease
Colorectal cancer screening*	Colorectal cancer or adenomatous polyps in first-degree relative younger than 60 years of age or in two or more first-degree relatives of any ages; family history of familial adenomatous polyposis or hereditary nonpolyposis colon cancer; history of colorectal cancer, adenomatous polyps, or inflammatory bowel disease
Fasting glucose testing	Obesity; first-degree relative with diabetes; member of a high-risk ethnic population (eg, African American, Hispanic, Native American, Asian, Pacific Islander); have delivered a baby weighing more than 9 lb or history of gestational diabetes mellitus; hypertensive; high-density lipoprotein cholesterol level no more than 35 mg/dL; triglyceride level of at least 250 mg/dL; history of impaired glucose tolerance or impaired fasting glucose
Fluoride supplementation	Live in an area with inadequate water fluoridation (<0.7 ppm)
Genetic testing/counseling	Exposure to teratogens; considering pregnancy at age 35 or older; patient, partner, or family member with history of genetic disorder or birth defect; African, Acadian, Eastern European Jewish, Mediterranean, or Southeast Asian ancestry
Hemoglobin level assessment	Caribbean, Latin American, Asian, Mediterranean, or African ancestry; history of excessive menstrual flow
Hepatitis A vaccination	International travelers; illegal drug users; people who work with nonhuman primates; chronic liver disease; clotting-factor disorders; sex partners of bisexual men; measles, mumps, and rubella nonimmune persons; food-service workers; health-care workers; day-care workers

(continued)

Table 3–1. High-Risk Factors *(continued)*

Intervention	High-Risk Factor
Hepatitis B vaccination	Intravenous drug users and their sexual contacts; recipients of clotting factor concentrates; occupational exposure to blood or blood products; patients and workers in dialysis units; persons with chronic renal or hepatic disease; household or sexual contact with hepatitis B virus carriers; history of sexual activity with multiple partners; history of sexual activity with sexually active homosexual or bisexual men; international travelers; residents and staff of institutions for the developmentally disabled and of correctional institutions
Hepatitis C virus (HCV) testing	History of injecting illegal drugs; recipients of clotting factor concentrates before 1987; chronic (long-term) hemodialysis; persistently abnormal alanine aminotransferase levels; recipient of blood from a donor who later tested positive for HCV infection; recipient of blood or blood-component transfusion or organ transplant before July 1992; occupational percutaneous or mucosal exposure to HCV-positive blood
Human immunodeficiency virus (HIV) testing	Seeking treatment for sexually transmitted diseases; drug use by injection; history of prostitution; past or present sexual partner who is HIV positive or bisexual or injects drugs; long-term residence or birth in an area with high prevalence of HIV infection; history of transfusion from 1978 to 1985; invasive cervical cancer; pregnancy. Offer to women seeking preconceptional care.
Influenza vaccination	Anyone who wishes to reduce the chance of becoming ill with influenza; resident in long-term care facility; chronic cardiopulmonary disorders; metabolic diseases (eg, diabetes mellitus, hemoglobinopathies, immunosuppression, renal dysfunction); health-care workers; day-care workers; pregnant women who will be in the second or third trimester during the epidemic season. Pregnant women with medical problems should be offered vaccination before the influenza season regardless of stage of pregnancy.

(continued)

Table 3–1. High-Risk Factors *(continued)*

Intervention	High-Risk Factor
Lipid profile assessment	Elevated cholesterol level; history of parent or sibling with blood cholesterol of at least 240 mg/dL; first-degree relative with premature (<55 years of age for men, <65 years of age for women) coronary heart disease; diabetes mellitus; smoking habit
Mammography	Women who have had breast cancer or who have a first-degree relative (ie, mother, sister, or daughter) or multiple other relatives who have a history of premenopausal breast or breast and ovarian cancer
Measles–mumps–rubella (MMR) vaccination	Adults born in 1957 or later should be offered vaccination (one dose of MMR) if there is no proof of immunity or documentation of a dose given after first birthday; persons vaccinated in 1963–1967 should be offered revaccination (2 doses); health care workers, students entering college, international travelers, and rubella-negative postpartum patients should be offered a second dose
Pneumococcal vaccination	Chronic illness such as cardiovascular disease, pulmonary disease, diabetes mellitus, alcoholism, chronic liver disease, cerebrospinal fluid leaks, functional or anatomic asplenia; exposure to an environment where pneumococcal outbreaks have occurred; immunocompromised patients (eg, HIV infection, hematologic or solid malignancies, chemotherapy, steroid therapy); pregnant patients with chronic illness. Revaccination after 5 years may be appropriate for certain high-risk groups
Rubella titer assessment	Childbearing age and no evidence of immunity
Sexually transmitted disease (STD) testing	History of multiple sexual partners or a sexual partner with multiple contacts, sexual contact with persons with culture-proven STD, history of repeated episodes of STD, attendance at clinics for STDs; routine screening for chlamydial and gonorrheal infection for all sexually active adolescents and other asymptomatic women at high risk for infection

(continued)

Table 3–1. High-Risk Factors *(continued)*

Intervention	High-Risk Factor
Skin examination	Increased recreational or occupational exposure to sunlight; family or personal history of skin cancer; clinical evidence of precursor lesions
Thyroid-stimulating hormone testing	Strong family history of thyroid disease; autoimmune disease (evidence of subclinical hypothyroidism may be related to unfavorable lipid profiles)
Tuberculosis skin testing	Human immunodeficiency virus infection; close contact with persons known or suspected to have tuberculosis; medical risk factors known to increase risk of disease if infected; born in country with high tuberculosis prevalence; medically underserved; low income; alcoholism; intravenous drug use; resident of long-term care facility (eg, correctional institutions, mental institutions, nursing homes and facilities); health professional working in high-risk health care facilities
Varicella vaccination	All susceptible adults and adolescents, including health care workers; household contacts of immunocompromised individuals; teachers; day-care workers; residents and staff of institutional settings, colleges, prisons, or military installations; international travelers; nonpregnant women of childbearing age

*For a more detailed discussion of colorectal cancer screening, see Byers T, Levin B, Rothenberger D, Dodd GD, Smith RA. American Cancer Society guidelines for screening and surveillance for early detection of colorectal polyps and cancer: update 1997. American Cancer Society Detection and Treatment Advisory Group on Colorectal Cancer. CA Cancer J Clin 1997;47:154–160.

American College of Obstetricians and Gynecologists. Primary and preventive care: periodic assessments. ACOG Committee Opinion 246. Washington, DC: ACOG, 2000

It is recognized that variations to routine assessments may be necessary to adjust to the needs of a specific patient. For example, certain risk factors may influence additional assessments and interventions. Caregivers need to be alert to high-risk factors, indicated by an asterisk in the boxes and further elucidated in Table 3–1. During evaluation, the patient should be made aware of high-risk conditions that require targeted screening or treatment.

Periodic Assessment

Ages 13–18 Years

SCREENING

History

- Reason for visit
- Health status: medical, surgical, family
- Dietary/nutrition assessment
- Physical activity
- Use of complementary and alternative medicine
- Tobacco, alcohol, other drug use
- Abuse/neglect
- Sexual practices

Physical Examination

- Height
- Weight
- Blood pressure
- Secondary sexual characteristics (Tanner staging)
- Pelvic examination (yearly when sexually active or beginning at age 18 years)
- Skin*

Laboratory Testing

Periodic

- Pap testing (yearly when sexually active or beginning at age 18 years)

*High-Risk Groups**

- Hemoglobin level assessment
- Bacteriuria testing
- Sexually transmitted disease testing
- Human immunodeficiency virus testing
- Genetic testing/counseling
- Rubella titer assessment
- Tuberculosis skin testing
- Lipid profile assessment
- Fasting glucose testing
- Cholesterol testing
- Hepatitis C virus testing
- Colorectal cancer screening†

EVALUATION AND COUNSELING

Sexuality

- Development
- High-risk behaviors
- Preventing unwanted/unintended pregnancy
  —Postponing sexual involvement
  —Contraceptive options
- Sexually transmitted diseases
  —Partner selection
  —Barrier protection

Fitness and Nutrition

- Dietary/nutrition assessment (including eating disorders)
- Exercise: discussion of program
- Folic acid supplementation (0.4 mg/d)
- Calcium intake

Psychosocial Evaluation

- Interpersonal/family relationships
- Sexual identity
- Personal goal development
- Behavioral/learning disorders
- Abuse/neglect
- Satisfactory school experience
- Peer relationships

Cardiovascular Risk Factors

- Family history
- Hypertension
- Dyslipidemia
- Obesity
- Diabetes mellitus

Health/Risk Behaviors

- Hygiene (including dental); fluoride supplementation*
- Injury prevention
  —Safety belts and helmets
  —Recreational hazards

(continued)

Periodic Assessment *(continued)*

Ages 13–18 Years

—Firearms

—Hearing

- Skin exposure to ultraviolet rays
- Suicide: depressive symptoms
- Tobacco, alcohol, other drug use

Immunizations

Periodic

- Tetanus–diphtheria booster (once between ages 11 years and 16 years)
- Hepatitis B vaccine (one series for those not previously immunized)

*High-Risk Groups**

- Influenza vaccine
- Hepatitis A vaccine
- Pneumococcal vaccine
- Measles–mumps–rubella vaccine
- Varicella vaccine

Leading Causes of Death

1. Motor vehicle accidents
2. Homicide
3. Suicide
4. Cancer
5. All other accidents and adverse effects
6. Diseases of the heart
7. Congenital anomalies
8. Chronic obstructive pulmonary diseases

Leading Causes of Morbidity

- Acne
- Asthma
- Chlamydia
- Depression
- Dermatitis
- Headaches
- Infective, viral, and parasitic diseases
- Influenza
- Injuries
- Nose, throat, ear, and upper respiratory infections
- Sexual assault
- Sexually transmitted diseases
- Urinary tract infections

*See Table 3–1.

†Only for those with a family history of familial adenomatous polyposis or 8 years after the start of pancolitis. For a more detailed discussion of colorectal cancer screening, see Byers T, Levin B, Rothenberger D, Dodd GD, Smith RA. American Cancer Society guidelines for screening and surveillance for early detection of colorectal polyps and cancer: update 1997. American Cancer Society Detection and Treatment Advisory Group on Colorectal Cancer. CA Cancer J Clin 1997;47:154–160.

American College of Obstetricians and Gynecologists. Primary and preventive care: periodic assessments. ACOG Committee Opinion 246. Washington, DC: ACOG, 2000

Periodic Assessment

Ages 19–39 Years

SCREENING

History

- Reason for visit
- Health status: medical, surgical, family
- Dietary/nutrition assessment
- Physical activity
- Use of complementary and alternative medicine
- Tobacco, alcohol, other drug use
- Abuse/neglect
- Sexual practices
- Urinary and fecal incontinence

Physical Examination

- Height
- Weight
- Blood pressure
- Neck: adenopathy, thyroid
- Breasts
- Abdomen
- Pelvic examination
- Skin*

Laboratory Testing

Periodic

- Pap testing (physician and patient discretion after three consecutive normal tests if low risk)

*High-Risk Groups**

- Hemoglobin level assessment
- Bacteriuria testing
- Mammography
- Fasting glucose testing
- Cholesterol testing
- Sexually transmitted disease testing
- Human immunodeficiency virus testing
- Genetic testing/counseling
- Rubella titer assessment
- Tuberculosis skin testing
- Lipid profile assessment
- Thyroid-stimulating hormone testing
- Hepatitis C virus testing
- Colorectal cancer screening

EVALUATION AND COUNSELING

Sexuality

- High-risk behaviors
- Contraceptive options for prevention of unwanted pregnancy
- Preconceptional and genetic counseling for desired pregnancy
- Sexually transmitted diseases
  - —Partner selection
  - —Barrier protection
- Sexual function

Fitness and Nutrition

- Dietary/nutrition assessment
- Exercise: discussion of program
- Folic acid supplementation (0.4 mg/d)
- Calcium intake

Psychosocial Evaluation

- Interpersonal/family relationships
- Domestic violence
- Work satisfaction
- Lifestyle/stress
- Sleep disorders

Cardiovascular Risk Factors

- Family history
- Hypertension
- Dyslipidemia
- Obesity
- Diabetes mellitus
- Lifestyle

Health/Risk Behaviors

- Hygiene (including dental)
- Injury prevention
  - —Safety belts and helmets

(continued)

Periodic Assessment *(continued)*

Ages 19–39 Years

—Occupational hazards

—Recreational hazards

—Firearms

—Hearing

- Breast self-examination
- Chemoprophylaxis for breast cancer (for high-risk women ages 35 years or older)†
- Skin exposure to ultraviolet rays
- Suicide: depressive symptoms
- Tobacco, alcohol, other drug use

Immunizations

Periodic

- Tetanus–diphtheria booster (every 10 years)

*High-Risk Groups**

- Measles–mumps–rubella vaccine
- Hepatitis A vaccine
- Hepatitis B vaccine
- Influenza vaccine
- Pneumococcal vaccine
- Varicella vaccine

Leading Causes of Death

1. Accidents and adverse effects
2. Cancer
3. Human immunodeficiency virus infection
4. Diseases of the heart
5. Homicide
6. Suicide
7. Cerebrovascular diseases
8. Chronic liver disease and cirrhosis

Leading Causes of Morbidity

- Asthma
- Back symptoms
- Breast disease
- Deformity or orthopedic impairment
- Depression
- Diabetes
- Gynecologic disorders
- Headache/migraines
- Hypertension
- Infective, viral, and parasitic diseases
- Influenza
- Injuries
- Nose, throat, ear, and upper respiratory infections
- Sexual assault/domestic violence
- Sexually transmitted diseases
- Skin rash/dermatitis
- Substance abuse
- Urinary tract infections
- Vaginitis

---

*See Table 3–1.

†The decision to use tamoxifen should be individualized. For a more detailed discussion of risk assessment and chemoprevention therapy, see American College of Obstetricians and Gynecologists. Tamoxifen and the prevention of breast cancer in high-risk women. ACOG Committee Opinion 224. Washington, DC: ACOG, 1999.

American College of Obstetricians and Gynecologists. Primary and preventive care: periodic assessments. ACOG Committee Opinion 246. Washington, DC: ACOG, 2000

Periodic Assessment

Ages 40–64 Years

SCREENING

History

- Reason for visit
- Health status: medical, surgical, family
- Dietary/nutrition assessment
- Physical activity
- Use of complementary and alternative medicine
- Tobacco, alcohol, other drug use
- Abuse/neglect
- Sexual practices
- Urinary and fecal incontinence

Physical Examination

- Height
- Weight
- Blood pressure
- Oral cavity
- Neck: adenopathy, thyroid
- Breasts, axillae
- Abdomen
- Pelvic examination
- Skin*

Laboratory Testing

Periodic

- Pap testing (physician and patient discretion after three consecutive normal tests if low risk)
- Mammography (every 1–2 years until age 50 years; yearly beginning at age 50 years)
- Cholesterol testing (every 5 years beginning at age 45 years)
- Yearly fecal occult blood testing plus flexible sigmoidoscopy every 5 years *or* colonoscopy every 10 years *or* double contrast barium enema (DCBE) every 5–10 years, with digital rectal examination performed at the time of each screening sigmoidoscopy, colonoscopy, or DCBE (beginning at age 50 years)
- Fasting glucose testing (every 3 years after age 45 years)

*High-Risk Groups**

- Hemoglobin level assessment
- Bacteriuria testing
- Fasting glucose testing
- Sexually transmitted disease testing
- Human immunodeficiency virus testing
- Tuberculosis skin testing
- Lipid profile assessment
- Thyroid-stimulating hormone testing
- Hepatitis C virus testing
- Colorectal cancer screening

EVALUATION AND COUNSELING

Sexuality†

- High-risk behaviors
- Contraceptive options for prevention of unwanted pregnancy
- Sexually transmitted diseases
  - —Partner selection
  - —Barrier protection
- Sexual functioning

Fitness and Nutrition

- Dietary/nutrition assessment
- Exercise: discussion of program
- Folic acid supplementation (0.4 mg/d before age 50 years)
- Calcium intake

Psychosocial Evaluation

- Family relationships
- Domestic violence
- Work satisfaction
- Retirement planning
- Lifestyle/stress
- Sleep disorders

Cardiovascular Risk Factors

- Family history
- Hypertension
- Dyslipidemia
- Obesity

(continued)

Periodic Assessment *(continued)*

Ages 40–64 Years

- Diabetes mellitus
- Lifestyle

Health/Risk Behaviors

- Hygiene (including dental)
- Hormone replacement therapy
- Injury prevention
  —Safety belts and helmets
  —Occupational hazards
  —Recreational hazards
  —Sports involvement
  —Firearms
  —Hearing
- Breast self-examination
- Chemoprophylaxis for breast cancer (for high-risk women)‡
- Skin exposure to ultraviolet rays
- Suicide: depressive symptoms
- Tobacco, alcohol, other drug use

Immunizations

Periodic

- Influenza vaccine (annually beginning at age 50 years)
- Tetanus–diphtheria booster (every 10 years)

*High-Risk Groups**

- Measles–mumps–rubella vaccine
- Hepatitis A vaccine
- Hepatitis B vaccine
- Influenza vaccine
- Pneumococcal vaccine
- Varicella vaccine

Leading Causes of Death

1. Cancer
2. Diseases of the heart
3. Cerebrovascular diseases
4. Accidents and adverse effects
5. Chronic obstructive pulmonary disease
6. Diabetes mellitus
7. Chronic liver disease and cirrhosis
8. Pneumonia and influenza

Leading Causes of Morbidity

- Arthritis/osteoarthritis
- Asthma
- Back symptoms
- Breast disease
- Cardiovascular disease
- Carpal tunnel syndrome
- Deformity or orthopedic impairment
- Depression
- Diabetes
- Headache
- Hypertension
- Infective, viral, and parasitic diseases
- Influenza
- Injuries
- Menopause
- Nose, throat, and upper respiratory infections
- Obesity
- Skin conditions/dermatitis
- Substance abuse
- Urinary tract infections
- Urinary tract (other conditions, including urinary incontinence)
- Vision impairment

*See Table 3–1.

†Preconceptional and genetic counseling is appropriate for certain women in this age group.

‡The decision to use tamoxifen should be individualized. For a more detailed discussion of risk assessment and chemoprevention therapy, see American College of Obstetricians and Gynecologists. Tamoxifen and the prevention of breast cancer in high-risk women. ACOG Committee Opinion 224. Washington, DC: ACOG, 1999.

American College of Obstetricians and Gynecologists. Primary and preventive care: periodic assessments. ACOG Committee Opinion 246. Washington, DC: ACOG, 2000

Periodic Assessment

Age 65 Years and Older

SCREENING

History

- Reason for visit
- Health status: medical, surgical, family
- Dietary/nutrition assessment
- Physical activity
- Use of complementary and alternative medicine
- Tobacco, alcohol, other drug use, and concurrent medication use
- Abuse/neglect
- Sexual practices
- Urinary and fecal incontinence

Physical Examination

- Height
- Weight
- Blood pressure
- Oral cavity
- Neck: adenopathy, thyroid
- Breasts, axillae
- Abdomen
- Pelvic examination
- Skin*

Laboratory Testing

Periodic

- Pap testing (physician and patient discretion after three consecutive normal tests if low risk)
- Urinalysis
- Mammography
- Cholesterol (every 3–5 years before age 75 years)
- Fecal occult blood testing plus flexible sigmoidoscopy every 5 years *or* colonoscopy every 10 years *or* double contrast barium enema (DCBE) every 5–10 years, with digital rectal examination performed at the time of each screening sigmoidoscopy, colonoscopy, or DCBE
- Fasting glucose testing (every 3 years)

*High-Risk Groups**

- Hemoglobin level assessment
- Sexually transmitted disease testing
- Human immunodeficiency virus testing
- Tuberculosis skin testing
- Lipid profile assessment
- Thyroid-stimulating hormone testing
- Hepatitis C virus testing
- Colorectal cancer screening

EVALUATION AND COUNSELING

Sexuality

- Sexual functioning
- Sexual behaviors
- Sexually transmitted diseases
  - —Partner selection
  - —Barrier protection

Fitness and Nutrition

- Dietary/nutrition assessment
- Exercise: discussion of program
- Calcium intake

Psychosocial Evaluation

- Neglect/abuse
- Lifestyle/stress
- Depression/sleep disorders
- Family relationships
- Work/retirement satisfaction

Cardiovascular Risk Factors

- Hypertension
- Dyslipidemia
- Obesity
- Diabetes mellitus
- Sedentary lifestyle

Health/Risk Behaviors

- Hygiene (general and dental)
- Hormone replacement therapy

(continued)

Periodic Assessment *(continued)*

Age 65 Years and Older

- Injury prevention
  - —Safety belts and helmets
  - —Prevention of falls
  - —Occupational hazards
  - —Recreational hazards
  - —Firearms
- Visual acuity/glaucoma
- Hearing
- Breast self-examination
- Chemoprophylaxis for breast cancer (for high-risk women)[†]
- Skin exposure to ultraviolet rays
- Suicide: depressive symptoms
- Tobacco, alcohol, other drug use

Immunizations

Periodic

- Tetanus–diphtheria booster (every 10 years)
- Influenza vaccine (annually)
- Pneumococcal vaccine (once)

High-Risk Groups *

- Hepatitis A vaccine
- Hepatitis B vaccine
- Varicella vaccine

Leading Causes of Death

1. Diseases of the heart
2. Cancer
3. Cerebrovascular diseases
4. Chronic obstructive pulmonary diseases
5. Pneumonia and influenza
6. Diabetes mellitus
7. Accidents and adverse effects
8. Alzheimer's disease

Leading Causes of Morbidity

- Arthritis/osteoarthritis
- Back symptoms
- Breast cancer
- Chronic obstructive pulmonary diseases
- Cardiovascular disease
- Deformity or orthopedic impairment
- Degeneration of macula retinae and posterior pole
- Diabetes
- Hearing and vision impairment
- Hypertension
- Hypothyroidism and other thyroid disease
- Influenza
- Nose, throat, and upper respiratory infections
- Osteoporosis
- Skin lesions/dermatoses/dermatitis
- Urinary tract infections
- Urinary tract (other conditions, including urinary incontinence)
- Vertigo

*See Table 3–1.

†The decision to use tamoxifen should be individualized. For a more detailed discussion of risk assessment and chemoprevention therapy, see American College of Obstetricians and Gynecologists. Tamoxifen and the prevention of breast cancer in high-risk women. ACOG Committee Opinion 224. Washington, DC: ACOG, 1999.

American College of Obstetricians and Gynecologists. Primary and preventive care: periodic assessments. ACOG Committee Opinion 246. Washington, DC: ACOG, 2000

Once a problem has been identified, intervention can take the form of behavior modification, treatment, or referral, as necessary. Therapeutic interventions that are commonly a part of the generalist's practice of preventive health care are described here. Other interventions are described in Part 4.

The leading causes of mortality and morbidity included in the boxes were derived from various sources. The leading causes of mortality are provided by the Mortality Statistics Branch at the National Center for Health Statistics. Data are from 1996, the most recent year for which data are available. The causes are ranked. The leading causes of morbidity are unranked estimates based on information from the following sources:

- National Health Interview Survey, 1994
- National Ambulatory Medical Care Survey, 1996
- National Hospital Discharge Survey, 1996
- U.S. Department of Justice National Crime Victimization Survey
- U.S. Centers for Disease Control and Prevention Sexually Transmitted Disease Surveillance, 1996
- U.S. Centers for Disease Control and Prevention HIV/AIDS Surveillance Report, 1997
- National Nursing Home Survey, 1995

The Women's Health Examination

The specialty of obstetrics and gynecology is devoted to the health care of women throughout their lifetime. It encompasses care of the whole patient in addition to focusing on the normal and abnormal processes of the female reproductive system, including the breast. A woman's first contact with an obstetrician–gynecologist is most often for a periodic health examination, family planning counseling, or pregnancy confirmation. The initial contact in most instances begins a long-term physician–patient relationship in which the obstetrician–gynecologist provides continuity of care through maintenance of a comprehensive medical record updated periodically by a history, physical examination, and appropriate laboratory procedures and through referral and integration of those medical services outside the purview of the obstetrician–gynecologist.

Medical History

Communication is the key to a successful medical history interview. The interviewer must make the patient comfortable enough to speak freely, and the questions must be easily understood and tailored to the individual patient. For patients who do not easily understand or speak the commonly used language(s) of the clinician, it is important that the clinician seek the help of a trained medical interpreter.

The goal of a medical history interview is to gather pertinent and basic information about the patient's health status (see box). An interviewer should consider all aspects of the patient's presentation and condition and prioritize areas for further evaluation. The interviewer should be aware of the influence of social, economic, and cultural factors in shaping the nature of the patient's concerns and her descriptions of health status and symptoms.

The "Five Vowels" Rule for Interviews

It is helpful to follow the rule of "five vowels" when conducting an interview. This rule states that a good interview contains the following elements:

- **A**udition
- **E**valuation
- **I**nquiry
- **O**bservation
- **U**nderstanding

Audition reminds the interviewer to listen carefully to the patient's story, *evaluation* refers to assessment of relevant versus irrelevant data, *inquiry* leads the interviewer to probe into significant areas that require more clarification, *observation* refers to the importance of nonverbal communication, and *understanding* refers to the concerns and apprehensions of the patient.

Modified from Swartz MH. Textbook of physical diagnosis: history and examination. 3rd ed. Philadelphia: W.B. Saunders, 1998;3–26

Conducting an Interview. The diagnostic process begins at the first moment of meeting a patient. The interviewer should greet the patient by name, make eye contact, shake hands, and smile. The interviewer should address the patient by her preferred name or title. The quality of the interview can be helped by the physical environment. If possible, the interview should take place in a quiet, private, well-lit room with comfortable and adequate space and seating, with the patient dressed.

As much as possible, allow the patient to express her story in her own words. Listen without interruption, and be aware that the presence of family members could be an impediment to an honest interview, especially in cases of domestic violence or when the patient is an adolescent. If the family is present, include time in the interview for a private conversation in the absence of family members.

Content of the Medical History. Several descriptions of the information contained in the medical history and its logical sequence exist in the medical literature. These include discussions of the chief complaint, present illness, past medical history, social history, sexual history, family history, and a review of systems. Because many patients are reluctant to volunteer problems of urinary and fecal incontinence, sexual dysfunction, or current or past domestic abuse or sexual assault, women should be asked routinely about these conditions. Direct and behaviorally specific questions generally result in more accurate responses for these sensitive issues.

To standardize health care delivery, the Joint Commission on Accreditation of Healthcare Organizations (JCAHO) has developed two documents that describe standards and intents for the generation of the health care document. The current standards are the 2000 edition of *Comprehensive Accreditation Manual for Hospitals* and the *2000–2001 Comprehensive Accreditation Manual for Ambulatory Care.* These documents provide a logical reference frame for delivery of health care throughout the duration of a patient's treatment.

In 1995 and 1997, the Health Care Financing Administration (currently known as the Centers for Medicare and Medicaid Services [CMS]) developed Medicare documentation guidelines for problem-oriented evaluation and management services. These guidelines were developed jointly by the American Medical Association (AMA) and CMS to provide physicians and claims reviewers with advice about preparing or reviewing documentation for the evaluation and management services provided under Medicare, but they are used more broadly. Either the 1995 or 1997 version can be used, and the difference between the two guidelines is in the examination only. Currently, the 1997 documentation guidelines for evaluation and management services recommend key threshold elements to determine the level of complexity related to the chief complaint, past history, and review of systems. These recommendations are currently being reviewed by the AMA, CMS, and other interested medical organizations. It is expected that the 1997 recommendations will be modified. Because these recommendations will substantially influence compensation for medical care, the recommendations presented here should be carefully compared with future guidelines published by the AMA and CMS.

Currently, many practices are modifying their medical records to reflect the requirements specified by CMS. These requirements are reflected in the Woman's Health Record produced by ACOG (Appendix G).

The levels of services described by CMS are based on four types of history (problem focused, expanded problem focused, detailed, and comprehensive). Each type of history includes some or all of the following elements:

- Chief complaint
- History of present illness
- Review of systems
- Past, family, and social history

The extent of history of present illness; review of systems; and past, family, and social history that is obtained and documented is dependent on clinical judgment and the nature of the presenting problem.

Chief Complaint. The chief complaint is a concise statement describing the symptom, problem, condition, diagnosis, physician-recommended return, or other factor that is the reason for the encounter. It usually is stated in the patient's words.

History of Present Illness. The history of present illness is a chronologic description of the development of the patient's present illness. It describes the illness from the first sign or symptom or from the previous encounter to the present.

Review of Systems. A review of systems is an inventory of body systems obtained throughout a series of questions seeking to identify signs and symptoms that the patient may be experiencing or has experienced. The ACOG Woman's Health Record (Appendix G) includes a review of those systems recognized by CMS.

Past, Family, and Social History. The past, family, and social history consists of a review of general medical and obstetric and gynecologic history, family health history, allergies, current medications, and sexual and social history (see Appendix G).

The General Examination

The general physical examination serves to detect abnormalities suggested by the medical history as well as unsuspected problems. Specific information given during the history should guide the practitioner to areas of physical examination that may not be surveyed in a routine screening. The extent of the examination is based on the practitioner's relationship with the patient, what is being medically managed by other clinicians, and what is medically indicated. Once a problem has been identified, intervention can take the form of behavior modification, treatment, or referral, as necessary. The focus of a preoperative examination will depend on the procedure (see "Ambulatory Gynecologic Surgery" in Part 3). Again, because these recommendations will substantially influence compensation for medical care, the recommendations presented here should be carefully compared with future guidelines published by the AMA and CMS.

The Breast Examination

The breast examination includes visual inspection and palpation. It should be a part of all initial obstetric and all complete gynecologic examinations. A visual examination should be performed while the patient is sitting or standing with her hands on her hips. The axillary and supraclavicular areas should be palpated to detect adenopathy. To assess any palpable dominant mass, the examiner should use the fingertips to palpate all of the breast tissue with the patient in both the upright and supine positions. The presence of nipple discharge should be ascertained by gentle pressure. The clinician is encouraged to review the principles of breast self-examination with the patient while performing the physical examination.

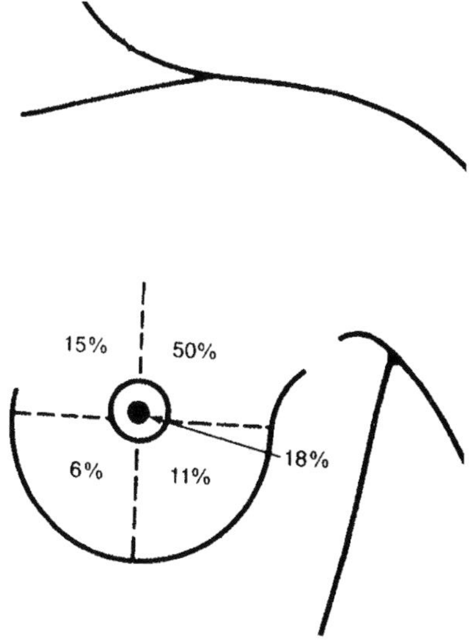

Fig. 3–1. Relative location of malignant lesions of the breast. (DiSaia PJ, Creasman WT. Clinical gynecologic oncology. 5th ed. St. Louis: Mosby, 1997)

A palpable mass requires evaluation, which may include a follow-up examination or additional diagnostic testing (see Fig. 3–1). Mammography may be useful to identify nonpalpable areas of suspicion but is not sufficient to rule out a malignancy. Sonography may be useful to define a cystic lesion. If a cyst is aspirated and the fluid is clear (transparent and not bloody) there is no need for cytology. If the cyst does not disappear after aspiration or recurs within 6 weeks, surgical follow-up should be considered. A solid, dominant, persistent mass requires tissue diagnosis by fine needle aspiration or biopsy.

The Pelvic Examination

After emptying her bladder, the patient should be assisted to the lithotomy position and properly draped. Other positions may be appropriate depending on the age or physical limitations of the patient (see "Pediatric Gynecology" and "Women with Disabilities" in Part 4). Careful inspection of the vulva and perianal area with adequate lighting is performed first.

The labia are then gently separated to allow visualization of the urethra and introitus. The clinician should carefully note and record any pertinent findings. After the external examination, a warm speculum of appropriate size should be gently inserted into the vagina, with posterior pressure against the perineal and levator muscles until the cervix can be visualized entirely. If the speculum does not pass easily, it may be moistened with water, but lubricant should not be used since it can interfere with the interpretation of results of cervical cytology as well as with the growth of microorganisms if a culture is taken.

If appropriate, cells for a cervical cytology test are obtained. If abnormal vaginal discharge is noted or if the history indicates, appropriate cultures and testing should be performed. After adequate inspection of the cervix and vaginal fornices, the speculum should be slowly removed so that the vaginal walls can be inspected. A bimanual examination is then carried out to evaluate the vagina and the cervix, and the size, shape, and position of the uterus. The adnexa are then examined for size, shape, and tenderness. When indicated, a rectovaginal examination should then be performed as the last part of the examination. This is important to evaluate the rectovaginal septum, the posterior uterine surface, the adnexal structures, the uterosacral ligaments, and the posterior cul-de-sac. The rectal finger examines for hemorrhoids, anal fissures, sphincter tone, and possible rectal polyps or carcinoma. If indicated, a stool specimen should be evaluated for occult blood.

All women who are or who have been sexually active or who have reached 18 years of age should undergo an annual cervical cytology test and pelvic examination. After a low-risk woman has had three or more consecutive, satisfactory annual examinations with normal findings, screening may be performed less frequently at physician and patient discretion.

Certain high-risk factors have been associated with the development of cervical intraepithelial neoplasia and cervical carcinoma, and ACOG recommends that when one or more of these risk factors is present, more frequent screening may be required. High-risk factors include:

- Women who have had multiple sexual partners or whose male sexual partners have had multiple partners

- Women who began sexual intercourse at an early age
- Women whose male sexual partners have had other sexual partners with cervical cancer
- Women with current or prior human papillomavirus (HPV) or condylomata or both
- Women with current or prior herpes simplex virus infections
- Women who are infected with human immunodeficiency virus (HIV)
- Women with a history of other sexually transmitted diseases (STDs)
- Women who are immunosuppressed (such as those who have received renal transplants)
- Smokers and abusers of other substances, including alcohol
- Women who have a history of cervical dysplasia or cervical, endometrial, vaginal, or vulvar cancer
- Women of lower socioeconomic status (low socioeconomic status appears to be a surrogate for a number of closely related risk factors that place these women at greater risk of cervical cancer)

The cost-effectiveness of cytologic screening for vaginal neoplasia after removal of the cervix for benign disease has not been demonstrated. Nonetheless, periodic cytologic evaluation of the vagina in such cases, based on the above risk factors, is warranted.

A cellular sample from the endocervical canal obtained with an endocervical brush and a scraping of the portio, to include the entire transformation zone, provides a reliable sample. An endocervical brush should be used to obtain the endocervical cell sampling because it is more reliable in terms of identifying cervical intraepithelial neoplasia, providing adequate cytology specimens, and limiting false-negative results.

Important measures in obtaining an adequate sample include the following steps:

- Cells should be collected prior to the bimanual examination.
- Care should be taken to avoid contaminating the sample with lubricant.

- If testing for STDs is indicated, the Pap smear should be taken first, followed by tests for STDs.
- Ideally, the entire portio should be visible when the sample is obtained.
- Vaginal discharge, when present in large amounts, should be removed before obtaining the sample so as not to disturb the epithelium. Small amounts of blood will not interfere with cytologic evaluation, but large amounts preclude cytologic sampling. If the patient has no signs or symptoms of a cervical disorder, consideration may be given to treating the vaginitis first and then obtaining a sample for cervical cytology.
- The portio sample should be obtained before the endocervical sample because of the frequency of bleeding from the endocervix when the brush is used and the concern that delays in fixing the endocervical sample may result in artifacts when the conventional Pap technique is used.
- The endocervical canal is best sampled by gently rotating a brush 180 to 360 degrees. Excessive manipulation should be avoided to prevent bleeding.
- For diethylstilbestrol-exposed patients, some practitioners take samples circumferentially from the upper two thirds of the vagina in addition to evaluating the cervix.

When performing conventional Pap tests, a single slide combining both the endocervical and ectocervical samples or two separate slides from the ectocervix and endocervix can be used. The most important consideration is rapid fixation; it should be appreciated that cellular samples, particularly those from the endocervical canal, can become air dried in a matter of seconds, underscoring the need for prompt fixation. The collected material should be applied uniformly to the slide with a rolling motion, without clumping, and should be rapidly fixed to avoid air drying. If spray fixatives are used, the spray should be held at least 10 inches away from the slide to prevent dispersal and destruction of the cells by the propellant.

Recently, several new screening techniques designed to improve the sensitivity of cervical cytology have been approved by the U.S. Food and Drug Administration for use in quality-control rescreening, primary screening, or both. The status of these systems, as well as that of others in development, is changing rapidly. No large, population-based, prospective study has been completed to determine whether any of these techniques lowers the incidence of invasive cervical cancer or improves the survival rate.

Human papillomavirus testing lacks the specificity necessary to be a useful screening test for cervical cancer or its precursors, because the vast majority of women with HPV DNA detected from cervical lavages would be cytologically normal. Human papillomavirus testing with identification of specific HPV types may be of value in the triage of certain subsets of patients. The utility of HPV testing in conjunction with cytology, however, must be evaluated prospectively in a clinical trial before it can be recommended for routine clinical use.

Suggested Reading

Agency for Health Care Policy and Research. Evaluation of cervical cytology. Rockville, Maryland: AHCPR, 1999

American College of Obstetricians and Gynecologists. Complementary and alternative medicine. ACOG Committee Opinion 227. Washington, DC: ACOG, 1999

American College of Obstetricians and Gynecologists. CPT coding in obstetrics and gynecology—2000. Washington, DC: ACOG, 2000

American College of Obstetricians and Gynecologists. ICD-9-CM diagnostic coding in obstetrics and gynecology—2000. Washington, DC: ACOG, 1999

American College of Obstetricians and Gynecologists. Physician responsibility under managed care: patient advocacy in a changing health care environment. In: Ethics in obstetrics and gynecology. Washington, DC: ACOG, 2002:64–68

American College of Obstetricians and Gynecologists. Primary and preventive care: periodic assessments. ACOG Committee Opinion 246. Washington, DC: ACOG, 2000

Centers for Disease Control and Prevention. 1998 guidelines for treatment of sexually transmitted diseases. MMWR Morb Mortal Wkly Rep 1998;47(RR-1):1–111

Health Care Financing Administration. Documentation guidelines for evaluation and management services. Baltimore, Maryland: HCFA, 1997

Joint Commission on Accreditation of Healthcare Organizations. Comprehensive accreditation manual for hospitals. Oakbrook Terrace, Illinois: JCAHO, 2000

Joint Commission on Accreditation of Healthcare Organizations. 2000–2001 comprehensive accreditation manual for ambulatory care. Oakbrook Terrace, Illinois: JCAHO, 1999

NCCLS. Papanicolaou technique: approved guideline. Villanova, Pennsylvania: NCCLS, 1994

U.S. Preventive Services Task Force. Guide to clinical preventive services: report of the U.S. Preventive Services Task Force. 2nd ed. Baltimore: Williams and Wilkins, 1996

CONTINUUM OF WOMEN'S HEALTH CARE

As women's health care physicians, obstetrician–gynecologists often serve as a woman's main source of continuity in health care throughout her lifetime. This section outlines areas of concern from adolescence onward, providing recommendations for patient care in the reproductive years, through menopause, for lesbians, for older women, and for end-of-life considerations. Some recommendations, such as those regarding reproductive health, lesbian health, and advance directives, may be applicable throughout adolescence and adulthood. Others may be more specific to stages of the life cycle.

Primary and preventive care for pediatric patients usually is not provided by an obstetrician–gynecologist. The obstetrician–gynecologist should be able to respond to a mother's health care concerns, however, and guide her to an appropriate source of care for her child. It is appropriate for an obstetrician–gynecologist to be a consultant to other physicians in the care of a female infant or child with a gynecologic problem or who has been sexually abused (see "Pediatric Gynecology" in Part 4).

Adolescence

Adolescence is a time of psychosocial, cognitive, and physical development as young people make the transition from childhood to adulthood. This transition includes sexual development and often entails behaviors that put young women at risk for pregnancy and STDs. Guidance from a physician, as well as needed reproductive health screening and care, can greatly facilitate a young woman's healthy transition to adulthood.

Health care professionals have an obligation to provide the best possible care to respond to the needs of their adolescent patients. This care should, at a minimum, include comprehensive reproductive health services, such as sexuality education, counseling, mental health assessment, diagnosis and treatment regarding pubertal development, access to contraceptives and abortion, pregnancy-related care, prenatal and delivery care, and the diagnosis and treatment of STDs. Every effort should be made to include male partners in such services and counseling.

Comprehensive services may be delivered to adolescents in a variety of sites, including schools, physician offices, and community-based and other health care facilities. Legal barriers that restrict the freedom of health care practitioners to provide these services should be removed. Institutional policies should be developed to require practitioners with views on confidentiality that restrict the provision of services to a minor to refer the patient to another practitioner.

Because the involvement of a concerned adult can contribute to the health and success of an adolescent, policies in health care settings should encourage and facilitate communication between a minor and her parent(s), when appropriate. However, concerns about confidentiality, as well as economic considerations, can be significant barriers to reproductive health care for some adolescents. The potential health risks to adolescents if they are unable to obtain reproductive health services are so compelling that legal barriers and deference to parental involvement should not stand in the way of needed health care for patients who request confidentiality. Therefore, laws and regulations that are unduly restrictive of adolescents' confidential access to reproductive health care should be revised.

Institutional procedures that safeguard the rights of their adolescent patients, including confidentiality during initial and subsequent visits and in billing, should be established.

Billing mechanisms for services and procedures for insurance and other third-party reimbursement should ensure adolescent confidentiality. When these mechanisms and procedures compromise a patient's request for confidentiality, policies should be implemented allowing payment alternatives such as reduced fees, sliding scales, and timed installment payments and patient referral to a practice or agency where subsidized care is offered or both.

An adolescent's initial visit for reproductive health guidance, screening, and provision of preventive services should take place around 13–15 years of age. The exact timing and scope of the initial visit will depend on the individual girl and her physical and emotional development. Gynecologic problems may necessitate a visit at an earlier age. Parents and adolescent females should be reassured that the initial visit at this age serves primarily to establish rapport between the obstetrician–gynecologist and the young woman, and generally does not include a pelvic examination. The provision of additional services beyond guidance and screening should be based on information obtained at this initial visit. If the patient has had intercourse, a pelvic examination, cervical cytology testing, and screening for STDs are appropriate. The timing of subsequent visits should be based on need but should include an annual visit for health guidance and assessment. This initial visit is an ideal opportunity to discuss normal adolescent development and concerns related to adolescence with both parent(s) and adolescents.

The rapid behavioral changes that occur during adolescence dictate frequent visits to screen for health risk behaviors and to provide health guidance. Health risk behaviors may, in some adolescents, coexist and be interrelated. Adolescents who are found to engage in one health risk behavior, therefore, should be asked about involvement in others. In her initial visit to her obstetrician–gynecologist, an adolescent should be given the opportunity to discuss the following high-risk areas: nutrition, eating disorders, physical activity, sexual activity, STDs, physical and sexual abuse, suicide and depression, unintended pregnancy and contraception, substance abuse, alcohol consumption and tobacco use, HIV, relationships, violence, and school performance. Lung cancer is a leading cause of early death in women. Smoking avoidance and cessation counseling should begin at an early age.

Adolescents are more likely to develop trusting relationships with their health care practitioners when the issue of confidentiality has been addressed. A confidential relationship, in turn, can facilitate the open disclosure of health histories and risky behaviors. The health and behavioral issues of adolescent patients can then be addressed with nonjudgmental counseling and medical intervention. Parental involvement should be encouraged, but confidentiality should be maintained, with the exception of a life-threatening emergency or grave risk to health (see "Human Resources" in Part 1).

In 1999, 49.9% of high school students reported that they had ever had sexual intercourse. It is estimated that nearly 4 million adolescents acquire an STD each year. Clinicians who care for adolescents should be aware of several issues that relate specifically to adolescents. The rates of many STDs are highest among adolescents (eg, the rate of gonorrhea is highest among females 15–19 years of age). Clinic-based studies have demonstrated that the prevalence of chlamydial infections, and possibly of HPV infections, also is the highest among adolescents. It is estimated that approximately 5% of the population has been infected with the hepatitis B virus (HBV), and adults and adolescents account for the majority of reported cases of acute hepatitis B. It is recommended that all children be administered the HBV vaccine, and that adolescents who have not been previously immunized receive one series of the hepatitis B vaccine. Adolescents are at greatest risk for STDs because they frequently have unprotected intercourse, are biologically more susceptible to infection, frequently have multiple sexual partners, and face multiple obstacles to the utilization of health care.

The adolescent pregnancy rate in the United States is still the highest of all developed countries, even though it has decreased over time. Of all births in the United States in 1998, more than 12% were to women 15–19 years of age. In 1998, approximately 9,400 babies were born to women younger than 15 years of age. From 1987 to 1995, the national ratio of abortions to live births steadily declined each year, reaching the lowest level since 1975. More than half of adolescent pregnancies result in live birth, nearly one third result in abortion, and the remainder resulted in miscarriages and stillbirths. Few adolescents choose adoption; most choose to parent their babies, resulting in many life-long consequences.

In the event of an unwanted pregnancy, the adolescent, as with any patient, should be counseled about her options: 1) continuing the pregnancy to term and keeping the infant, 2) continuing the pregnancy to term and placing the infant for legal adoption, or 3) terminating the pregnancy. The discussion with the patient also should determine her wishes as to what counseling should be offered to her partner or information given to her parents (if she is a dependent adolescent). Some states require parental notification or consent before a minor can obtain an abortion. In some states, pregnancy in women younger than a certain age is considered child abuse and must be reported. All health care professionals should be aware of their state laws in this regard. Rates of unintended pregnancy are higher for adolescents than for any other age group.

Contraception, STDs, and pregnancy are major health issues in sexually active adolescent patients. These factors underscore the need for comprehensive, age-appropriate sexuality education in both the home and in schools. The American College of Obstetricians and Gynecologists supports the inclusion of age-appropriate sexuality education from kindergarten through 12th grade as an integral part of comprehensive health education in schools and communities. The American College of Obstetricians and Gynecologists encourages its members to advocate for and participate in such education.

Efforts to encourage young people to delay becoming sexually active are components of almost all sexuality education programs. These programs typically are described as "abstinence-only," "abstinence-based," "abstinence-plus," and "abstinence-centered." One particular form of "abstinence-only" education is characterized by a definition of abstinence included in recent federal welfare reform law that narrowly describes its contents and purposes. This federal law, along with other factors, has contributed to a growing emphasis by some on limiting sexuality education so as to exclude accurate instruction about contraception, abortion, and sexual orientation. A recent report indicates that as of 1999, 4 in 10 sexuality education teachers in secondary public schools either teach that birth control and condoms are ineffective means of preventing pregnancy and STDs or do not cover birth control or condoms at all. Abstinence "based/plus/centered" programs, by contrast, not only promote abstinence but also incorporate reproductive health information, including both the risks and benefits of various methods of contraception, STD prevention, and forms of sexual expression alternative to intercourse.

Sexuality education programs, in general, have not been well evaluated. In particular, the impact on behavior of "abstinence-only" programs has not yet been documented through appropriate research. However, some "abstinence-based" programs that include positive messages and promote contraceptive use among those who are sexually active have shown modest success in delaying the initiation of sexual activity and increasing the use of contraception. Communities planning appropriate sexuality education for adolescents should consider the following points which are supported by ACOG:

- Parental involvement in their child(ren)'s sexuality education
- The goal of promoting healthy lifestyles for adolescents and their families. This includes the following objectives:
  —Promote abstinence from sexual intercourse as the preferred responsible behavior for adolescents
  —Increase effective use of contraceptives, including latex condoms, by sexually active adolescents
  —Support increased availability of confidential reproductive health services, including family planning and services for the prevention, diagnosis, and/or treatment of STDs
- All sexuality education programs should provide scientifically accurate information about sexuality, STDs, contraception, and preventive health care.

- Ongoing rigorous evaluation of the effectiveness of a variety of forms of sexuality education in terms of their effect on sexual behavior, as well as unintended pregnancy and abortion rates.

The Reproductive Years

Every encounter with the health care system should be viewed as an opportunity to reinforce reproductive awareness in women of childbearing age. Patient awareness of reproductive risks, health-enhancing behaviors, and family planning options are essential to improving the outcome of pregnancy. That about only half of pregnancies in the United States are planned suggests the need for a new approach to reproductive awareness. Because unintended pregnancies and reproductive health hazards—including the use of alcohol, tobacco, and other drugs—occur across all socioeconomic groups, the target group for reproductive awareness must include all women of childbearing age. New reproductive awareness messages, and strategies to deliver them, also should be developed for men. Marketing techniques may be effective in changing attitudes and behaviors among both women and men. To implement this new strategy, health practitioners should ask one basic question: is the patient in her reproductive years? If the answer is yes, a dialogue about reproductive awareness should take place. Reproductive health screening should be used by all health care professionals serving women in their reproductive years.

Family Planning

At any given time, approximately two thirds of American women of reproductive age wish to avoid or postpone pregnancy. Despite this, the United States has one of the highest unintended pregnancy rates among developed nations. Women should be counseled about the need for family planning and options for contraception, including emergency contraception.

Initial Evaluation. The initial visit for family planning provides an opportunity to assess the health status of the woman and to enlist her involvement in overall health maintenance. This also may be a time to initiate age- and risk-appropriate testing (eg, mammography, serum lipids, cervical cytology, and urinalysis) or to suggest referrals for psychosocial needs, nutritional counseling, and weight control. Physicians who wish to increase the availability and use of emergency contraception may offer patients an advance prescription for emergency contraception.

For all women of reproductive age, a contraceptive and sexual history should be obtained to assess the need for contraceptive services. Women requesting contraception should have a general medical and gynecologic history, physical examination, and laboratory studies as indicated to identify relative and absolute contraindications to the various family planning methods.

The general physical examination should be consistent with that described for asymptomatic women (see "Primary and Preventive Care" in Part 3). After review of the patient's medical history and clinical situation, the clinician may elect to defer the physical examination at the request of a woman, including an adolescent, choosing oral contraceptives.

For women who do not have risk factors and have been receiving care on a regular basis, additional laboratory tests are not needed prior to prescribing contraception. Women with identified risk factors (eg, multiple sexual partners) should be evaluated for STDs. Women with a family history of early-onset cardiovascular disease should undergo lipid analysis, including high-density lipoprotein (HDL) cholesterol and triglycerides, prior to initiating oral contraception. Patients who have significant risk factors for diabetes, including hypertension, ethnicity, abnormal serum HDL cholesterol or triglyceride levels, obesity, diabetes in a first-degree relative, or glucose intolerance or macrosomia during a prior pregnancy, should undergo either fasting or random blood glucose testing. Combination oral contraceptives should be prescribed with caution, if ever, to women who are older than 35 years of age and are smokers.

Major coronary heart disease is rare during oral contraceptive use; it is related to the combined effects of age, smoking, diabetes, hypertension, and other risk factors. In patients with dyslipidemia, treatment of the dyslipidemia should be instituted, and use of oral contraceptives may be based on low-density lipoprotein (LDL) cholesterol and triglyceride levels, the presence of other risk factors for heart disease, and age. There is no universal agreement on a set of risk factors for coronary heart disease that are absolute contraindications for oral contraceptives.

In the absence of contraindications, the patient's choice of a method of contraception or family planning should be the principal factor for prescribing one more than another. The health care practitioner should fully explain the efficacy as well as potential side effects and risks for all methods, including failure rates. A comparison with the risks of pregnancy may be valuable. Noncontraceptive benefits also should be addressed.

Counseling. Appropriate counseling is an essential element of the initial encounter with a patient who desires or needs contraception. The contraindications and relative contraindications, serious sequelae, and adverse side effects of contraceptive choices are outlined in Table 3–2. The desired characteristics affecting the choice of contraceptive methods are summarized in Table 3–3 and the efficacy of contraceptive methods is shown in Table 3–4. Information regarding birth-related and method-related deaths is shown in Table 3–5.

Patients should be counseled regarding the need for the use of barrier methods to protect against STDs combined with hormonal methods (see "Routine Detection and Prevention of Disease" in Part 3). The availability of emergency contraception should be discussed.

Sexually active adolescents deserve special attention because of the high incidence of unintended pregnancy in this population and a tendency of the adolescent not to adhere to methods of contraception requiring action on the part of the patient. The efficacy of a method requiring minimal patient activity, such as subdermal implants and injectable progestins, must be balanced against the relatively high frequency of side effects that adolescents may find particularly objectionable, such as abnormal uterine bleeding, weight gain, and acne. Adolescents also require additional counseling regarding the prevention of STDs because of the high incidence in this population.

Prevention of unintended pregnancy assumes increasing importance during the perimenopausal years. About 75% of pregnancies in women older than 40 years of age are unintended. It may be difficult to know when it is safe to change from oral contraception to postmenopausal hormone treatment. Assessment of follicle-stimulating hormone levels to determine when older oral contraceptive users have become menopausal and thus no longer need contraception is expensive and may be misleading. Until a well-validated tool to confirm menopause is available, an alternative approach is for women to discontinue oral contraceptives routinely between 50 and 55 years of age, because the likelihood that a woman has reached menopausal status by 55 years of age is 85%.

A woman considering that her family is complete should be informed about the option of vasectomy as well as female sterilization. As a part of informed consent, the patient should be told that the procedure is intended to be permanent, that there is a small chance of failure, and that the success of any attempts for subsequent surgical restoration of fertility is uncertain. Although most women do not regret their decision to have tubal sterilization, women who are 30 years of age or younger at the time of sterilization are more likely than those older than 30 years of age to express regret about the procedure. The advantages of vasectomy (eg, less invasive surgery, local anesthesia, lower cost, the potential of establishing efficacy) also should be discussed. If the patient requests sterilization and her physician agrees to perform this surgery, consultation with another physician or with her partner is not necessary. Physicians need to be aware of applicable federal and state informed consent legal requirements. If there is any question about the patient's competence to authorize the procedure, the physician should seek consultation to ensure that legal requirements are met.

Periodic Reassessment. If a patient is a first-time user of a contraceptive method, contact with her health care practitioner within the first few months of her initial visit provides an opportunity to evaluate major and minor contraceptive side effects, check blood pressure, reinstruct the patient regarding appropriate use, and dispel any fears or concerns the

Table 3–2. Contraindications, Serious Sequelae, and Side Effects of Contraceptives*

Method	Contraindications	Relative Contraindications —Use with Caution	Serious Sequelae†	Adverse Side Effects
Combination oral contraceptives	Active thrombophlebitis or thromboembolic disorders Past history of deep-vein thrombophlebitis or thromboembolic disorders Cerebral vascular or coronary artery disease Breast carcinoma Endometrial carcinoma Other estrogen-dependent neoplasia Unexplained abnormal genital bleeding Cholestatic adenoma or carcinoma	Nonresponsive hyperlipidemia Migraines with focal neurologic signs Diabetes mellitus Impaired liver function Smokers over age 35 Hypertension Morbid obesity Gallbladder disease Lactation	Thromboembolism Cerebrovascular accident Myocardial infarction Benign hepatic adenoma Cholelithiasis Hypertension (reversible on discontinuation) Glucose intolerance	Irregular bleeding Amenorrhea Nausea Weight gain Breast tenderness Depression Headache (common and migraine)
Levonorgestrel subdermal implants, injectable medroxyprogesterone acetate, and progestin-only oral contraceptives	Active thrombophlebitis or thromboembolic disorders Unexplained abnormal genital bleeding Benign or malignant liver tumors Breast carcinoma	History of depression	No serious adverse sequelae to progestin noted to date Infection at implant site Implant removal difficulties	Prolonged bleeding Irregular bleeding Amenorrhea Headache (common and migraine) Anxiety Depression Weight gain Acne or dermatitis Hirsutism Dizziness

<table>
<tr>
<td>IUD</td>
<td>History of salpingitis (PID)
Acute cervical, vaginal, or tubal infection
Known or suspected pregnancy
Postpartum endometritis or infected abortion in past 3 months
Uterine abnormalities with distortion or incomplete involution of the uterus
Known or suspected uterine or cervical malignancy
Abnormal genital bleeding
Multiple sexual partners
Immunosuppressive disorders
Genital actinomycosis
Wilson disease (copper-containing IUDs)
Allergy to copper (copper-containing IUDs)
History of ectopic pregnancy or a condition that predisposes to ectopic pregnancy (progesterone and levonorgestrel IUDs)
Acute liver disease or liver tumor (levonorgestrel IUDs)
Known or suspected carcinoma of the breast (levonorgestrel IUDs)
Hypersensitivity to product (levonorgestrel IUDs)
Presence of or a history of STD (progesterone IUDs)
IV drug use (progesterone IUDs)</td>
<td>Nulliparity
Severe dysmenorrhea
Small uterine size
Menorrhagia
Valvular heart disease
Corticosteroid treatment
Anemia
Coagulopathy or receiving anticoagulants
Diabetes mellitus</td>
<td>Salpingitis, pelvic abscess
Uterine perforation
Septic abortion (if pregnancy occurs)
Ectopic pregnancy</td>
<td>Heavy menses
Irregular menses
Dysmenorrhea
Vaginal discharge</td>
</tr>
</table>

(continued)

Table 3–2. Contraindications, Serious Sequelae, and Side Effects of Contraceptives* *(continued)*

Method	Contraindications	Relative Contraindications —Use with Caution	Serious Sequelae†	Adverse Side Effects
Diaphragm	History of hypersensitive reaction to product History of toxic shock	Uterine prolapse or retroflexion Vaginal wall relaxation Recurrent cystitis	Toxic shock (rare, no increased risk with proper use) Acute and recurrent cystitis	Hypersensitive reaction to product or spermicide
Cervical cap	History of hypersensitive reaction to product	Abnormal cervical anatomy Recurrent PID	—	Cervicitis Vaginal odor Hypersensitive reaction to product or spermicide
Condom (latex)	History of hypersensitive reaction to product	—	—	Hypersensitive reaction to product
Condom (nonlatex, polyurethane male or female condom)	History of hypersensitive reaction to product	—	—	Hypersensitive reaction to product
Spermicide	History of hypersensitive reaction to product	—	—	Hypersensitive reaction to product

*IUD indicates intrauterine device; PID, pelvic inflammatory disease; STD, sexually transmitted disease; IV, intravenous

†All forms of contraception carry some risk of failure. See Table 3–4, "Contraception Failure Rates During the First Year of Use," for failure rates by method.

Table 3–3. Desired Characteristics Affecting the Choice of Contraceptive Methods*

Characteristics Desired	Method
High-efficacy contraceptives	Combination oral contraceptives Levonorgestrol subdermal implant Injectable medroxyprogesterone IUD Sterilization
Limited or no side effects	Barrier methods Spermicides Natural family planning
Coitally independent or minimal patient activity to use	Subdermal implants Injectable medroxyprogesterone IUD Sterilization
Minimal risk to future fertility	Oral contraceptives Subdermal implants Injectable medroxyprogesterone Barrier methods Spermicides Natural family planning
Partial protection against infections	
Cervical gonorrhea, *Chlamydia*	Barrier methods
PID	Barrier methods Oral contraceptives
HIV infection	Barrier methods Spermicides
Noncontraceptive health benefits Increased menstrual cycle regularity Decreased menstrual blood loss and anemia Decreased incidence of dysmenorrhea, ovarian cysts, benign breast disease,endometrial and ovarian cancer	Oral contraceptives

*IUD indicates intrauterine device; PID, pelvic inflammatory disease; HIV, human immunodeficiency virus.

Adapted from the American Fertility Society. Guideline for practice: contraceptive choices. Birmingham, Alabama: AFS, 1994

Table 3–4. Contraception Failure Rates During the First Year of Use

Method	Percentage of Women Experiencing an Unintended Pregnancy Within the First Year of Use		Percentage of Women Continuing Use at One Year‡
	Typical Use*	Perfect Use†	
Chance§	85	85	
Spermicides‖	26	6	40
Periodic Abstinence	25	—	63
Calendar	—	9	
Ovulation Method	—	3	
Symptothermal¶	—	2	
Postovulation	—	1	
Cap#			
Parous women	40	26	42
Nulliparous women	20	9	56
Diaphragm#	20	6	56
Withdrawal	19	4	
Condom**			
Female (Reality)	21	5	56
Male	14	3	61
Pill	5	—	71
Progestin only	—	0.5	
Combined	—	0.1	
Intrauterine device			
Progesterone T	2	1.5	81
Copper T 380A	0.8	0.6	78
Depot medroxyprogesterone acetate	0.3	0.3	70
Levonorgestrel implant	0.05	0.05	88

(continued)

Table 3–4. Contraception Failure Rates During the First Year of Use *(continued)*

Method	Percentage of Women Experiencing an Unintended Pregnancy Within the First Year of Use		Percentage of Women Continuing Use at One Year‡
	Typical Use*	Perfect Use†	
Female sterilization	0.5	0.5	100
Male sterilization	0.15	0.10	100

Emergency Contraceptive Pills: Treatment initiated within 72 hours after unprotected intercourse reduces the risk of pregnancy by at least 75%.†† The Copper T intrauterine device also has been described as a means of emergency contraception (99% efficacy if inserted within 5 days of unprotected intercourse).

Lactational Amenorrhea Method: LAM is a highly effective, *temporary* method of contraception.‡‡

*Among typical couples who initiate use of a method (not necessarily for the first time), numbers reflect the percentage who experience an accidental pregnancy during the first year if they do not stop use for any other reason.

†Among couples who initiate use of a method (not necessarily for the first time) and who use it perfectly (both consistently and correctly), numbers reflect the percentage who experience an accidental pregnancy during the first year if they do not stop use for any other reason.

‡Among couples attempting to avoid pregnancy, the percentage who continue to use a method for one year.

§The percentages becoming pregnant in Column 2 (Typical Use) and Column 3 (Perfect Use) are based on data from populations where contraception is not used and from women who cease using contraception in order to become pregnant. Among such populations, about 89% become pregnant within one year. This estimate was lowered slightly (to 85%) to represent the percentage who would become pregnant within one year among women now relying on reversible methods of contraception if they abandoned contraception altogether.

||Foams, creams, gels, vaginal suppositories, and vaginal film.

¶Cervical mucus (ovulation) method supplemented by calendar in the preovulatory and basal body temperature in the postovulatory phases.

#With spermicidal cream or jelly.

**Without spermicides.

††The treatment schedule is one dose within 72 hours after unprotected intercourse, and a second dose 12 hours after the first dose. The doses are described in Table 3-6.

‡‡However, to maintain effective protection against pregnancy, another method of contraception must be used as soon as menstruation resumes, the frequency or duration of breastfeeds is reduced, bottle feeds are introduced, or the baby reaches 6 months of age.

—Data not reported.

Trussell J. Contraceptive efficacy. In: Hatcher RA, Trussell J, Stewart F, Cates W Jr, Stewart GK, Guest F, et al. Contraceptive technology. 17th revised edition. New York: Ardent Media, 1998:779–844

Table 3–5. Annual Number of Birth-Related or Method-Related Deaths Associated with Contraception

Method	Annual No. of Birth-related or Method-related Deaths (per 100,000 nonsterile women) Among Women by Age				
	15–19	20–24	25–29	30–34	35–39
No fertility-control methods*	7.0	7.4	9.1	14.8	25.7
Oral contraceptives					
Nonsmoker†	0.3	0.5	0.9	1.9	13.8
Smoker†	2.2	3.4	6.6	13.5	51.1
Intrauterine device†	0.8	0.8	1.0	1.0	1.4
Condom*	1.1	1.6	0.7	0.2	0.3
Diaphragm/spermicide*	1.9	1.2	1.2	1.3	2.2
Periodic abstinence*	2.5	1.6	1.6	1.7	2.9

*Deaths are birth related.

†Deaths are method related.

Reproduced with the permission of The Alan Guttmacher Institute. Adapted from Ory HW. Mortality associated with fertility and fertility control: 1983. Fam Plann Perspect 1983;15:57–63

patient may have developed since the initial counseling. The rates of pregnancy and discontinuation are highest in the first few months after the initiation of contraception, making this primarily educational visit most appropriate. Once the patient has gained a comfort level with her method of contraception, annual follow-up examinations, including cervical cytology and consideration of STD testing based on risk factors, should be conducted in accordance with age-specific recommendations for asymptomatic women.

Emergency Contraception. Combination or progestin-only oral contraceptives for emergency contraception, as outlined in Table 3–6, should be offered to women who experience unprotected sexual intercourse or sexual assault within 72 hours of intercourse. Because the progestin-only

Table 3–6. Brands of Oral Contraceptives That Can Be Used for Emergency Contraception in the United States

Brand*	Pills per Dose†	Ethinyl Estradiol per Dose (μg)	Levonorgestrel per Dose (mg)‡
Plan B	1 white pill	0	0.75
Preven	2 blue pills	100	0.50
Ovral	2 white pills	100	0.50
Ogestrel	2 white pills	100	0.50
Alesse	5 pink pills	100	0.50
Levlite	5 pink pills	100	0.50
Nordette	4 light-orange pills	120	0.60
Levlen	4 light-orange pills	120	0.60
Levora	4 white pills	120	0.60
Lo/Ovral	4 white pills	120	0.60
Low-Ogestrel	4 white pills	120	0.60
Triphasil	4 yellow pills	120	0.50
Tri-Levlen	4 yellow pills	120	0.50
Trivora	4 pink pills	120	0.50
Ovrette	20 yellow pills	0	0.75

*Plan B and Preven are the only dedicated products specifically marketed for emergency contraception. Ovral, Ogestrel, Alesse, Levlite, Nordette, Levlen, Levora, Lo/Ovral, Low-Ogestrel, Triphasil, Tri-Levlen, and Trivora have been declared safe and effective for use as emergency contraceptives by the U.S. Food and Drug Administration.

†The treatment schedule is one dose within 72 hours after unprotected intercourse and another dose 12 hours later.

‡The progestin in Ovral, Ogestrel, Lo/Ovral, Low-Ogestrel, and Ovrette is norgestrel, which contains two isomers, only one of which (levonorgestrel) is bioactive; the amount of norgestrel in each dose is twice the amount of levonorgestrel.

Adapted from Trussell J, Koenig J, Ellertson C, Stewart F. Preventing unintended pregnancy: the cost-effectiveness of three methods of emergency contraception. Am J Public Health 1997;87:932–937

method produces less nausea and may be more effective than the combination oral contraceptive method, this regimen should be strongly considered. To minimize nausea and vomiting with combination oral contraceptive products, an antiemetic agent should be prescribed and the patient should take it 1 hour before the first dose. If possible, emergency contraception should be used within the first 24 hours after unprotected intercourse because efficacy may be greatest if used within 24 hours after exposure. Patients should be evaluated for pregnancy if menses have not begun within 21 days following emergency contraceptive treatment. A 75% reduction in risk of pregnancy has been estimated for the combined regimen, and the progestin-only method appears to be even more effective in preventing pregnancy.

Physicians who wish to increase the availability and use of emergency contraception may offer patients an advance prescription at a routine gynecologic visit. There are two approved packages of oral contraceptives (Preven and Plan B) labeled specifically for use as emergency contraception (see box). The copper-T intrauterine device also has been described as a method of emergency contraception.

Contraceptive Failures. There is no substantive evidence that the use of any contraception during early pregnancy is associated with fetal anomalies. If a patient becomes pregnant while using a contraceptive method, she should be counseled about any specific risks. If a pregnancy occurs while a hormonal method of contraception is being used, the method should be discontinued. If a patient becomes pregnant while using an intrauterine device, the device should be removed, if possible, because of the increased risk of spontaneous abortion, infection, preterm rupture of membranes, and preterm delivery.

Emergency Contraception Information

The web site ec.princeton.edu/ offers information on emergency contraception. It includes a directory of physicians and clinics that offer prepackaged emergency contraception and how to join the directory.

Preconceptional Care

Women who are contemplating pregnancy should be encouraged to undergo a comprehensive preconceptional examination and counseling. Preconceptional counseling can identify women who might be at risk from pregnancy (eg, women with heart disease, diabetes mellitus, hypertension, renal disease) and those who may be at risk for having a newborn with a birth defect (eg, women who have a family history of inherited disorders, have diabetes, or are taking anticonvulsants). When pregnancy is planned, a woman can use the months preceding conception to evaluate her health status and to make changes that will benefit her own health status, that of her baby, and that of family members.

During a preconceptional evaluation, the clinician may make recommendations that may reduce the chance of having a baby with a birth defect, determine whether any maternal medical problems are present and provide recommendations for treatment, and provide information about nutrition, exercise, and other means of achieving optimum physical and psychologic health. This visit is an opportunity for women to learn about fertility issues and what to expect during pregnancy.

History. At the preconceptional visit, information that may have a bearing on a future pregnancy should be obtained. The following components serve as a guide to preconceptional care:

- Systematic identification of preconceptional risks through assessment of reproductive, family, and medical histories; nutritional status; drug, alcohol, and tobacco exposures; environmental exposures at work and at home; and social concerns of all fertile women
- Provision of education regarding any identified risks
- Discussion of possible effects of pregnancy on existing medical conditions for both the prospective mother and the fetus and introduction of interventions, if appropriate and desired
- Discussion of genetic concerns and referral, if appropriate and desired
- Determination of immunity to rubella, hepatitis, and varicella and immunization, if indicated

- Laboratory tests, as indicated
- Discussion of physical activity and exercise
- Nutritional counseling on appropriate weight for height, recommendation for folic acid supplementation, and avoidance of excessive vitamin supplementation; referral for in-depth counseling, if appropriate and desired
- Discussion of social, financial, and psychological issues and social supports in preparation for pregnancy and parenting
- Discussion regarding desired birth spacing and real and perceived barriers to achieving these goals, including problems with contraceptive use
- Emphasis on the importance of early and continuous prenatal care and discussion of how care may be structured based on the woman's risks and concerns
- Recommendation to patient to keep a menstrual calendar
- Human immunodeficiency virus counseling and testing, if desired

Medical History. Conditions that may have an effect on pregnancy should be covered in the medical history. Information should be obtained about chronic conditions, such as diabetes; hypertension; epilepsy; anemia and disorders of coagulation; herpes and other STDs, including HIV; heart disease; kidney disease; endocrine disease; and reactive airway disease. The history also should include menstrual history, surgical history, contraceptive methods previously used and any complications, past accidents, allergies, childhood disease history, and immunization history (including rubella). The patient should be questioned about specific conditions related to ethnic background and family history suggestive of genetic disorders such as muscular dystrophy, hemophilia, Tay–Sachs disease, sickle cell disease, cystic fibrosis, thalassemia, consanguinity, mental retardation, anatomical birth defects, Down syndrome, and other chromosomal abnormalities.

Medication and Substance Abuse. Patients should be asked about prescription or over-the-counter medications that they take regularly or as needed. Patients should be asked specifically about medications that they may be reluctant to mention, such as sedatives or tranquilizers, herbal supplements, or appetite suppressants. Use of tobacco, alcohol, and illegal drugs should be determined. The preconceptional interview allows for timely education about drug use and abuse in pregnancy, informed decision making about the risks of conception, and the introduction of interventions for those who abuse substances. A summary of steps for integrating an effective smoking cessation screening and treatment protocol into routine obstetric–gynecologic practice has been outlined (see "Suggested Reading" at the end of this section). Patients should be reassured of the confidentiality of this information, in an attempt to ensure a candid response; however, a few states require health care practitioners to report drug use by pregnant women. Use of tobacco and alcoholic beverages should be determined and discouraged, especially during pregnancy. This is a good opportunity to offer smoking cessation programs.

Reproductive History. Patients should be asked about conditions that may affect future pregnancy. These include a history of therapy or surgery on the cervix, ovaries, uterus, or fallopian tubes; in-utero exposure to diethylstilbestrol; and prior adverse pregnancy outcomes.

Nutrition. The patient's height and weight and a general assessment of her dietary habits should be recorded. Information about her use of dietary supplements, efforts to control weight, any history of eating disorders such as bulimia or anorexia, and prior obesity should be obtained in the inquiry.

The preconceptional ingestion of folic acid has been shown to reduce the risk of neural tube defects. The U.S. Public Health Service has advocated that all women of reproductive age who are capable of becoming pregnant take 0.4 mg of folic acid daily to prevent neural tube defects. For this reason, the recommended dietary allowance for folic acid has been increased to 0.4 mg as well. Although grain is now fortified with folic acid, it is unlikely that a daily intake of 0.4 mg can be achieved through diet alone. Therefore, daily supplementation with 0.4 mg is recommended for all women of reproductive age. To be of value, folic acid supplementation must be taken early in pregnancy, even before pregnancy has been identified. Those patients at high risk for neural tube defects (eg, those who have a history of neural tube defects, had an affected infant, or who are taking anticonvulsants) should ingest 4 mg of folic acid daily, preferably starting 1 month prior to the time they plan to become pregnant and continuing through the first 3 months of pregnancy. Increasing the doses of multivitamin preparations to reach these levels is not advised because of the potential for ingesting excessive amounts of other vitamins.

Environmental Factors. The clinician should inquire about the patient's occupation, working conditions, number of hours worked per week, physical activity required at work, and possible exposure to toxic substances such as lead, certain solvents, insecticides, or irradiation. Similar inquiries should be made regarding the patient's home environment. Information about exercise habits, pets (especially cats), and hobbies should be elicited. Although there is a paucity of data on the effects of toxic hazards during pregnancy, information may be obtained from company physicians or toxicology hotlines if toxic hazards may be an issue (see box).

Other aspects of an individual's home environment also may be an area of concern. Fear and abuse are problems for many women. It is important to determine if the woman feels safe and what options she may have if she does not feel safe (see "Routine Detection and Prevention of Disease" in Part 3 and "Domestic or Intimate Partner Violence" in Part 4).

Physical Assessment. After a history is obtained, a complete physical assessment of the patient should be performed, with emphasis on conditions that might adversely affect pregnancy. A pelvic examination should be conducted to detect possible reproductive anomalies that may influence conception and pregnancy. Cervical cytology testing and screening for STDs should be performed when appropriate. Human immunodeficiency virus screening should be offered.

Counseling. After the history and physical assessment are completed, the patient should be counseled regarding risk factors and lifestyle changes appropriate to a successful pregnancy. It should be stressed to the patient

Sources of Current Teratogen Information

Several sources of useful current information regarding potential teratogens are available, including numerous teratogen information services available throughout the United States to serve specific geographic areas. For information on the teratogen service in a particular area, contact:

Eastern United States

Massachusetts Teratogen Information Service
Boston, Massachusetts
(781) 466-8474

or

Western United States

Pregnancy Riskline
Salt Lake City, Utah
(801) 328-2229

The following computerized teratology and reproductive risk databases provide up-to-date summaries of electronic resource teratology information:

Micromedex, Inc.
REPRORISK (REPROTEXT, REPROTOX, Shepard's Catalog of Teratogenic Agents and TERIS)
Englewood, CO
800-525-9083

National Library of Medicine, MEDLARS Service Desk
GRATEFUL MED (TOXLINE, TOXNET, and MEDLINE)
Bethesda, MD
888-346-3656

Reproductive Toxicology Center
REPROTOX
Bethesda, MD
(301) 657-5984

TERIS and Shepard's Catalog of Teratogenic Agents
Seattle, WA
(206) 543-2465

that a healthy lifestyle will not only improve her chances of having a healthy pregnancy but also have long-term benefits for her and her family; however, patients should be informed that ideal physical health prior to pregnancy does not prevent all complications of pregnancy. Pregnancy complications or discomforts may necessitate changes in lifestyle, such as cessation of work or prolonged bedrest, that are not predictable before or in early pregnancy.

Measures should be taken to modify behavior that may be detrimental, such as smoking, alcohol consumption, or poor nutrition. If the patient has known high-risk factors, such as diabetes or hypertension, these conditions should be assessed and controlled prior to conception.

Couples with identifiable risks of having a child with heritable abnormalities and couples with genetic concerns should be counseled appropriately or referred to genetic counseling services. Genetic counseling includes in-depth assessment of risks, as well as discussion of availability and limitations of prenatal diagnosis and options. Recognizing positive carrier status before conception allows couples to understand the risks outside the emotional context of pregnancy, allows time for thorough family evaluation, when indicated, and prepares the couple for prenatal diagnostic procedures during pregnancy if desired (see "Genetics" in Part 4).

Women with metabolic diseases, such as phenylketonuria and diabetes mellitus, should be counseled regarding the importance of appropriate diet and metabolic control before conception and during pregnancy. Women should be asked whether they have phenylketonuria or whether they were placed on a special diet during childhood, because some women are not aware they were diagnosed with phenylketonuria. Dietary restrictions that result in lower maternal phenylalanine levels appear to reduce the risk of fetal abnormalities. Good glycemic control reduces the risk of miscarriage, fetal anomalies, and other adverse pregnancy outcomes in women with diabetes. To be most effective, appropriate dietary modifications should be made before conception.

Women should be educated regarding pregnancy outcome with advancing maternal age, especially beyond 35 years of age. The ability to conceive and carry a pregnancy to viability decreases slightly after 30 years of age, decreases more rapidly after 35 years of age, and decreases still more rapidly beyond 40 years of age. Although any woman may give birth to a child with Down syndrome or other trisomy, the risk of autosomal trisomy increases with advancing maternal age. At about 35 years of age, the procedure-related risk of pregnancy loss from invasive prenatal diagnostic studies is almost equivalent to the risk of aneuploidy. Other complications of pregnancy more common in older pregnant women include gestational diabetes, hypertensive disorders, cesarean delivery, maternal mortality, and possibly perinatal mortality and neural tube defects.

Patients should be counseled regarding the possibility of postpartum depression. This is more common in women with a history of depression prior to pregnancy, previous postpartum depression, or other emotional disorders.

Lesbian Health

Lesbians are found among all age, racial and ethnic groups, and socioeconomic strata. There has been, however, relatively little research on the health care needs of this subgroup of women. Estimates of the numbers of lesbians in the United States vary considerably, primarily based on the definition used for identification.

Lesbians are not at higher risk for any specific health problems simply because of their sexual orientation. They share the same risk factors for physical and mental health as all women. Although limited data are available, some risk factors may be more common among this population, such as nulliparity, decreased use of oral contraceptives, more frequent smoking or alcohol use or both, and increased weight. These combined risk factors may increase the risk for breast cancer, lung cancer, cardiovascular disease (CVD), and type 2 diabetes.

Despite what some clinicians and some lesbians believe about lack of risk, lesbians are at risk for STDs and HIV based on the same risk factors as other women, including number of partners and unprotected sex with an infected partner. Some lesbians may have had, or continue to have, sex with male partners and skin-to-skin transmission of HPV and herpes can occur with both male–female and same-sex sexual contact. Therefore, even among women who have sex only with women, standard comprehensive gynecologic care, including cervical cytology testing and STD testing as indicated, is recommended.

Lesbians experience disproportionate barriers to health care access. Lesbians desiring pregnancy may have difficulty accessing artificial insemination and may encounter barriers to insurance coverage for these procedures. Many states do not permit spousal benefits for unmarried partners, and lesbians report higher levels of uninsurance than married heterosexual women. Lack of recognition of lesbian relationships makes it more difficult for a partner to obtain medical information or provide permission for medical care under certain circumstances. Assigning a durable power of attorney to the partner may help with this issue.

Finding accepting, supportive, and culturally competent health and mental health practitioners may be difficult. For this reason, lesbians may forgo needed health care or they may not disclose their sexual identity to health care professionals. Some who have disclosed their sexual identity have reported negative responses from clinicians, including shock, embarrassment, ostracism, and breached confidentiality. Some of those who do not disclose their sexual identity have reported a lack of trust and communication, irrelevant health education, and inappropriate care because of assumptions about heterosexuality. Studies of health care professionals suggest that few physicians are knowledgeable or have been trained about the health care needs of lesbians.

Clinicians should develop the requisite skills to query patients about sexual health including discussions of differing lifestyles. There are nonjudgmental methods for inquiring about sexual orientation and behavior. Questions should be framed in ways that do not make assumptions and use language that is inclusive, allowing the patient to decide when and what she wishes to disclose about her sexual behaviors and orientation. Examples include the following questions:

- "Are you single, partnered, married, widowed, or divorced?"

- "Do you have a primary relationship?"
- "Who is in your immediate family?"

If a woman discloses that she is a lesbian, a response could be "Do you have any questions about your sexual activity?" Counseling and health maintenance plans then can be developed to include individual risk factors. To more fully address the health care needs of lesbians, clinicians should educate themselves and examine their own biases, developing responses to disclosure that are positive, respectful, and therapeutic.

Menopause

Menopause is the permanent cessation of menstruation that occurs after the loss of ovarian activity. In North America the median age of menopause is 51 years. Medical intervention in menopausal women should focus on primary–preventive health care and counseling and address diet, fitness, use of alcohol, smoking cessation, cancer screening, and the role of hormone replacement therapy (HRT) (see "Primary and Preventive Care" and "Routine Detection and Prevention of Disease" in Part 3).

Most women go through a period of irregular menstrual function prior to menopause. Common symptoms of menopause include vasomotor symptoms (hot flashes or flushes) and vaginal dryness. Atrophic changes of the external genitalia commonly occur with time. Certain medical conditions occur more often in the absence of estrogen. These include osteoporosis, coronary artery disease, stroke, and possibly Alzheimer's disease and adult macular degeneration.

Counseling

Counseling should be provided as described in "Primary and Preventive Care" and "Routine Detection and Prevention of Disease" in Part 3. The following recommendations are of particular importance.

Patients in the perimenopausal period should be given information about the normal events of aging, including specific information regarding the reduction of ovarian hormonal function and the manifestations of these changes. Patients should be advised about the benefits of HRT in protecting against osteoporosis and the potential benefits in protecting against CVD and colon cancer and preserving central nervous system function. Patients should be aware of other medications that are effective in preventing osteoporosis. In addition, modifications in lifestyle such as changes in dietary habits, social habits, and exercise patterns that may benefit the overall health of women during menopause should be discussed. Smoking cessation, lipid monitoring, blood pressure monitoring, and annual health care maintenance should be reemphasized.

Menopausal women should be counseled about the benefits of exercise in retarding osteoporosis. They also should be informed about special dietary needs, including the importance of calcium intake. The National Institutes of Health's current recommendation for optimal calcium intake in postmenopausal women is 1,000 mg/d for those receiving estrogen therapy and 1,500 mg/d for those not receiving hormone therapy. Because of the risk of fractures, women should be informed of the importance of accident prevention and safety issues. Recommendations for cancer screening procedures, such as cervical cytology testing and mammography, should be reviewed. Discussions regarding elder abuse and domestic violence should be considered.

Hormone Replacement Therapy

Estrogen replacement therapy provides effective treatment of menopausal symptoms, such as hot flushes and vaginal dryness, and can help relieve stress incontinence (see "Hormone Replacement Therapy" in Part 4). For a woman who still has her uterus, the addition of a progestin is recommended to decrease the risk of endometrial cancer.

The two main uses for long-term therapy—CVD and osteoporosis prevention—often are asymptomatic. Most epidemiologic studies have shown a dramatic cardiovascular protective effect of exogenous estrogens. The presumed cardiovascular benefits of estrogen are based on several factors. Estrogen therapy has been shown to reduce serum levels of LDL cholesterol and to increase serum levels of HDL cholesterol in a dose-dependent fashion, although only 25–50% of the risk reduction is thought to be secondary to changes in lipid patterns. Other proposed mechanisms of action of estrogen in the prevention of CVD include direct vasodilation and reduced platelet adhesiveness. Some progestins, such as medroxyprogesterone acetate, have an opposite effect on lipids; however, studies have not shown that this effect negates the cardiovascular protection.

The widely held assumption that HRT will protect women against heart disease is being questioned by the findings of four key studies: the Heart and Estrogen/Progestin Replacement Study, the Nurses' Health Study, the Estrogen Replacement and Atherosclerosis trial, and the Women's Health Initiative. All four of these studies have found either a lack of benefit or association with poorer outcomes during the first 2–3 years after commencing HRT. The Heart and Estrogen/Progestin Replacement Study, a clinical trial of conjugated estrogens/medroxyprogesterone acetate versus placebo in women with heart disease, showed an almost 50% increase in coronary heart disease in the active treatment group during the first year, followed by no effect in the second year, and a trend towards benefit in subsequent years. Following the publication of the Heart and Estrogen/Progestin Replacement Study's findings in 1998, 1 year later the Nurses' Health Study investigators reported a similar pattern of early harm and later benefit in the observational study data of women with heart disease. More recently, the Estrogen Replacement and Atherosclerosis trial investigators reported no effect of conjugated estrogens or conjugated estrogens/medroxyprogesterone acetate on coronary atherosclerosis in a 3-year angiography trial.

All of these studies involved women with existing disease, and the findings may have been dismissed as being of less relevance to healthy women. However, in 2000 the Women's Health Initiative investigators alerted the more than 27,000 women in that study about a small increase in heart attacks, strokes, and blood clots the first 2 years in the group on active treatment (either conjugated estrogens or conjugated estrogens/medroxyprogesterone acetate) compared with placebo. Participants were notified that the excess events appear to diminish expectations of benefit for CVD, at least for the first year or two after commencing HRT. It remains possible that longer term treatment will decrease risk for CVD, as suggested by dozens of observational studies. The Women's Health Initiative trial and a similar trial in the United Kingdom are continuing, in the hope of providing more definitive data on this issue.

Patients who are candidates for HRT should be evaluated and treated on an individual basis. Concerns about hormone therapy as they pertain to each patient should be reviewed in detail:

- Endometrial neoplasia—Unopposed estrogen use increases the risk of endometrial cancer by four to eight times. Treatment with a combination of progestin and estrogen diminishes the risk of endometrial cancer to less than that for women not treated with estrogen.
- Ovarian neoplasia—No relationship between estrogen replacement therapy and ovarian cancer has been proven.
- Breast neoplasia—Some data suggest a minimally increased risk of breast cancer for women who used estrogen for more than 10–20 years. Recent studies report a modestly increased risk for the development of breast cancer among women using estrogen–progestin combination HRT compared with women using estrogen-only HRT. These studies also showed increased risk with fewer years of use (4–8 years). Additional research is needed to better define the balance of risks and benefits of HRT use.
- Cholelithiasis—There may be a slight, but as yet unconfirmed, increase in the incidence of gallstones in women who receive estrogen.
- Thromboembolic disease—Recent studies have shown a twofold to fourfold increase in the risk of venous thromboembolism in users of estrogen-only and combined estrogen–progestin HRT. Because the absolute risk of venous thromboembolism in both users and nonusers of estrogen is low, there is only a modest increase in the morbidity associated with HRT, and this increased risk must be weighed against documented benefits.
- Hypertension—Hormone replacement therapy modestly lowers blood pressure; however, in a few women it may induce or exacerbate hypertension. Routine blood pressure monitoring is appropriate.

- Cardiovascular disease—Some data suggest that HRT may be associated with an initial increase in morbidity in women who have had a prior cardiovascular event. Within several years of the start of therapy, however, the risk of morbidity drops to below the baseline risk.

Contraindications to estrogen therapy include the following:

- Unexplained vaginal bleeding
- Active liver disease
- Chronic impaired liver function
- Recent vascular thrombosis (with or without emboli)

Relative contraindications include the following conditions:

- Seizure disorders
- Very high levels of triglycerides and lipids in the blood
- Migraine headache
- Atraumatic thrombophlebitis
- Current gallbladder disease
- Breast and endometrial cancer

The use of estrogen in women known to have had endometrial or breast cancer is undergoing evaluation and is controversial. Each patient's needs should be considered on an individual basis in consultation with the oncologist and the patient, who should be fully informed of the known risks and benefits and alternative therapies.

After a thorough discussion regarding the risks and benefits of HRT, the patient should undergo a medical evaluation prior to the initiation of treatment. At least three treatment regimens are used for administration of HRT:

1. Cyclic—Estrogen is given for 25 days or more per month with the addition of a cyclic progestin.
2. Combined—Estrogen and a low dose of progestin are given daily.
3. Estrogen only—Estrogen is given for 25 or more days per month.

A dose of 0.625 mg of conjugated estrogen or its equivalent is thought to provide protection against bone disease. The estrogen dose that may protect against CVD remains to be established. A progestin should be added when a woman has an intact uterus. It is unclear, at present, whether the addition of a progestin diminishes any cardiovascular protection of estrogen. Women who cannot tolerate progestins may benefit from unopposed estrogen therapy if closely monitored.

Endometrial sampling is not necessary prior to instituting therapy in asymptomatic patients. It should be performed annually, however, in women who are taking estrogen without progestin. An endometrial biopsy also should be performed if a patient bleeds at unpredictable times.

New HRT strategies that could reduce the risk of breast cancer currently are being developed. A number of selective estrogen receptor modulators (SERMs) have been studied as chemopreventive agents. Raloxifene, a newer SERM, has been developed to treat osteoporosis and may have antineoplastic activity against breast cancer. Current evidence suggests that SERMs do not alleviate vasomotor symptoms and may not protect against CVD or prevent bone demineralization as well as HRT. Presently, SERMs are not first-line agents for HRT, but offer positive effects for bone demineralization. Tamoxifen, another SERM, has been shown to reduce the risk for breast cancer in women at high risk. The decision to use tamoxifen to reduce the risk of breast cancer in women at high risk for the disease should be individualized.

Older Women

By the year 2010, 13.2 % of the U.S. population will be older than 65 years of age. By the year 2030, those older than 65 years of age will be fully 20% of the population and it is estimated that 50% of health care expenditures will be focused on the care of older women. Obstetrician–gynecologists and other clinicians who care for older women can play an important role in promoting health and preventing disease by ensuring that the recommended preventive screening is performed (see box on page 132 "Periodic Assessment: Age 65 Years and Older") and by addressing the special needs of older women.

Communication Issues

Communication with elderly women can present special challenges. Effective and sensitive communication can be facilitated by asking for concerns rather than complaints and by remembering that older people may have multiple chronic conditions and show atypical presentations of disorders. Loquacity is a common trait, and the clinician may have to allow extra time or schedule additional appointments to best meet the needs of older patients. It is important to maintain an unhurried pace as many elderly will function poorly if rushed. Closed-ended questions should be used when necessary, and the availability of previous medical records, as well as an accompanying family member, can be helpful. Some topics may be difficult to discuss, but are very important to proper care. These include sexuality, incontinence, abuse, depression, long-term care, terminal care and death, and cognitive and functional impairment. These issues are addressed in more depth later in this part and in Part 4.

Visual and hearing deficits may influence communication with the elderly. It is important to ask early in the visit whether the patient can hear adequately. Speaking clearly and directly, enunciating consonants particularly, and increasing volume can help.

Although memory for short, logically associated material usually is good, the elderly learn more complex and logically unassociated material less well. Comprehension can be improved by screening out distractions, using attention-getting signals, such as gestures, pauses, touch, or questions, and by alerting the patient to changes of subject. Memory can be aided by stating clearly the important information to be learned, keeping new information brief and relevant, providing written instructions (in a size print easily seen by the elderly person), using logical relationships, tying new information to old knowledge, and using repetition.

Functional Assessment

Although there is a wide variation in the mental, social, and physical status of older women, they often have multiple medical problems made more complex by the physiologic changes in almost every organ system that accompany aging. These changes manifest as altered height, weight, and posture; changes in common laboratory values; and altered regulation of homeostasis. These changes can affect a woman's metabolism of drugs, susceptibility to and visible signs of infection, as well as her ability to recover from surgery.

In the elderly woman, multiple chronic conditions may interact in ways that impact on her ability to manage independently. The assessment of the woman's ability to function in the arena of everyday life is critical. Evaluation of functional assessment, coupled with appropriate management or referrals, can assist the elderly woman to maintain health. For the patient approaching a medical intervention or surgery, functional assessment is critical. Patients who are at a borderline level of function may not be able to tolerate the impact of the treatment and may become dependent as a result of medical or surgical intervention (see also "Ambulatory Gynecologic Surgery" in Part 3).

Functional assessment includes an evaluation of the following:

- Cognitive and affective mental functions
- Vision
- Hearing
- Motor function
- Gait and balance
- Bowel and bladder function
- Activities of daily living
- Environmental risks and support systems

Numerous screening and assessment tools for functional assessment have been developed and tested. These tools are simple, reasonably time-efficient, sensitive, and valid in their ability to detect significant impairment.

The cognitive changes in aging women are subject to significant variation. Some may be age-related while others can be related to underlying, often unidentified, illnesses and/or medications. The two most common dementias are Alzheimer's disease and dementia associated with a previously documented cerebrovascular disease. There also are a number of noncortical dementias, including those related to drug toxicity and interaction; alcohol and other substance abuse; systemic infections; renal failure; heart failure; or metabolic diseases, such as malnutrition, iron deficiency, hypothyroidism, and B_{12} and folate deficiencies. Dementia also can be related to social and family isolation, inactivity, elder abuse, and neglect.

Delirium, although often confused with dementia, is a transient condition that usually is associated with a treatable medical condition. The risk factors for development of delirium include disturbance of consciousness due to recent anesthesia or surgery, sleep medication or change in environment, or an underlying medical condition. Delirium is characterized by an acute and fluctuating course and is an impairment of cognition that is not attributable to prior or progressive dementia.

Hearing disorders afflict more than a third of people older than 65 years of age and visual defects are almost universal. Early identification and management can reduce the resulting emotional and physical morbidity. Primary visual symptoms common in the elderly include night blindness, reading difficulty, eye pain, blurred central vision, and diminished awareness of peripheral objects. Hearing difficulties may appear as tinnitus, difficulty understanding women and children (high frequency hearing loss), difficulty locating the source of sounds, and vertigo.

Loss of the ability to perform the activities of daily living is one of the greatest fears of older people. Identification, prevention, and minimization of disorders associated with decreased mobility can be of appreciable help in addressing these problems. Osteoporosis-related disability is more common in elderly women. Falls, particularly in older women, are associated with prolonged restriction of mobility, so special effort should be made to prevent them.

Incontinence is one of the most common disorders for aging women. In addition to causes intrinsic to the lower urinary tract, delirium, infection, atrophic urethritis/vaginitis, medications, depression, excessive urine output (eg, from congestive heart failure or hyperglycemia), restricted mobility, and stool impaction can be involved. Bacteruria in the elderly is common and does not require treatment if asymptomatic.

About 20% of elderly people are affected by increasing dissatisfaction with bowel habit. Normal bowel habits include formed stools every 1–3 days. Constipation can be related to a low-fiber diet, medications, low fluid intake, colorectal dysmotility, irritable bowel syndrome, obstruction, hypothyroidism, or inadequate toilet facilities. Diarrhea may result from infection, medications, laxative abuse, irritable bowel syndrome, or interventions to alleviate bowel impaction.

Common Medical Conditions

Certain medical conditions are more common in the elderly. These include CVD, fractures, cancer, and infections. In addition, nutritional deficiencies may be present.

Cardiovascular disease is the leading cause of death among women. Symptoms of CVD in women may be subtler than those in men, and recognition requires higher awareness (see "Routine Detection and Prevention of Disease" in Part 3). Late onset of hypertension, especially isolated systolic hypertension, has an influence on stroke and myocardial infarction; therefore, detection and treatment are important.

Fracture is a major health hazard in women 65 years of age and older. Vertebral and hip fractures are common and are associated with morbidity and mortality. These complications often lead to placement in a long-term care facility. Osteoporosis increases risk for fractures, and hormone replacement has proved to be a preventive factor. Other medications are available for therapy. Frequent falls is another risk, and older women should be counseled about the need to reduce their risk for falls and injuries and to make their homes as safe as possible.

Cancer is the second leading cause of death in women 65 years of age or older. Screening and preventive counseling should take place (see box on page 132 "Periodic Assessment: Age 65 Years and Older" and "Routine Detection and Prevention of Disease" in Part 3). Screening for breast cancer has been particularly controversial. Although there are insufficient data regarding women aged 70 years and older to make a definitive recommendation about screening for breast cancer, the incidence of this condition does increase with age. Therefore, ACOG continues to recommend annual screening in this age group.

Infections account for about one third of mortality in older women. The most commonly encountered infections in the elderly include urinary tract infections, pneumonia, influenza, herpes zoster, and tuberculosis, especially in institutionalized women. Clinicians should recommend appropriate immunizations as indicated (see box on page 133 "Periodic Assessment: Age 65 Years and Older").

Alterations in nutrient requirements and changes in metabolism, as well as medical problems, can lead to nutritional deficiencies in elderly women. Because many foods containing complex carbohydrates (ie, starches such as grains, legumes, potatoes, fruit) also contain large amounts of vitamins and minerals, elderly individuals should consume a larger proportion of complex carbohydrates (55–60%) to increase their nutrient intake. Aging women should be evaluated for a decline in their need for caloric intake, and their diet should be adjusted accordingly. Women should be encouraged to maintain weight in the normal range and to follow a regular exercise program for weight regulation and other health benefits. Often, a dietary history or serial measures of weight will reveal problems, but additional diagnostic testing may be warranted. Management includes an evaluation of financial and support resources with social service referrals, as necessary, nutritional counseling, and correction of any underlying medical conditions.

Common Psychosocial Concerns

In addition to variations in cognitive function, many older women are at increased risk for psychosocial concerns. Depression is very common in elderly women and often is unrecognized and untreated. Women should be screened for suicide risk factors, symptoms of depression, abnormal bereavement, and changes in cognitive function. Sleep disorders in aging women are associated with dementia and depression, sleep apnea, daytime medication use, and pain syndromes.

Alcoholism, sexual dysfunction, and complications arising from multiple medication use increase and often are undiagnosed in this age group. Signs of physical or emotional abuse, as well as neglect, should be sought. The woman's social support system is critical for her recovery and functioning. Patients should be asked about family and other support systems, as well as whether she has formal or informal help in her home.

Medication Use

Older women experience adverse events relating to drug therapy more frequently and in more unexpected ways than do younger women. Polypharmacy, or many drugs from many sources, is not uncommon. Over-the-counter medications often are not included by women in their recall of medications. Asking a patient or a family member to bring in a paper bag everything the woman takes, including vitamins and over-the-counter medications, to the clinical visit is one method for determining medication use.

Often, older women have poor medication compliance due to multiple medications, misunderstanding of instructions, diminished hearing, impaired vision, or poor short-term memory. Additional difficulties may result from a lack of access to a pharmacy, inability to pay for medications, or difficulty opening medications. Additionally, borrowed medication can make up a significant percentage of medication taken by older women.

The physiologic changes that accompany aging result in alterations in the processes of drug absorption, distribution, metabolism, and elimination (pharmacokinetics), and can alter drug bio-availability. Additionally, the biochemical and physiologic effects of drugs and their mechanisms of action (pharmacodynamics) appear to change in aging women. The elderly often are more sensitive or responsive to the effects of a drug and require smaller doses. This altered responsiveness ranges from increased therapeutic effects to serious adverse drug reactions. Adverse effects in the elderly may present atypically as subtle changes in mental status or an acute decline in functional status. Serious drug reactions in the elderly are most commonly caused by psychotropic drugs, diuretics, and cardiovascular agents.

An attempt to minimize the number of drugs prescribed may minimize adverse drug reactions. Medical conditions should be managed without medications whenever appropriate. It is critical to monitor for multiple medications prescribed by different physicians and to develop a coordinated medication plan for elderly patients. The cornerstone of a medication plan is an accurate list of everything the patient is taking, including over-the-counter and borrowed medications. This requires frequent updating and an evaluation of adherence and drug-taking patterns. Many new drugs have not been thoroughly evaluated in elderly women and may need to be used with caution.

There are a variety of techniques that may improve a patient's adherence to medication regimens. These include actively involving the patient in the decision to use a medication, simplifying the dosing regimen as much as possible, eliminating unnecessary medications, evaluating the woman's functional ability to take the medications, using assistance devices such as easy to open bottles and prefilled medication boxes, and encouraging the woman to report any adverse reaction immediately.

End-of-Life Considerations

Medical advances have made it possible to keep patients alive by sustaining the vital functions of people who are terminally ill or who exist in a persistent vegetative state. Regardless of a patient's age, the opportunity to determine advance directives allows her to express her choices about the treatment she would like to receive in the event she becomes unable to participate in decisions concerning her care.

As the aging population increases, many more clinicians will be caring for patients at the end of their lives. Familiarity with the ethical, legal, and emotional aspects of providing end-of-life care will assist clinicians in providing the most appropriate care to their patients.

The first step in caring for a dying patient is to identify her management goals. These goals are properly identified through a process of shared and ongoing communication between the patient and clinician. Explicit discussion about the goals of care is important for a number of reasons, which include:

- Assumptions about the objectives of care shape perceptions about appropriate treatment.

- These objectives may be understood differently by the patient and her caregivers.
- Unarticulated commitments to certain goals may lead to misunderstanding and conflict.
- The goals of care may evolve and change in response to clinical or other factors.

Comprehensive and ongoing communication not only advances patient self-determination but also helps establish a moral common ground that may prevent ethical conflict and crisis. Clinicians should be especially careful not to impose their own conception of benefits and risks on a patient or coerce her to achieve goals that she does not share. The harms associated with prolonged attempts at cure may not be acceptable to the dying patient.

Improving discussions about death will be difficult. Repeated attempts to improve physician–patient communications have been made over the years, but there is little evidence that educational reforms have improved care. Ultimately, caregivers need feedback on how well they are doing with such discussions. This might come in the form of consultation or courses addressing communication skills. From an ethical and practical viewpoint, it is always preferable to restrict life-sustaining interventions with the agreement of the patient and family, rather than trying to limit interventions against their wishes.

Many clinicians are uncomfortable with the prospect of providing care for a patient at the end of her life. The ethos that has shaped American medical research and practice for the past half century regards the use of intervention to promote cure and prolong life as the clinician's primary obligation. But palliative strategies such as pain relief, attentive and responsive communication with the patient about her health status, and the facilitation of communication with the patient's family also are essential components of care. It is important to note that neither the presence of a "Do Not Resuscitate" order nor specific directives regarding limitation of other treatments remove the responsibility for providing palliative care. For the generalist whose patient is or has been under the care of a specialist, palliative care often is the most valuable service that can be offered. The expression "nothing more can be done" improperly equates care with cure and undervalues the considerable importance of the clinician in providing comfort to the dying patient.

Legal Rights

The federal Patient Self-Determination Act of 1990 requires, as of December 1991, that all hospitals and other medical programs receiving federal Medicare and Medicaid money create a formal procedure to inform patients, on admission to the facility or at the time of enrollment, about their rights under state law regarding health care decision making. This includes the rights to refuse treatment and to formulate advance directives. Facilities also are required to document in the patient's record whether or not an advance directive was executed. Noncompliance with these requirements can mean the loss of eligibility to receive Medicaid and Medicare funds. Every state and the District of Columbia also have laws allowing for advance directives. State law will determine what an advance directive may contain and how and when it is followed.

A living will and a health care power of attorney are the two most common types of advance directives. Depending on the laws in a particular state, a patient may decide that either a living will or a health care power of attorney is better suited to her needs. She also may have both types of directives or a single document that combines the aspects of both. Clinicians and patients should be familiar with the laws in their states. Although legal advice to prepare an advance directive is not necessary, patients may want to consult with an attorney for guidance.

A living will is a written statement that tells the health care team and family in advance what types of health care the patient would accept or refuse if she were unable to express her wishes. The laws about living wills vary from state to state, but, in general, living wills address the following issues:

- Life-sustaining treatments, including cardiopulmonary resuscitation and respirators

- Artificial nutrition and hydration as the main treatment to keep patients alive
- The degree of pain relief
- Major surgery

Laws in some states are more strict than in others regarding when a living will can be used. Most states limit the rights of pregnant patients to refuse certain treatments to protect the developing fetus. A knowledge of local regulations is important. Additionally, although most physicians will honor a patient's living will, they may not be required to do so if they believe in good faith that the request is not sound.

A living will goes into effect only if the patient has a terminal condition and cannot make decisions for herself. Until this time, the patient can change her mind at any time about what she has written.

Forms for living wills are simple to fill out and usually are available from hospitals, insurance companies, physician offices, and health departments. When using a standard form, it is important to confirm that the form is valid under state law and follow the instructions, including those about witnesses.

In a health care power of attorney, the patient authorizes a health care agent to make medical decisions for her. A patient may indicate in her health care power of attorney her wishes about her medical care, but her agent is not required to follow them, because the power to make decisions becomes the agent's. In a health care power of attorney, the patient might specify what powers she is giving her agent. These may include the power to choose physicians, the right to decide whether to hospitalize the patient, and the right to accept or refuse treatment. The health care power of attorney is more flexible than a living will.

After a living will, health care power of attorney, or both are completed, several copies should be made to provide to physicians, an attorney, and to someone such as a family member or a friend. If the patient has a health care power of attorney, this individual should have copies of all advance directives. Patients should keep the original(s) in a secure place and provide a copy to the hospital when admitted. Patients also might want to keep in their wallet or purse a small card indicating that they have an advance directive, where the advance directive can be found, and the name and address of their health care agent, if any.

Unfortunately, only a small number of adults have prepared advance directives. Most patients do not want to think about becoming ill and being unable to care for themselves. It is best to prepare an advance directive when healthy. No one knows when a serious accident will happen. For these reasons, it is important that the medical team make the options of advance directives known and available to patients. A good opportunity to initiate the discussion of end-of-life caregiving goals is during well-woman care at the time of the periodic examination. To facilitate these discussions, the patient history form could contain questions about a patient's execution of an advance directive.

Because a patient's wishes regarding care might change over time or under different conditions of illness, these discussions should include occasional reevaluation of values and goals and, if necessary, updating of the advance directive. Decision making should be treated as a process rather than as an event.

It is important for clinicians caring for women to recognize the gender disparity that exists in honoring patients' decisions about end-of-life care. In a review of "right to die" cases, Miles and August found that courts honored the previously stated treatment decisions of men in 75% of cases, whereas they respected the prior choices of women in only 14% of cases. Given the persistence and pervasiveness of social attitudes that take women's moral choices less seriously than men's, clinicians caring for women must prevent these biases from undermining their care of and advocacy for female patients. Likewise, this evidence should motivate women to make their treatment wishes as explicit as possible.

Terminal Care

Provisions for Care (Hospital, Hospice, Home). Several options for the provision of terminal care commonly exist for dying patients and their families. Among the levels of care available are care in the hospital, care in a residential hospice, and care in the home with or without hospice support.

Seriously ill people generally seek out hospital care in the hope of avoiding death. However, when death is imminent, the anticipation of a "hospitalized death" may be accompanied by the fear that medical care is less focused on human suffering and dignity than on medical logic and vital functions. In 1989, the Study to Understand Prognosis and Preferences for Outcomes and Risks of Treatment was undertaken in an effort to understand the characteristics of dying in American hospitals. The baseline study showed that much terminal care in the United States is inappropriate. Many patients died after prolonged hospitalization or intensive care; many suffered from unrelieved pain. Several reasons exist for these problems. Clinicians may be uncertain about patient prognosis, do not know the patient's preferences regarding life-sustaining interventions, or have failed to discuss care options with patients and families.

Hospitalized patients and their families should be granted real decision-making powers concerning terminal care. Recommendations to grant patients more powers in these decisions include the following suggestions:

- Patients and families should be provided with explicit prognostic information.
- Discussions about life-sustaining care need to occur frequently. Typically, patients want physicians to take the lead in these discussions.
- The quality of discussions about life-sustaining interventions should be improved. These discussions should include information about providing or withholding therapy, with special attention to the patient's values and concerns.

Hospice refers to a concept of care rather than a specific place for care. Hospice care provides support for people in the last phases of incurable diseases in the hope that they will live as fully or comfortably as possible. Care is provided in both home-based and facility-based settings. No specific supportive therapy is excluded from consideration, and treatments generally are based on agreements among the patient, the physician, and the hospice team. The expected outcome is relief from symptoms and enhancement of quality of life. The patient's and family's needs should be considered when deciding between home-based or residential hospice care.

The core team providing hospice care typically consists of the patient's attending and hospice physicians, registered nurses, social workers, spiritual counselors, and trained volunteers. Hospice also uses specialized team members to meet specific patient care needs. These team members may include allied therapists, art and music therapists, dieticians, pharmacists, nurses, and nursing assistants.

The hospice interdisciplinary team collaborates with the patient's attending physician to develop a patient-directed individualized plan of care. The plan of care is based on team assessments that recognize the patient's and family's psychologic and social values. At a minimum the plan generally includes the following parameters:

- Problems and needs of the patient and her family
- Realistic and achievable goals and objectives
- Agreed-on outcomes
- Required medical equipment
- The use of advance directives in care plan development

Medicare coverage includes hospice benefits. Today, many private insurers and Medicaid also offer hospice benefits, recognizing the compassion associated with hospice care and its cost-effective delivery.

Pain Management. Pain often is undertreated, and this is particularly true at the end of life. Current protocols often specify principles such as that no terminal patient should be in pain. Concerned family members are generally satisfied with life-sustaining treatment decisions, but their primary concerns are with failures in communications and pain control. Pain relief is one of the primary goals for terminal care for both the family and the patient (see "Pain Management" in Part 4).

Suggested Reading

Alliance for Aging Research, National Heart, Lung, and Blood Institute. A clinical guide: controlling high blood pressure in older women. Bethesda, Maryland: National Institutes of Health, 1998

American Academy of Pediatrics. Policy reference guide of the American Academy of Pediatrics: a comprehensive guide to AAP Policies issued through January 2000. 13th ed. Elk Grove Village, Illinois: AAP, 2000

American Academy of Pediatrics, American College of Obstetricians and Gynecologists. Guidelines for perinatal care. 4th ed. Elk Grove Village, Illinois: AAP; Washington, DC: ACOG, 1997

American Academy of Pediatrics Committee on Adolescence: Homosexuality and adolescence. Pediatrics 1993;92:631–634

American College of Obstetricians and Gynecologists. Adolescent pregnancy facts. Washington, DC: ACOG, 2000

American College of Obstetricians and Gynecologists. Adolescent victims of sexual assault. ACOG Educational Bulletin 252. Washington, DC: ACOG, 1998

American College of Obstetricians and Gynecologists. Adolescents' right to refuse long-term contraceptives. ACOG Committee Opinion 139. Washington, DC: ACOG, 1994

American College of Obstetricians and Gynecologists. Confidentiality in adolescent health care. ACOG Educational Bulletin 249. Washington, DC: ACOG, 1998

American College of Obstetricians and Gynecologists. Emergency oral contraception. ACOG Practice Bulletin 25. Washington, DC: ACOG, 2001

American College of Obstetricians and Gynecologists. End-of-life decision making: understanding the goals of care. In: Ethics in obstetrics and gynecology. Washington, DC: ACOG, 2002:10–15

American College of Obstetricians and Gynecologists. Health maintenance for perimenopausal women. ACOG Technical Bulletin 210. Washington, DC: ACOG, 1995

American College of Obstetricians and Gynecologists. Maternal phenylketonuria. ACOG Committee Opinion 230. Washington, DC: ACOG, 2000

American College of Obstetricians and Gynecologists. Medical futility. In: Ethics in obstetrics and gynecology. Washington, DC: ACOG, 2002:49–52

American College of Obstetricians and Gynecologists. Oral contraceptives for adolescents: benefits and safety. ACOG Educational Bulletin 256. Washington, DC: ACOG, 1999

American College of Obstetricians and Gynecologists. Prevention of adolescent suicide. ACOG Committee Opinion 190. Washington, DC: ACOG, 1997

American College of Obstetricians and Gynecologists. Primary and preventive health care for female adolescents. ACOG Educational Bulletin 254. Washington, DC: ACOG, 1999

American College of Obstetricians and Gynecologists. Smoking and women's health. ACOG Educational Bulletin 240. Washington, DC: ACOG, 1997

American College of Obstetricians and Gynecologists. The use of hormonal contraception in women with coexisting medical conditions. ACOG Practice Bulletin 18. Washington, DC: ACOG, 2000

American Medical Association. Council on Ethical and Judicial Affairs. Reports on end-of-life care. Chicago: AMA, 1998

American Medical Association, The Robert Wood Johnson Foundation. EPEC: education for physicians on end-of-life care: participant's handbook. Chicago: AMA; Princeton, New Jersey: RWJF, 1999

Brody H, Campbell ML, Faber-Langendoen K, Ogle KS. Withdrawing intensive life-sustaining treatment—recommendations for compassionate clinical management. N Engl J Med 1997;336:652–657

Canadian Consensus Conference on Menopause and Osteoporosis: part I: consensus statements. J SOGC 1998;20:1243–1272

Carroll NM. Optimal gynecologic and obstetric care for lesbians. Obstet Gynecol 1999;93: 611–613

Cassel CK, Vladeck BC. ICD-9 code for palliative or terminal care. N Engl J Med 1996;335: 1232–1234

Darroch JE, Landry DJ, Singh S. Changing emphasis in sexuality education in U.S. public secondary schools, 1988–1999. Fam Plann Perspect 2000;32:204–211, 265

Dying well in the hospital: the lessons of SUPPORT. Hastings Cent Rep 1995;25(6):S1–S36

Gorelick PB, Sacco RL, Smith DB, Alberts M, Mustone-Alexander L, Rader D, et al. Prevention of a first stroke: a review of guidelines and a multidisciplinary consensus statement from the National Stroke Association. JAMA 1999;281:1112–1120

Health care needs of gay men and lesbians in the United States. Council on Scientific Affairs, American Medical Association. JAMA 1996;275:1354–1359

Hillis SD, Marchbanks PA, Tylor LR, Peterson HB. Poststerilization regret: findings from the United States. Collaborative Review of Sterilization. Obstet Gynecol 1999;93:889–895

Institute of Medicine. Committee on Lesbian Health Research Priorities. Lesbian health: current assessment and directions for the future. Washington, DC: National Academy Press, 1999

Miles SH, August A. Courts, gender and the "right to die." Law Med Health Care 1990;18: 85–95

National Hospice Organization. Standards of a hospice program of care. Arlington, Virginia: NHO, 1993

Program for Appropriate Technology in Health. Emergency contraception: a resource manual for providers. Seattle: PATH, 1997

Roberts JA, Brown D, Elkins T, Larson DB. Factors influencing views of patients with gynecologic cancer about end-of-life decisions. Am J Obstet Gynecol 1997;176:166–172

ROUTINE DETECTION AND PREVENTION OF DISEASE

Periodic assessments provide an excellent opportunity to counsel patients about preventive care. The assessments recommended in *Guidelines for Women's Health Care* are intended to prevent disease and identify disease at the earliest opportunity.

Personal behavioral characteristics are important aspects of a woman's health. Major preventable problems are obesity, inactivity, and smoking. Approximately one fourth of the women in the United States are obese. Cigarette smoking is on the rise in young women. Considering the impact of these behaviors on the long-term health of women, counseling regarding diet and smoking cessation should be offered during the office visit. Positive behaviors, such as exercise, also should be reinforced.

Assessment of a patient's health status and factors about her lifestyle that could have an implication for her health should be considered in each patient encounter. Weight checks, immunization schedules, blood pressure assessments, and inquiry about habits that affect the health of patients and their families can be tied to periodic women's health evaluations. Routine visits are opportunities for health care professionals to educate and counsel patients regarding illness and accident prevention behavior and to stress the importance of health maintenance habits not only for the patient but also for her family. Women often are responsible for much of a family's interaction with the health care system and can exert a major influence on the health of family members.

A self-assessment inventory for patients can help give the clinician insight into the patient's lifestyle and risks to which patients could be exposed (see Appendix G). The patient should be counseled regarding those areas of her lifestyle that place her at risk for illness or injury. She also should be encouraged to modify her behavior to reduce risks and promote health benefits. Conditions that have a high prevalence in the general population are CVD, diabetes, cancer, and STDs. Counseling, preventive care, and behavior modification can have a major beneficial impact on these disorders.

The clinician should provide access to a variety of community resources. Nurse practitioners, clinical nurse specialists, physician assistants, or certified nurse–midwives often are qualified to intervene with patients who need education and counseling regarding nutrition, stress management, detrimental health habits, and issues of sexuality. These practitioners also may make appropriate referrals for patients who are victims of or threatened with violence in their homes, need marriage and family counseling, or are exposed to health hazards in the workplace.

Fitness

Patients should be assessed for general fitness and encouraged to exercise and eat a healthy diet. Adjustments may be necessary based on the presence of risk factors and the woman's current lifestyle and condition. Efforts should focus on weight control, cardiovascular fitness, and reduction of risk factors associated with CVD and diabetes.

Fitness has a positive effect on longevity and quality of life. For instance, exercise and diet can help prevent osteoporosis. Education should begin in the adolescent age group to encourage adequate weight-bearing exercise as well as adequate calcium intake because the baseline calcium content and bone structure can be influenced at that time.

Weight for Height

Different methods have been used to establish a healthy weight for a given height. There are height and weight tables that suggest different weights for men and women based on body frame sizes—small, medium, and large. The table developed by the U.S. Department of Agriculture often is used to determine what is a healthy weight (see Table 3–7). This table shows only one range for both men and women based on height and age. Individuals who weigh 5% or more below the suggested range are underweight. Individuals who weigh 5–20% more than the suggested range are overweight. People who are 20% heavier than the top weight in the range are considered obese.

Table 3–7. U.S. Department of Agriculture Suggested Weights for Adults

	Weight in pounds†, ‡	
Height*	**19–34 years**	**≥35 years**
5'0"	97–128	108–138
5'1"	101–132	111–143
5'2"	104–137	115–148
5'3"	107–141	119–152
5'4"	111–146	122–157
5'5"	114–150	126–162
5'6"	118–155	130–167
5'7"	121–160	134–172
5'8"	125–164	138–178
5'9"	129–169	142–183
5'10"	132–174	146–188
5'11"	136–179	151–194
6'0"	140–184	155–199

*Height is without shoes.

†Weight is without clothes.

‡The higher weights generally apply to men, who tend to have more muscle and bone. The lower weights more often apply to women, who have less muscle and bone.

Adapted from the U.S. Department of Agriculture, U.S. Department of Health and Human Services. Nutrition and your health: dietary guidelines for Americans. 5th ed. Washington, DC: USDA; USDHHS, 2000

Increasingly, body mass index (BMI) is being used in establishing reference levels for body weight for women and men. Body mass index is computed as follows:

$$\frac{\textit{Weight in kilograms}}{(\textit{Height in meters})^2}$$

Using pounds and inches, multiply the division results by 700. Charts are available to eliminate the need to calculate BMI (Table 3–8). Charts also have been developed to measure BMI for adolescents. In recent clinical guidelines from the National Heart, Lung, and Blood Institute, BMI cutoff values to determine weight classification are as follows:

- Underweight (<18.5)
- Normal weight (18.5–24.9)
- Overweight (25.0–29.9)
- Obese (≥30.0)

Table 3–8. Body Mass Index Chart

BMI	19	20	21	22	23	24	25	26	27	28	29	30	31	32
Height (inches)	Weight (pounds)													
58	91	96	100	105	110	115	119	124	129	134	138	143	148	153
59	94	99	104	109	114	119	124	128	133	138	143	148	153	158
60	97	102	107	112	118	123	128	133	138	143	148	153	158	163
61	100	106	111	116	122	127	132	137	143	148	153	158	164	169
62	104	109	115	120	126	131	136	142	147	153	158	164	169	175
63	107	113	118	124	130	135	141	146	152	158	163	169	175	180
64	110	116	122	128	134	140	145	151	157	163	169	174	180	186
65	114	120	126	132	138	144	150	156	162	168	174	180	186	192
66	118	124	130	136	142	148	155	161	167	173	179	186	192	198
67	121	127	134	140	146	153	159	166	172	178	185	191	198	204
68	125	131	138	144	151	158	164	171	177	184	190	197	203	210
69	128	135	142	149	155	162	169	176	182	189	196	203	209	216
70	132	139	146	153	160	167	174	181	188	195	202	209	216	222
71	136	143	150	157	165	172	179	186	193	200	208	215	222	229
72	140	147	154	162	169	177	184	191	199	206	213	221	228	235
73	144	151	159	166	174	182	189	197	204	212	219	227	235	242
74	148	155	163	171	179	186	194	202	210	218	225	233	241	249

Adapted from Clinical guidelines on the identification, evaluation, and treatment of overweight and obesity in adults: the evidence report. Bethesda, Maryland: National Heart, Lung, and Blood Institute, 1998

Nutrition

Primary care practitioners should furnish patients with general nutritional information and question them about their diet and lifestyle (see box). If they cannot provide indicated long-term therapy, appropriate consultation should be arranged.

Assessment of the patient's height and weight as compared with general norms, including calculating BMI, will give valuable information about the patient's nutritional status. Patients who are above or below the normal range require more extensive evaluation and counseling and should

Sample Questions for Basic Nutrition and Lifestyle History

- What did you eat and drink yesterday?
- Do you avoid any foods for religious reasons? For health reasons? Which ones?
- Do you drink alcoholic beverages? How often? How much?
- How many cigarettes or other tobacco products have you used in the past month?
- Are you on any medication?
- Have you used any street drugs in the past month?
- Do you exercise? What kind? How often?
- Do you take any vitamin, mineral, or food supplements? What kind? How much?
- Has your weight changed in the past 5 years? How?
- Do you have a decreased sense of smell or taste?
- Are you trying to lose (or gain) weight? How? Why?
- How often do you skip meals?
- Do you eat breakfast?
- Does it bother you to know that you are going to be weighed?
- Do you ever force yourself to vomit? Use laxatives or diuretics to lose weight?
- Do you have unusual food or other cravings?
- Are you on a special diet? What kind? Why?
- Do you have problems with planning and preparing meals for yourself or your family? If so, for what reasons:
  —Too little time?
  —Poor access to shopping?
  —Financial constraints?
  —Lack of equipment and space for storing food or preparing meals?
  —Lack of appetite?
  —Physical problems with preparing or eating food?
  —Anything else?

be assessed for systemic disease or an eating disorder. Anorexia nervosa and some forms of bulimia may require hospitalization or long-term care. Often obesity requires behavior modification for correction. A referral network to ensure proper access to behavior modification therapists is essential if the primary practitioner cannot render long-term therapy.

Recent clinical guidelines from the National Heart, Lung, and Blood Institute recommend the use of waist circumference as an independent predictor of risk for type 2 diabetes, dyslipidemia, hypertension, and CVD, over and above that of BMI, especially for patients categorized as normal or overweight on the BMI scale (BMI<30). A waist circumference of >88 cm (>35 in) in women with a BMI between 25.0 and 34.9 is associated with increased risk. Waist circumference adds little predictive power to determinations of disease risk for women with a BMI of 35.0 or higher.

The Food Guide Pyramid developed by the U.S. Department of Agriculture helps women to choose food from five groups to provide needed nutrients. The pyramid stresses eating a variety of foods to get adequate energy, protein, vitamins, minerals, and fiber. It also stresses a diet that is high in vegetables, fruits, and grain products (Fig. 3–2).

Fat intake is considered excessive in traditional American diets. Excessive fat intake has been associated with elevated plasma lipids and an increase in coronary artery disease. It also is suspected of increasing the risk of certain malignancies, especially of the breast and colon. Fats should make up no more than 20–30% of the total calories in an adult diet.

Daily sodium requirements will vary with an individual's size and physical activity, which affect salt loss. Average recommended intake of salt is in the range of 6 g or less per day for normal individuals who do not have a need for salt restriction. Patients should be advised about the value of limiting salt intake, and efforts should focus on education and eliminating barriers to compliance.

Fiber content of the diet is being studied for its potential role in the prevention of several disorders, particularly colon cancer. Currently it is recommended that the average diet contain 20–30 g of fiber per day. Foods high in dietary fiber include whole-grain breads and cereals, green and yellow vegetables, citrus fruits, and some legumes.

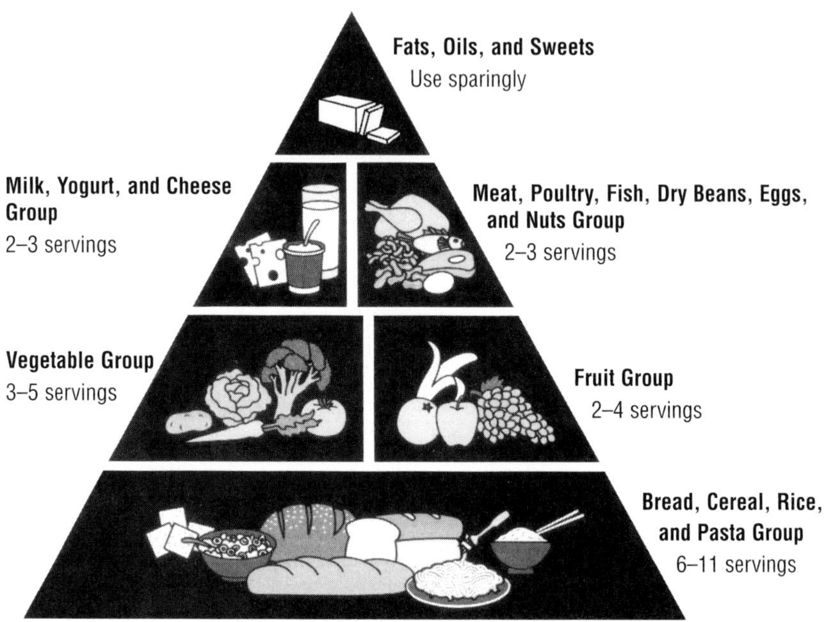

Serving Sizes:

Bread, Cereal, Rice, and Pasta:
1 slice of bread
1 ounce of ready-to-eat cereal
1/2 cup of cooked cereal, rice, or pasta

Vegetable:
1 cup of raw leafy vegetables
1/2 cup of other vegetables, cooked or chopped raw
3/4 cup of vegetable juice

Fruit:
1 medium apple, banana, orange
1/2 cup of chopped, cooked, or canned fruit
3/4 cup of fruit juice

Milk, Yogurt, and Cheese:
1 cup of milk or yogurt
1 1/2 ounces of natural cheese
2 ounces of processed cheese

Meat, Poultry, Fish, Dry Beans, Eggs, and Nuts:
2–3 ounces of cooked lean meat, poultry, or fish
1/2 cup of cooked dry beans, 1 egg, or 2 tablespoons of peanut butter count as 1 ounce of lean meat

Fig. 3–2. Food guide pyramid. (Modified from the U.S. Department of Agriculture and U.S. Department of Health and Human Services.)

Lifelong adequate calcium intake is important in the prevention of osteoporosis. Adult women should receive 1,000 mg/d, and adolescents should receive 1,300 mg/d. Women older than 51 years of age should receive 1,200 mg/d. A postmenopausal woman who is not taking estrogen should receive 1,500 mg/d. There is no evidence that moderate caffeine intake causes osteoporosis when calcium intake is adequate. Because it is difficult to ingest 1,500 mg of calcium daily in an average diet, the use of supplements may be required.

A daily dosage of 0.4 mg of folic acid, taken before conception and for the early part of pregnancy, has been shown to aid in the prevention of neural tube defects. In the United States, however, approximately 50% of pregnancies are unplanned, making preconceptional use of folic acid difficult to achieve. In addition, few women will be able to obtain the equivalent of 0.4 mg of folic acid from dietary sources of folate. Grain currently is being fortified at a level of 140 μg of folic acid per 100 g of grain, but fortification alone has not yet been shown to meet the requirements for 0.4 mg/d. Therefore, daily supplementation with 0.4 mg of folic acid is recommended for all women of reproductive age to prevent neural tube defects (see "Continuum of Women's Health Care" in Part 3). For those women who have a history of neural tube defects or who have had previous children with neural tube defects, higher levels are recommended.

The Committee on Diet and Health of the National Research Council have issued general nutritional guidelines for all women. Some of these recommendations follow:

- Total fat intake should be 30% of calories or less. Saturated fatty acid intake should be less than 10% of calories, and the intake of cholesterol should be less than 300 mg daily.
- Every day, five or more servings of a combination of vegetables and fruits, especially green and yellow vegetables and citrus fruit, should be eaten. The daily intake of starches and other complex carbohydrates should be increased by eating six or more servings of a combination of breads, cereals, and legumes.
- Protein intake should be maintained at moderate levels (less than 1.6 g/kg of body weight).

- Alcoholic beverages should be limited to less than 1 oz of absolute alcohol per day (equivalent to two cans of beer, two small glasses of wine, or two average cocktails).
- Total daily intake of salt should be limited to 6 g or less.
- Vitamin–mineral supplement intake should not exceed the recommended dietary intake per day (Table 3–9).

Exercise

Properly conducted exercise can have a positive influence on promoting health and well-being by controlling or preventing disease in women of all ages. It also can be one mechanism for relieving stress. Before beginning an exercise program, it is advisable for patients to have a physical examination to rule out any risk factors.

Patients should receive information on the benefits of physical activity and assistance in developing an exercise program. Factors that should be considered include medical limitations, such as obesity or arthritis, as well as activities that promote health and enhance compliance. Women should be counseled about safety guidelines for exercise (see box on page 204). Individuals who require additional direction or supervision may be referred to a fitness center or exercise specialist.

Emphasis should be placed on regular physical activity (eg, 30 min/d) rather than episodic vigorous exercise, especially for individuals with sedentary lifestyles. A 30-minute program of exercise should be continuous and sufficient to increase heart rate. A variety of self-directed, moderate-level physical activities (eg, gardening, raking leaves, walking, taking the stairs) can be incorporated easily into an individual's daily routine.

High-impact exercise is not necessary to achieve benefits, and it may be harmful. Regular low-impact or moderate aerobic exercise has been associated with improved long-term compliance and with adequate health maintenance benefits.

Measurement of heart rate during exercise is an excellent method by which to evaluate cardiovascular fitness. As conditioning improves, the heart rate stabilizes at a fixed level. The heart rate at which conditioning will develop is called the target heart rate. The formula for calculating the target heart rate is 220 minus the patient's age multiplied by 0.75. For example, the target heart rate for a 50-year-old woman would be 119 ($220 - 50 = 170 \times 0.75 = 119$). Exceeding this target may be dangerous and should only be done under supervision.

Postmenopausal women may partially retard bone loss with a moderate exercise program coupled with adequate calcium supplementation. Prolonged forms of strenuous exercise can be associated with hypoestrogenic chronic anovulation and its potential long-term problems similar to those of menopause: CVD and osteoporosis. Proper counseling is in order for women with amenorrhea. The interaction of exercise and emotional status should be recognized not only from the perspective of benefit but also from the perspective of counseling when exercise is excessive.

Cardiovascular Disorders

Patients should be counseled about factors that increase their risk of CVD: family history of CVD, dyslipidemia, hypertension, obesity, lack of exercise, and smoking. Those at risk should be encouraged to modify their lifestyle to reduce these risks by eating a low-fat, low-salt diet; controlling hypertension; exercising to promote weight loss and cardiovascular fitness; and smoking cessation. Menopausal patients should be informed of the possible cardiovascular benefits of HRT. For patients with risk factors, such as obesity or hyperlipidemia, diet and exercise help prevent CVD at any age and constitute the first line of management prior to initiating drug therapy.

Cardiovascular disease is the leading cause of death in American women. Cardiovascular disease often presents differently and has a higher mortality rate in women than in men. The obstetrician–gynecologist can educate, screen, monitor, and treat women to reduce their risk of morbidity and mortality from CVD, such as myocardial infarction and stroke (see "Cholesterol" and "Hypertension" in Part 4). A consensus panel statement, "Guide to Preventive Cardiology for Women," has been endorsed by ACOG and is included in Appendix H.

Table 3–9. Dietary Reference Intakes and Recommended Dietary Allowances for Adolescent and Adult Nonpregnant Women*

Nutrient (unit)†	14–18 y	19–30 y	31–50 y	51+ y
Calcium (mg/d)‡	1,300	1,000	1,000	1,200
UL	2,500	2,500	2,500	2,500
Phosphorus (mg/d)	1,250	700	700	700
UL	4,000	4,000	4,000	4,000
Magnesium (mg/d)	360	310	320	320
UL (from nonfood sources)	350	350	350	350
Vitamin D (μg/d)	5	5	5	10
UL	50	50	50	50
Fluoride (mg/d)	3	3	3	3
UL	10	10	10	10
Thiamin (mg/d)	1.0	1.1	1.1	1.1
(No established UL)				
Riboflavin (mg/d)	1.0	1.1	1.1	1.1
(No established UL)				
Niacin (mg/d)	14	14	14	14
UL	30	35	35	35
B_6(mg/d)	1.2	1.3	1.3	1.5
UL	80	100	100	100
Folate (μg/d)	400	400	400	400
UL	800	1,000	1,000	1,000
B_{12} (μg/d)	2.4	2.4	2.4	2.4
(No established UL)				
Pantothenic acid (mg/d)	5	5	5	5
(No established UL)				
Biotin (μg/d)	25	30	30	30
(No established UL)				
Choline (mg/d)	400	425	425	425
UL	3,000	3,500	3,500	3,500
Vitamin A (μg/d)	700	700	700	700
UL	2,800	3,000	3,000	3,000

(continued)

Table 3–9. Dietary Reference Intakes and Recommended Dietary Allowances for Adolescent and Adult Nonpregnant Women* *(continued)*

Nutrient (unit)†	14–18 y	19–30 y	31–50 y	51+ y
Vitamin E (mg/d)	15	15	15	15
UL	800	1,000	1,000	1,000
Vitamin K (μg/d)	75	90	90	90
(No established UL)				
Vitamin C (mg/d)	65	75	75	75
UL	1,800	2,000	2,000	2,000
Iron (mg/d)	15	8.1	8.1	5
UL	45	45	45	45
Zinc (mg/d)	9	8	8	8
UL	34	40	40	40
Iodine (μg/d)	150	150	150	150
UL	900	1,100	1,100	1,100
Selenium (μg/d)	55	55	55	55
UL	400	400	400	400

*Dietary reference intakes (DRIs) encompass a variety of recommendations for nutrients, including the well-known recommended dietary allowances (RDA). They are being developed by the Institute of Medicine in an ongoing fashion.

†Values for nutrients reflect recently established DRIs. Nutrients shown in bold type are given as RDAs, while those shown in italic type are given as adequate intakes (AIs). The RDA is the value used in guiding individuals to achieve adequate nutrient intake. The RDAs are given separately for specified life-stage groups; they are intended to apply to healthy individuals. The RDA for each nutrient is set at a value that should be adequate for 97–98% of all individuals in a life-stage group, given a specified definition of adequacy. An AI is based on observed or experimentally determined estimates of the average nutrient intake, by a defined population, that appears to be sufficient for sustenance. The AI is used as a reference value when sufficient data are not available to estimate an average requirement. Healthy individuals with an intake at or above the AI are assumed to have a low risk of insufficient intake. Tolerable upper intake levels (ULs) have been established for some nutrients. The UL is defined as the highest level of daily nutrient intake that is likely to pose no risks of adverse health effects to almost all individuals in the general population.

‡For postmenopausal women who do not take estrogen replacement therapy, the recommended daily dietary intake of calcium is 1,500 mg.

Data from Institute of Medicine. Dietary reference intakes for calcium, phosphorous, magnesium, vitamin D, and fluoride. Washington, DC: National Academy Press, 1997; Institute of Medicine. Dietary reference intakes for thiamin, riboflavin, niacin, vitamin B6, folate, vitamin B12, pantothenic acid, biotin, and choline. Washington, DC: National Academy Press, 1998; Institute of Medicine. Dietary reference intakes for vitamin C, vitamin E, selenium, and carotenoids. Washington, DC: National Academy Press, 2000; and Institute of Medicine. Dietary reference intakes for vitamin A, vitamin K, arsenic, boron, chromium, copper, iodine, iron, manganese, molybdenum, nickel, silicon, vanadium, and zinc. Washington, DC: National Academy Press, 2001

Safety Guidelines for Exercise

The following guidelines are useful for counseling the average woman seeking to improve her physical fitness through exercise without incurring excessive risk of injury.

GUIDELINES FOR AEROBIC DANCE AND SIMILAR EXERCISE

1. It is recommended that exercise routines involving repeated foot impacts be limited to 30 minutes in duration at intensities not exceeding 75% of maximal heart rate. There should be a day of rest between such sessions.
2. A resilient floor should be selected for exercise that involves repeated foot impacts. If such a surface is not available, the exercise routines should be modified to ensure that the feet remain close to the floor throughout the program.
3. Aerobic exercise should be preceded by a gentle warm-up routine that uses the full range of motion of the joints. This increases the elasticity of the muscles and will help prevent potentially injurious movements.
4. Muscles that are used repeatedly during aerobic exercise must be stretched carefully before and afterward.
5. To reduce the severity of impact shock on the lower extremities, repetitive jumping on the same foot should not exceed four consecutive jumps.
6. Extremes of joint flexion and extension (such as deep knee bends and ballistic hyperextension of the knee) should be avoided.
7. The feet should be moved repeatedly to prevent cramping in the intrinsic muscles of the foot.
8. Trunk rotation should be avoided while on the feet with hips or lower spine flexed. Rotational activity in this position subjects the intervertebral disks to very high mechanical stress.
9. Intense physical activity always should be followed by a cool-down period of at least 10 minutes of lighter activity to prevent pooling of blood in the extremities. Hot showers and baths should be avoided immediately after intense physical activity.
10. Participants should be given a specific means of assessing physical status and progress. Working heart rate should be measured during peak levels of exercise to ensure that the intensity of activity is within the desired range. Regular measurement of the recovery heart rate will motivate participants by documenting their progress. Failure to progress as measured by this method may indicate the need for more intense activity during the aerobic phase or may signal the presence of other problems.

(continued)

Safety Guidelines for Exercise *(continued)*

Guidelines for Strengthening Exercises

1. Strengthening exercises should not be performed on the same muscles on consecutive days.
2. A general warm-up routine should be performed before muscles are made to work against resistance.
3. Exercises should be preceded and followed by stretching exercises that are specific for the muscles that are made to work against resistance.
4. All strengthening exercises should be performed in a slow and controlled manner. Ballistic (rapid or jerky) movements increase the risk of injury.
5. The most efficient way to improve strength is to allow brief rest periods between bouts of vigorous exercise. Repetitions should be limited to short sets (10 or fewer) that are repeated later.
6. When the strength of one muscle or muscle group is disproportionate to that of the antagonist(s) for that muscle or group, the weaker muscle should be strengthened to restore balance around the joint.
7. Participants should not hold their breath during strength-training exercises. Exhalation should take place during the exertion phase of each repetition.

Guidelines for Stretching Exercises

1. Stretching exercises may be performed as often as desired, preferably at least once a day.
2. A general warm-up routine should be performed before muscles are stretched.
3. Stretching routines should be performed statically, without holding the breath. Rapid, jerky movements should be avoided.
4. Each stretch should be held long enough so that relaxation will occur sufficiently to achieve the maximum benefit of the stretch. This can vary from as little as 6 seconds in some individuals to 20 seconds in others.
5. Muscles should be stretched only to the point of tension. Pain should be regarded as a signal that a stretch has gone too far.

Nonmodifiable risk factors for CVD include age more than 55 years, first-degree male relative with coronary heart disease before 55 years of age or first-degree female relative with coronary heart disease before age 65, and African-American ancestry. Risk factors that can be modified include cigarette smoking, lack of exercise, obesity, high-fat diet, excessive alcohol consumption, excessive stress, and medical conditions such as diabetes, hypertension, hyperlipidemia, and hypertriglyceridemia. In menopausal women, some retrospective studies indicate that HRT may reduce a woman's overall risk of CVD by 50%, but these findings have been called into question (see "Continuum of Women's Health Care" in Part 3 and "Hormone Replacement Therapy" in Part 4).

The clinician should address the following issues with patients as indicated, depending on age, risk factors, and medical history:

- Educate patients regarding risk factors for and symptoms of CVD
- Educate patients regarding heart attack symptoms: sudden, intense pressure or pain in the chest; shortness of breath; chest pain that spreads to the shoulders, neck, or arms; feelings of light-headedness, fainting, sweating, or nausea
- Counsel patients regarding lifestyle modifications:
  —Diet low in saturated fat
  —Exercise (five times per week for 30 minutes)
  —Smoking cessation
  —Weight control (maintain body mass index <25)
  —Benefits and risks of small-to-moderate alcohol intake
- Screen for hypertension (systolic blood pressure >140 mm Hg, diastolic blood pressure >90 mm Hg, or both on two or more occasions within 2 months)
- Screen for levels of total cholesterol and HDL cholesterol
- Counsel patients with diabetes on the need to maintain normoglycemia
- Counsel patients on the benefits and risks of postmenopausal HRT
- Treat or refer when risk factors are identified

Hypertension

High blood pressure, or hypertension, is known to contribute to other medical conditions and their complications, including congestive heart failure and renal, cerebrovascular, and coronary artery disease. African-American women are at greater risk of developing hypertension.

In 1997, the National Heart, Lung, and Blood Institute released its *Sixth Report of the Joint National Committee on Prevention, Detection, Evaluation, and Treatment of High Blood Pressure*, endorsing an optimal blood pressure as being less than 120/80 mm Hg and calling for more aggressive treatment of patients with high normal blood pressure, especially when complicated by other conditions (Table 3–10). The report also included guidelines classifying patients by blood pressure level and the presence of risk factors (eg, organ damage or high blood cholesterol), intended to identify which patients need medication or other treatment (see "Hypertension" in Part 4). Guidelines for blood pressure screening in adolescents have been developed by the National Heart, Lung, and Blood Task Force on High Blood Pressure in Children and Adolescents.

Proper technique is crucial to measuring blood pressure accurately. The method recommended by the Joint National Committee is shown in the box. Particularly important is proper assessment of Korotkoff sounds. Phase I Korotkoff sounds usually are easily identified as the time sound

Table 3–10. Classification of Blood Pressure for Adults Age 18 Years and Older*

Category	**Systolic (mm Hg)**		**Diastolic (mm Hg)**
Optimal†	<120	and	<80
Normal	<130	and	<85
High normal	130–139	or	85–89
Hypertension‡			
Stage 1 (mild)	140–159	or	90–99
Stage 2 (moderate)	160–179	or	100–109
Stage 3 (severe)	≥180	or	≥110

*All measurements are in patients who are not acutely ill and not taking antihypertensive medications. If measurements fall in two different categories, then the highest category should be used for classification purposes. Additionally, clinicians should specify presence or absence of target organ disease and additional risk factors.

†Optimal blood pressure with respect to cardiovascular risk is below 120/80 mm Hg. However, unusually low readings should be evaluated for clinical significance.

‡Based on the average of two or more readings taken at each of two or more visits after an initial screening.

Sixth Report of the Joint National Committee on the prevention, detection, evaluation, and treatment of high blood pressure. Bethesda, Maryland: National Heart, Lung, and Blood Institute, 1997

Recommended Techniques for Blood Pressure Measurement

- Patients should be seated in a chair with their backs supported and their arms bared and supported at heart level. Patients should refrain from smoking or ingesting caffeine during the 30 minutes preceding the procedure.
- Measurement should begin after at least 5 minutes of rest.
- The appropriate cuff size must be used to ensure accurate measurement. The bladder within the cuff should encircle at least 80% of the arm. Many adults will require a large adult cuff.
- Measurements should be taken preferably with a mercury sphygmomanometer; otherwise, a recently *calibrated* aneroid manometer or a *validated* electronic device can be used.
- Both systolic blood pressure and diastolic blood pressure should be recorded. The first appearance of sound (phase 1) is used to define systolic blood pressure. The disappearance of sound (phase 5) is used to define diastolic blood pressure.
- Two or more readings separated by 2 minutes should be averaged. If the first two readings differ by more than 5 mm Hg, additional readings should be obtained and averaged.

Sixth Report of the Joint National Committee on the prevention, detection, evaluation, and treatment of high blood pressure. Bethesda, Maryland: National Heart, Lung, and Blood Institute, 1997

becomes audible. Phase IV and V sounds are more difficult to identify. Phase IV Korotkoff sounds are defined as the point when muffling occurs, and phase V sounds are defined by sound disappearance. Phase I and phase V Korotkoff sounds should be used when possible.

Hypertension is generally defined as blood pressure greater than 140/90 mm Hg. Most affected individuals have essential hypertension; perhaps 5% of affected patients have secondary (associated with other diseases) or malignant hypertension. Therapeutic intervention normally should be based on elevated readings taken from the average of two or more readings taken at each of two or more visits after an initial screening. "White coat" hypertension, associated with the stress sometimes experienced during a visit to a health care practitioner, is common. Initially elevated blood pressure returns to normal during the visit in 23% of patients. Laboratory workup and management recommendations for hypertensive patients are found in Part 4.

Cholesterol

Cholesterol has been firmly linked to atherosclerosis and cardiovascular and cerebrovascular disease. However, standards as to the identification of candidates for testing and frequency of testing differ between organizations. Furthermore, the value of cholesterol screening in women without definite risk factors (tobacco use, hypertension, diabetes, or a family history of CVD) remains disputed. Current ACOG guidelines recommend that women without risk factors have their cholesterol level evaluated every 5 years, beginning at age 45 years.

Recently, the National Cholestrol Education Program Expert Panel on Detection, Evaluation, and Treatment of High Blood Cholesterol in Adults (Adult Treatment Panel III) released revised recommendations for screening for high blood cholesterol. The panel recommends that a fasting lipoprotein profile (total cholesterol, LDL cholesterol, HDL cholesterol, and triglyceride) be obtained for all adults 20 years of age or older, once every 5 years. Optimal levels are <100 mg/dL for LDL cholesterol, <200 mg/dL for total cholesterol, and ≥60 mg/dL for HDL cholesterol (see box). The recommended level of LDL cholesterol is based on risk factors (see "Cholesterol" in Part 4).

The U.S. Preventive Services Task Force strongly recommends that clinicians routinely screen women 45 years of age and older for lipid disorders and treat abnormal lipids in women who are at increased risk of coronary heart disease. The task force recommends routinely screening younger women (20–45 years of age) for lipid disorders if they have other risk factors for coronary heart disease. Although the task force recommends that screening for lipid disorders include measurement of total cholesterol and HDL cholesterol, it concludes that evidence is insufficient to recommend for or against triglyceride measurement as a part of routine screening for lipid disorders. The task force finds that nonfasting or fasting samples can be used.

Complicating the issue of cholesterol screening are both individual and laboratory variations. Blood lipid measurements in one person may vary by 4–11%; cholesterol trends over a period of time rather than a single measurement are probably a more accurate indicator of a woman's condi-

Classification of LDL, Total, and HDL Cholesterol (mg/dL)

LDL CHOLESTEROL

<100	Optimal
100–129	Near optimal/above optimal
130–159	Borderline high
160–189	High
≥190	Very high

TOTAL CHOLESTEROL

<200	Desirable
200–239	Borderline high
≥240	High

HDL CHOLESTEROL

<40	Low
≥60	High

Executive Summary of The Third Report of the National Cholesterol Education Program (NCEP) Expert Panel on Detection, Evaluation, and Treatment of High Blood Cholesterol In Adults (Adult Treatment Panel III). JAMA 2001;285:2486–2497

tion. Laboratory variations exist for cholesterol readings as well. Even well-maintained laboratory services do not always meet national standards. Office laboratory analyzers are so difficult to maintain that their use is not recommended. Recommendations effective in limiting individual and laboratory variance are shown in the box.

Diabetes

Diabetes mellitus is a group of disorders that share hyperglycemia as a common feature. Even when symptoms are not present, the disease can cause long-term complications so it should be detected and treated in its early stages. The American Diabetes Association recommends, and ACOG agrees, that all individuals be screened regularly beginning at 45 years of age (see box on page 212). Testing should begin at a younger age or be more frequent in those with risk factors.

Recommendations for Obtaining Blood for Lipid Testing

- Normal diet should be consumed in the days before sampling
- Patient should fast for 12 hours before drawing specimen
- There should be no exercise during fasting period and before venipuncture
- Alcohol intake before sampling (ie, several days) should be constant
- Tobacco use and caffeine intake should be at normal levels before obtaining samples, but should not be ingested the day of sampling
- Individual should be sitting quietly for 15 minutes before obtaining sample
- Sampling should be obtained within 2 minutes of tourniquet time
- Finger stick determinations should be avoided because of contamination by interstitial fluids and lymph

Modified from American College of Obstetricians and Gynecologists. Primary & preventive care. 2nd ed. Precis: an update in obstetrics and gynecology. Washington, DC: ACOG, 1999;153–164

Diabetes can be diagnosed on the basis of several criteria (see box on page 213). Although the oral glucose tolerance test and fasting plasma glucose are both suitable tests, fasting plasma glucose is recommended because it is easier and faster to perform, more convenient and acceptable to patients, more reproducible, and less expensive. The American Diabetes Association also recognizes an intermediate group of individuals whose glucose levels, although not meeting the criteria for diabetes, are nevertheless too high to be considered altogether normal. This group, those with impaired fasting glucose, is defined as having fasting plasma glucose levels greater than or equal to 110 mg/dL but less than 126 mg/dL *or* 2-hour values in the oral glucose tolerance test of greater than or equal to 140 mg/dL but less than 200 mg/dL. Thus, the categories of fasting plasma glucose values are as follows:

- Fasting plasma glucose less than 110 mg/dL = normal fasting glucose
- Fasting plasma glucose greater than or equal to 110 mg/dL and less than 126 mg/dL = impaired fasting glucose
- Fasting plasma glucose greater than or equal to 126 mg/dL = provisional diagnosis of diabetes (the diagnosis must be confirmed [see box on page 213])

Criteria for Testing for Diabetes in Asymptomatic, Undiagnosed Individuals

1. Testing for diabetes should be considered in all individuals 45 years of age and older and, if normal, it should be repeated at 3-year intervals.
2. Testing should be considered at a younger age or be carried out more frequently in individuals who:

- Are obese (≥120% desirable body weight or a body mass index ≥27 kg/m^2)
- Have a first-degree relative with diabetes
- Are members of a high-risk ethnic population (eg, African American, Hispanic, Native American, Asian, Pacific Islander)
- Have delivered a baby weighing >9 lb or have been diagnosed with gestational diabetes mellitus
- Are hypertensive (≥140/90 mm Hg)
- Have a high-density lipoprotein cholesterol level ≤35 mg/dL, a triglyceride level ≥250 mg/dL, or both
- On previous testing, had impaired glucose tolerance or impaired fasting glucose

The oral glucose tolerance test or fasting plasma glucose test may be used to diagnose diabetes; however, in clinical settings the fasting plasma glucose test is greatly preferred because of ease of administration, convenience, acceptability to patients, and lower cost.

Modified from The Expert Committee on the Diagnosis and Classification of Diabetes Mellitus. Report of the Expert Committee on the diagnosis and classification of diabetes mellitus. Diabetes Care 2000;23(suppl 1):S4–S19

The corresponding categories when the oral glucose tolerance test is used are:

- 2-h postload glucose less than 140 mg/dL = normal glucose tolerance
- 2-h postload glucose greater than or equal to 140 mg/dL and less than 200 mg/dL = impaired glucose tolerance
- 2-h postload glucose greater than or equal to 200 mg/dL = provisional diagnosis of diabetes (the diabetes must be confirmed [see box])

Because the 2-hour oral glucose tolerance test cutoff of 140 mg/dL will identify more people as having impaired glucose homeostasis than will the fasting cutoff of 110 mg/dL, it is essential that investigators always report which test was used.

Criteria for the Diagnosis of Diabetes Mellitus

1. Symptoms of diabetes plus casual plasma glucose concentration ≥200 mg/dL (11.1 mmol/L). Casual is defined as any time of day without regard to time since last meal. The classic symptoms of diabetes include polyuria, polydipsia, and unexplained weight loss.

or

2. Fasting plasma glucose ≥126 mg/dL (7.0 mmol/L). Fasting is defined as no caloric intake for at least 8 h.

or

3. 2-h postload glucose ≥200 mg/dL during an oral glucose tolerance test. The test should be performed as described by the World Health Organization, using a glucose load containing the equivalent of 75-g anhydrous glucose dissolved in water.

In the absence of unequivocal hyperglycemia with acute metabolic decompensation, these criteria should be confirmed by repeat testing on a different day. The third measure (oral glucose tolerance test) is not recommended for routine clinical use.

Modified from The Expert Committee on the Diagnosis and Classification of Diabetes Mellitus. Report of the Expert Committee on the diagnosis and classification of diabetes mellitus. Diabetes Care 2000;23(suppl 1):S4–S19

Previously, persons with diabetes were classified as being either insulin dependent (type I) or noninsulin dependent (type II). In 1997, however, the American Diabetes Association changed the system of nomenclature to type 1 and type 2 and dropped the terms *insulin dependent* and *noninsulin dependent.* In either case, the goal of management is to ensure adequate glucose control. If symptoms are present, immediate drug therapy may be necessary; otherwise, dietary control, weight loss, and active exercise programs should be instituted, and the patient should be educated about her disease. The patient's condition should be assessed to detect complications of the disease, such as organ damage from vascular changes.

Nutritional control is an integral component of care for women with existing or potential diabetes. Patients should be educated about the importance of sufficient fiber and limiting saturated fats and refined sugars. Women with diabetes need significant dietary counseling and may need the services of a dietitian with experience in diabetic diet education.

Cancer

Cancer is currently the second leading cause of death in women, following CVD. Because cancer is such a significant cause of morbidity and mortality in women, every obstetrician–gynecologist should be able to provide basic cancer evaluation and screening. Evaluation of risk for cancer includes assessment of high-risk habits and family history. The estimated number of women in the United States who will develop various malignancies and the number expected to die of these cancers in 2001 is shown in Table 3–11. Even though breast cancer is the most frequent cancer in women, with 192,200 new cases expected in 2001, lung cancer is the most common cause of cancer deaths in the United States.

From currently available information, the most important factors in the development of cancer appear to be tobacco, diet, infectious agents,

Table 3–11. The Most Common Malignancies in American Women (2001)

Site of Malignancy	New Cases	Deaths
Breast	192,200	40,200
Lung	78,800	67,300
Colon	52,000	25,100
Uterine	38,300	6,600
Lymphoma	28,600	13,100
Ovary	23,400	13,900
Skin, including melanoma	24,700	3,500
Rectum	16,100	3,900
Bladder	15,100	4,100
Pancreas	15,000	14,800
Thyroid	14,900	800
Cervix	12,900	4,400

Data from Greenlee RT, Hill-Harmon MB, Murray T, Bolden S, Thun M. Cancer statistics, 2001. CA Cancer J Clin 2001;51:15–36

alcohol, and geographic location. The most well-understood of these factors is tobacco, which is thought to cause approximately 30% of cancer deaths in developed countries. The second major cause of cancer is the more complex aspects of diet and nutrition, with 35% of cancer deaths associated with dietary practices. Recent research has identified clear associations between cancer risk and certain infectious agents, such as some types of HPV, and cervical and vulvar cancer. In addition, striking associations also exist between hepatitis viruses and liver cancer and Epstein-Barr virus and nasopharyngeal cancer, as well as Hodgkin's disease. Current estimates suggest that at least 10% of human cancers may be the result of infection, and it is expected that with further research in this area, this estimate will increase significantly. Most of the other proposed causes of cancer, including alcohol, industrial products, food additives, and other constitutional and geographic factors, account for much smaller proportions of cancer deaths.

The American College of Obstetricians and Gynecologists recommends that every woman should have a general health evaluation annually, or as appropriate, and that this should include evaluation for cancer and an examination to detect signs of premalignant or malignant conditions. This examination should include annual pelvic and breast examinations and also may include evaluation of the skin, lymph nodes, thyroid gland, oral cavity, anus, and rectum. Cancer screening components currently recommended by ACOG take into account the recommendations of major national organizations and are summarized in the box.

Lung cancer is a leading cause of death from malignancy for women 40–64 years of age. No available techniques are currently suitable for routine screening. The only effective way to reduce mortality is to promote smoking cessation. A health care practitioner can make a major contribution to the long-term health of women who smoke by identifying all women who smoke and counseling them to stop. A concrete smoking cessation plan, coupled with the use of pharmacotherapy aids when indicated, and proper follow-up care can help women quit smoking and avoid relapse. Legislative and voluntary measures to reduce the risk of secondary exposure to smoke also are important current efforts to reduce the incidence of this disease.

Suggested Cancer Screening Guidelines

General health counseling and cancer evaluation	All women should have a general health evaluation annually or as appropriate, which should include evaluation for cancer and examination to detect signs of premalignant or malignant conditions
Breast cancer	Mammography should be performed every 1–2 years for women 40–49 years of age and then annually thereafter
Cervical cancer	All women who are or who have been sexually active or who have reached 18 years of age should undergo an annual Pap test and pelvic examination. After a woman has had three or more consecutive, satisfactory, annual cytologic examinations with normal findings, the Pap test may be performed less frequently on a low-risk woman at the discretion of her physician
Endometrial cancer	Screening all women for endometrial cancer and its precursors is neither cost-effective nor warranted
Ovarian cancer	No screening techniques that have proved to be effective in reducing the disease-specific mortality of ovarian cancer are currently available
Colorectal cancer	Beginning at age 50 years, one of three screening options should be selected: yearly fecal occult blood testing plus flexible sigmoidoscopy every 5 years *or* colonoscopy every 10 years *or* double contrast barium enema (DCBE) every 5–10 years. A digital rectal examination should be performed at the time of each screening sigmoidoscopy, colonoscopy, or DCBE
Lung cancer	No available techniques are currently suitable for routine screening

American College of Obstetricians and Gynecologists. Routine cancer screening. ACOG Committee Opinion 247. Washington, DC: ACOG, 2000

The incidence of breast cancer increases with age. The following factors also increase the risk of breast cancer:

- Previous history of breast cancer
- Nulliparity

- Delayed childbearing (after 30 years of age)
- Early menarche (before 12 years of age)
- Late menopause (after 53 years of age)
- Family history of breast cancer (first-degree relatives)
- Biopsy-proven ductal or lobular hyperplasia, particularly with atypia
- Higher socioeconomic status
- Obesity

Mammography may be used as either a screening device or an adjunct in the diagnosis of a palpable mass. A palpable mass, in the presence of a negative mammogram, requires tissue assessment. At present, mammography is the only screening method available to detect subclinical or occult breast cancer, the stage least likely to have spread to regional lymph nodes and beyond. The American College of Obstetricians and Gynecologists recommends mammography screening every 1–2 years for women 40–49 years of age and annually for women 50 years of age and older. Patients 19 years of age or older should be counseled regarding breast self-examination.

Recently, the U.S. Food and Drug Administration granted approval of tamoxifen for the purpose of reducing the incidence of breast cancer in women at high risk for the disease. The decision to use tamoxifen should be individualized.

Endometrial cancer is the most common genital cancer in women 45 years of age and older. Routine screening of asymptomatic women for endometrial cancer and its precursors is not cost-effective. Women with a history or evidence of abnormal vaginal bleeding and women taking unopposed estrogen are at increased risk for endometrial cancer and should be evaluated.

Ovarian cancer is the leading cause of death from gynecologic pelvic malignancies. More women die from ovarian cancer than from cervical and endometrial cancers combined. Many different techniques, including peritoneal fluid profiles, investigation of tumor-associated antigens, ultrasonography, and computed tomography imaging have been or are being investigated as possible screening tools for ovarian cancer. To date, none of these techniques has proved practical or effective.

Colon cancer causes nearly as many deaths among women as all gynecologic pelvic malignancies combined. In most cases, it is preceded by adenomatous polyps. Both adenomatous polyps and early colonic cancer can be detected by routine screening. Although testing of stool for blood is limited in sensitivity and specificity, it can aid in early detection. Flexible sigmoidoscopy, colonoscopy, double contrast barium enema, and rectal examinations performed at specified intervals can increase the ability to detect asymptomatic lesions and are recommended for patients in the age ranges indicated. More comprehensive assessments should be undertaken on the basis of risk factors.

Sexually Transmitted Diseases

Sexually transmitted diseases include a variety of infectious diseases that involve both the upper and the lower genital tract, as well as a number of other infectious diseases such as HBV and HIV infection. Sexually transmitted diseases are considered public health issues, and clinicians should be aware of local and state statutes and regulations governing their need to be reported. The hallmark for the management of these diseases is prevention.

Multiple diseases can be transmitted through sexual activity. For some diseases (eg, syphilis, bacterial vaginosis, *Trichomonas vaginalis*, gonorrhea, chlamydial infection, and herpes), sexual activity is almost the only method of transmission, whereas for other diseases (eg, HIV infection and *Candida* species infections), other methods of transmission also are common. For other diseases (eg, HBV), sexual activity is a less common (30–60%) although frequent method of transmission.

Risk Factors

Certain behaviors are associated with an increased risk of genital infections. Women who have had multiple sexual partners and those who use illicit drugs have an increased risk of exposure to one or more infectious agents. Multiple STD infections are common. Two thirds of Americans who acquire STDs are younger than 25 years of age.

A history of recurrent genital tract infections also may indicate other serious medical disease. Recurrent, difficult-to-treat yeast infections also may be an early sign of HIV infection or diabetes mellitus. Abnormal vaginal bleeding may be associated with upper genital infection (chronic endomyometritis). The diagnosis of one STD indicates screening for others.

Prevention

Strategies for prevention include safe sex, partner notification and treatment, and in some cases, immunization. Recommended immunizations are described in the boxes on pages 126–133 in "Primary and Preventive Care" in Part 3.

Evaluation

Screening should be done on the basis of risk factors. Cultures or nucleic-acid detection tests from the vagina or cervix add little useful information except in cases of gonorrhea and chlamydial infection. In most cases, treatment should conform with guidelines issued by the Centers for Disease Control and Prevention (see "Sexually Transmitted Diseases" in Part 4).

Gonorrhea. Although the most common site for detection of infection with *Neisseria gonorrhoeae* in women is the uterine cervix, swab samples also should be obtained from the urethra, periurethral glands, and rectum. A significant number of cases can be identified from a rectal swab alone. If the patient has had oral sex with a suspected infected partner, swabs of the oral pharynx are recommended.

Rapid tests for the detection of *N gonorrhoeae* by nucleic-acid detection tests are available and have greater sensitivity and specificity than culture. Culture, however, remains a common method of detection. Cultures often must be handled in a special manner and transported quickly to the laboratory. Health care workers should be thoroughly familiar with the method of collection and transport suggested by their laboratory. Women with gonorrhea also should have a serologic test for syphilis and HBV and be offered confidential counseling and testing for HIV. Nonimmune individuals should be offered HBV immunization.

An ever-increasing number of cases of gonorrheal infection are caused by organisms that are resistant to penicillin. Therefore, penicillin is no longer used as primary therapy for treatment of *N gonorrhoeae.* Rather, treatment should be accomplished through the use of drugs for which no (or minimal) resistance has been documented. Because gonorrheal infections commonly coexist with infections of *Chlamydia trachomatis*, treatment that is effective against *C trachomatis* also should be prescribed when treating gonorrhea.

Chlamydia. Infections with *C trachomatis* are common in women younger than 35 years of age. They may be asymptomatic. Routine screening for chlamydia is not recommended for all women but should be done for sexually active adolescents and any patient with risk factors (see "Primary and Preventive Care" in Part 3). *C trachomatis* infection should be treated when detected even if asymptomatic. Nucleic acid detection tests are most sensitive and specific for detection of a *C trachomatis* infection. Chlamydial infections are commonly associated with gonorrheal infections, and concomitant screen for gonorrhea should be obtained.

Pelvic Inflammatory Disease. Pelvic inflammatory disease (PID), a leading cause of infertility, is associated with STDs. Minimum criteria for diagnosis of PID have been delineated by the U.S. Centers for Disease Control and Prevention. Minimum criteria for a clinical diagnosis include lower abdominal tenderness, bilateral adnexal tenderness, or cervical motion tenderness. Supportive criteria include fever, nausea and vomiting, abnormal cervical or vaginal secretions, elevated erythrocyte sedimentation rate or C-reactive protein and positive screen for gonococcus or chlamydia. Definitive criteria include sonography demonstrating tuboovarian abscess, histopathologic evidence of endometritis, and laparoscopic abnormalities consistent with PID. Treatment considerations include broad-spectrum antibiotic coverage for *C trachomatis*, gonococcus, anaerobes, and gram-negative rods.

The routine use of laparoscopy to diagnose PID is not indicated because of cost and operative risk. However, if the diagnosis is uncertain, the patient fails to respond to therapy, or symptoms recur soon after adequate therapy, diagnostic laparoscopy then may be indicated.

Treatment of PID varies greatly, depending on the patient's initial symptoms. Many clinicians treat all PID with outpatient antibiotics. Such treatment involves the use of broad-spectrum antibiotics that cover *N gonorrhoeae, C trachomatis*, and anaerobes. Others routinely treat PID as an inpatient disease with the use of intravenous antibiotics. In different populations both of these widely divergent practices have been shown to cure the signs and symptoms of PID. The decision of whether hospitalization is necessary should be based on the discretion of the clinician.

Syphilis. The prevalence of syphilis is decreasing yet high prevalence exists in areas of high frequency of drug use and prostitution. Most cases of syphilis are detected through serologic screening tests. Screening for present or past syphilitic infections is commonly done at several points in life. Most states require a syphilis test prior to marriage and also during pregnancy. Health departments provide diagnostic laboratories but may use a variety of tests. Clinicians should be familiar with the sensitivity and specificity of the tests commonly used in their area.

Penicillin remains the treatment of choice for syphilis. In nonpregnant penicillin-allergic individuals, several other medications, including erythromycin, may be used; however, in pregnancy erythromycin transports poorly across the placenta and will not reliably prevent congenital syphilis. Therefore, penicillin is the only therapy for syphilis in pregnant women. In pregnant women who have a documented allergy to penicillin, rapid desensitization and treatment with penicillin is required.

Trichomonas. *Trichomonas vaginalis* causes only infections of the vagina. Vaginitis caused by the organism *T vaginalis* is a commonly occurring infection in the United States. It is diagnosed by the microscopic observation of the motile organisms on a saline wet mount or by culture and may be reported on routine cervical cytology.

Trichomonas infections are routinely treated with metronidazole, with all sexual partners being treated concomitantly. Strains of *T vaginalis* are becoming relatively resistant to metronidazole; however, most of these organisms respond to higher doses of metronidazole.

Herpes Simplex Virus. Herpes simplex virus (HSV) infection of the genital tract is one of the most common viral STDs. Approximately 45 million adolescent and adult Americans have been infected with genital herpes. Initial contact with HSV usually occurs early in childhood and involves HSV-1. Herpes simplex virus type 1 causes most nongenital herpetic lesions. The female genital tract can be infected with HSV-1 or HSV-2. In the United States, most genital infection is from HSV-2.

There are three stages of HSV infection based on clinical presentation and serology. Primary infections are those in which no HSV-1 or HSV-2 antibodies are present. In nonprimary first-episode disease, HSV-1 antibodies are present in the woman who has HSV-2 infection or HSV-2 antibodies are present in the woman who has HSV-1 infection. In recurrent infections, homologous antibodies are present. In the absence of systemic symptoms, the distinction between first-episode and recurrent herpetic infections is difficult to ascertain.

Initial genital infection due to herpes may be either asymptomatic or associated with severe symptoms. With symptomatic primary infection, lesions may occur on the vulva, vagina, or cervix, or on all three between 2 and 14 days following exposure to infectious virus. These lesions are larger in number and size than those observed in patients with recurrent disease and patients who have had prior infection with HSV-1. The initial vesicles rupture and subsequently appear as shallow and eroded ulcers. Inguinal lymphadenopathy is demonstrated readily as the consequence of virus replication in the sites of lymphatic drainage. When systemic symptoms (malaise, myalgia, and fever) occur, they are most commonly restricted to presumed primary herpetic infections. Local symptoms of pain, dysuria, and soreness of the vulva and vagina are common in both primary and recurrent infections.

A nonprimary first episode can be identified as a first clinically recognized genital HSV infection that does not behave clinically like a symptomatic primary infection. There are fewer systemic manifestations, less pain, a briefer duration of viral shedding, and a more rapid resolution of the clinical lesions in the nonprimary infection.

Recurrences of genital HSV infection can be symptomatic or subclinical, and there is significant variation from patient to patient in the frequency, severity, and duration of symptoms and amount of viral shedding. Confinement of the ulcers to the genital area is more common in recurrent forms of the disease. The ulcers tend to be limited in size, number, and duration. Local symptoms predominate over systemic symptoms, with many patients indicating increased vaginal discharge or pain.

Systemic antiviral drugs partially control the symptoms and signs of herpes episodes when used to treat first clinical episodes or recurrent episodes or when used as daily suppressive therapy.

Although the lesions of HSV infection are relatively typical, even experienced examiners may overdiagnose the disease. Because of significant social and medical implications, confirmatory testing is recommended. Because of patient discomfort, however, it is recommended that oral antiviral therapy be initiated at the time of clinical diagnosis while awaiting test reports.

Human Papillomavirus. Infection with one or more HPV subtypes is extremely common. It is estimated that up to 30% of all young sexually active men and women are infected with this organism. Some subtypes (particularly 6 and 11) are associated with the development of genital warts. In most cases, external warts can be treated with the topical application of podofilox, imiquimod, trichloroacetic or bichloroacetic acid or podophyllin resin, or the use of cryotherapy, laser, or electrocautery. Treatment using general anesthesia should be reserved for those cases in which bulky lesions are present. In cases that are resistant to local therapy, interlesional injections of interferon have been found to be of some use. Patients who fail to respond to treatment may be immunosuppressed and should be counseled about and tested for HIV infection.

Infections of the cervix often are diagnosed through assessment of cervical cytology. The diagnosis is relatively specific for the presence of HPV if the cytologist adheres strictly to the cytologic criteria, which include the presence of koilocytosis and nuclear changes. Most cervical intraepithelial neoplasias and carcinomas can be demonstrated to contain HPV DNA. Although millions of women are infected with HPV, only a few will ever develop significant cervical neoplasia. It is not clear that all women with evidence of HPV alone on a cervical cytology specimen should undergo colposcopic evaluation.

Laboratory tests for the detection and typing of HPV infections are currently available in many areas of the country. It does not appear at this time that such testing is clinically useful.

Bacterial Vaginosis. The term *bacterial vaginosis* encompasses those entities previously referred to as nonspecific vaginitis, *Gardnerella* vaginitis, and *Haemophilus* vaginitis. This infection is associated with profuse malodorous vaginal discharge that has a fishy odor when exposed to an alkaline substance. Often vaginal epithelial cells seen in a wet mount are coated with bacteria (clue cells). Although these infections often are associated with bacterial growths of *Gardnerella vaginalis* and *Mobiluncus* species, the presence of these organisms is not pathognomonic for bacterial vaginosis.

Bacterial vaginosis is an overgrowth of facultative and obligate anaerobic bacteria derived from the patient's own endogenous vaginal flora. Therefore, the intent of treatment is not to eradicate these bacteria but to reduce their numbers and allow for the lactobacilli to become dominant. Treatment of bacterial vaginosis generally involves the use of metronidazole or clindamycin orally or intravaginally. In general, treatment of asymptomatic partners is not recommended, although in some cases of recurrent disease such therapy might be considered.

Candidal Vaginitis. Various yeast and fungal organisms often infect the vagina. One or more of these organisms can be found in approximately 10–15% of all asymptomatic women. In some cases yeast overgrows and produces a thick, very white discharge that causes profound itching. In these cases, patients usually seek treatment.

If yeast vaginitis does not respond quickly to a topical or oral antifungal agent, or if recurrent infections have occurred in a short period of time, one of several abnormalities may be present. Diabetes mellitus is associated with recurrent yeast infections, and women with such complaints should be evaluated for glucose intolerance. Recurrent yeast infections are common among women taking antibiotics on a daily or cyclic basis. Intractable recurrent yeast infections also are associated with infection with HIV.

A few yeast organisms are resistant to treatment by some topical medications. Although wet mount is the usual method of detection of candida, a large number of other organisms (eg, *Candida glabrata* [formerly classified as *Torulopsis glabrata*]) are identified by culture. In these cases a longer duration of therapy than that used for mild-to-moderate, sporadic, or nonrecurrent infection may be required. Medications that are specific for action against the offending organism should be used.

Hepatitis B. Although infection with HBV is more often contracted by other routes of exposure, some studies have suggested that up to 30–60% of all such infections result from sexual transmission. Women who have active HBV infections or women who are HBV carriers should be counseled to have their partners use condoms during intercourse. Oral–genital contact should be avoided. Patients with STDs, and all adolescents not previously immunized, should be offered hepatitis B vaccination.

Human Immunodeficiency Virus. Heterosexual contact is the leading mode of transmission of HIV in women. Women with ulcerated or nonulcerated STDs have an increased risk of infection.

Women should be routinely counseled regarding HIV infection. The ACOG guidelines on counseling and testing should be followed (see “Human Immunodeficiency Virus” in Part 4).

Clinicians who recommend HIV testing should be prepared to provide both pretest and posttest counseling. Some clinicians have the experience to perform such counseling themselves; others may prefer to refer the patient to a clinician specifically trained in HIV and its related diseases. Individuals who have positive test results should undergo posttest counseling. In the event of a negative test result, counseling may be necessary to discuss those lifestyle factors that place the patient at high risk for HIV.

Each clinician should be thoroughly familiar with the local and state statutes and regulations applicable to HIV testing. In general, testing for HIV may not be performed without a patient’s specific knowledge and consent. Clinicians also should be aware of state laws protecting confidentiality of test results.

Counseling

The safest sex occurs between two individuals who have no other sexual partners and are free of infections. Other preventive measures are limiting the number of sex partners, routine use of barrier contraceptives, and avoiding the exchange of bodily fluids. If it is unclear whether a partner is infected, barrier protection should be used during intercourse. Condoms should be used with each sexual encounter, even if the woman is using another form of contraception. Latex male condoms are the method that is most likely to protect against STDs. The female condom has been less well studied but offers some protection. Polyurethane male condoms are available and may provide an alternative for those allergic to latex, although the effectiveness of these condoms in the prevention of STDs is unknown. Diaphragms and cervical caps offer some protection from infection with *N gonorrhoeae* and *C trachomatis* but do not protect against other infections. Counseling regarding the prevention of STDs should be offered as part of routine gynecologic care for all adolescent and adult patients.

Noncoital sexual activity also should be practiced in a safe manner. Oral–genital sex and anal intercourse are known to be the method of transmission of several forms of STDs. Digital–genital activity may be responsible for transmission of some infections, although this association has not been well studied.

Psychosocial Issues

A woman's health and well-being is affected by psychosocial factors. In many cases, early detection of unhealthy situations and therapeutic intervention can improve her quality of life and, in some situations, prevent harm. These are areas both clinicians and patients often are uncomfortable discussing. Communication and counseling skills are an important aspect of women's health care, as psychosocial well-being is an important element of overall health. Some of the more significant psychosocial issues are discussed here.

Sexuality

Sexuality is a major consideration in women's health. Mutual trust and respect in the patient–clinician relationship will allow appropriate discussion of questions and concerns about sexuality. A nonjudgmental approach by the clinician, as well as awareness by the clinician of his or her own biases, is essential for effective counseling.

History and Orientation. A sexual history should be a part of an evaluation of the patient's general health and well-being. The use of broad, open-ended questions in a routine history can help disclose problems that require further exploration. Inquiry about the partner's sexual function and level of satisfaction may elicit more specific information and give an indication of the couple's level of communication.

Sexual practices vary widely and are influenced by personal and cultural preferences. Sexuality involves a broad range of expressions of intimacy, and the clinician should not make assumptions about the woman's behavior. Sexual practices may be influenced by race and education. The clinician should keep in mind the possibility of cultural and personal variation in sexual practices when counseling patients. Discussions of sexuality are best accomplished in a confidential and supportive setting.

Although most women report that their sexual partners are men, a percentage of women have sex exclusively with other women, and others may have partners of both sexes. Use of phrases such as "partner" instead of "husband," and "sexual activity" instead of "sexual intercourse" are appropriate. An understanding of nonheterosexual sexuality will assist in both open communication and assessment of any difficulties (see also "Continuum of Women's Health Care" in Part 3).

Sexual Function and Dysfunction. Clinicians should be familiar with the most commonly recognized pattern of sexual response (desire, arousal, orgasm, and resolution) and should understand that variations may occur. Sexual dysfunction may be related to relationship difficulties, psychologic factors, or physical or biological factors. Sexual function also is influenced by a person's health and emotional well-being, history of sexual violence, fatigue, stress, depression, and use of alcohol and other drugs. If a problem is identified, it may be appropriate for the partner to be involved in therapy. Sometimes the patient's concerns are related to the sexual health of her partner. Treatment may be within the scope of obstetric–gynecologic practice or referral may be appropriate, depending on the nature and extent of the problem (see "Sexual Dysfunction" in Part 4).

The importance of a nurturing environment should not be overlooked, especially when the patient's dissatisfaction with any aspect of sexual activity is explored. Deliberate inquiries should be made to assess the quality of the interpersonal relationship between the patient and her partner, including mutual satisfaction with their sexual relationship.

There are several common causes of sexual dissatisfaction. Some basic questions, which should be posed in a gender-neutral fashion, are:

1. "Are you sexually active?"
2. "Are you sexually satisfied?"
3. "Do you think your partner is satisfied?"
4. "Do you have questions or concerns about sexual functioning?"

If an examination is performed, the patient should be informed of what it will entail. The presence of a chaperon is strongly recommended, regardless of the sex of the health care practitioner.

Interruption or absence of any stage in the sexual response cycle (desire, arousal, orgasm, resolution) can result in sexual dysfunction. Vaginismus and dyspareunia also can be factors in sexual dysfunction. Some forms of sexual dysfunction may be related to age, emotional factors, medical conditions, or use of medications such as antihypertensives, antipsychotics, and antidepressants.

Lack of desire can be attributed to interpersonal causes or to a conditioned response that causes a woman to interpret a sexual encounter in terms of success or failure. Although most women with low sexual desire have some difficulty experiencing arousal or orgasm, some are capable of achieving these states but have little interest in initiating the process.

Desire may be blunted by previous negative experiences. Repeated failures to progress to subsequent stages in the response cycle decrease desire.

Androgens have been proposed for some women as treatment for certain types of sexual dysfunction. Although androgen therapy has been prescribed for sexual dysfunction for many years, data regarding its safety and efficacy are incomplete and physiologic androgen replacement therapy has not been shown to consistently affect the libido.

Lack of arousal may be caused by insufficient foreplay, use of objectionable forms of stimulation, absence of desired stimulation, or emotional or physical distraction. Sensate focus exercises can help couples develop nonverbal means to communicate to each other their desired types of stimulation.

Lack of orgasm may not be a problem unless the patient or partner perceives it to be. The loss of the ability to achieve orgasm may be a symptom of an underlying problem. More than 90% of women are able to experience orgasm, often through a combination of techniques. Lack of orgasm may be attributable to arousal phase dysfunction. Self-stimulation techniques may be beneficial for the patient.

Vaginismus may occur following major trauma, such as sexual abuse, rape, or an injury to the vagina. It also may follow less severe problems such as episodes of painful intercourse occurring as the result of vaginal infection. Dyspareunia can occur during entry, with deep thrusting, or after intercourse. Dyspareunia at the time of penetration may be secondary to a functional problem such as vaginismus or a physical condition such as vaginal septae or vestibulitis. Dyspareunia with deep penetration can be related to abnormalities of the upper genital tract, such as endometriosis or pelvic inflammation. Treatment by desensitizing exercises can be effective for vaginismus, whereas specific therapy is necessary for organic causes.

After menopause, women often experience a lack of vaginal lubrication that makes intercourse painful. The use of estrogen and lubricants can ease the problem. Although more common in the elderly, women of any age may experience personal illness or illness in a partner that interferes with sexual function. They should be counseled about the effects of illness or medication on sexuality and encouraged to experiment with alternative forms of sexual expression to accommodate their or their partner's physical limitations.

Emotional issues can be the basis for sexual dysfunction. The physician should attempt to identify any factors that could affect sexual function and provide education and counseling about them. Events that may have occurred in the past and can affect sexual function are childhood inhibitions or sexual abuse. Patients with complex sexual problems of a psychologic nature may benefit from referral to professionals who can provide appropriate services in an ethical, effective manner. When emotional problems are clearly limited to unsatisfactory sexual experiences, referral to a qualified sex therapist may be appropriate. If the difficulty involves issues other than sexuality, referral to a counselor skilled in marital and other relationship problems may be preferable. Individuals with sexual dysfunction resulting from a history of sexual victimization should be referred to mental health professionals with an expertise in abuse-related problems.

Male factors include low desire and erectile dysfunction, which may be based on organic or psychologic factors. Acknowledgment and support from the woman's physician will assist the patient in helping her partner seek counseling and treatment.

Abuse

Violence and abuse are significant problems affecting women, often resulting in serious short- and long-term health consequences. Abuse can take the form of domestic or intimate partner violence, child abuse, rape or sexual assault, or elder abuse or neglect. Clinicians should be alert to signs of exposure to violence or abuse. However, because patients may be asymptomatic, it is important that physicians conduct screening for past and present abuse with all patients. Universal screening can be conducted while obtaining a woman's health history. Practitioners should ask patients directly about current or past domestic violence, rape or sexual assault, and childhood physical/sexual abuse. Screening should be done in a comfortable and private environment. Arrangements should be made for referral to appropriate community services as needed. Clinicians should be familiar with any local and state requirements to report domestic violence, child abuse or assault (physical or sexual), and neglect or abuse of the incapacitated elderly.

Domestic or Intimate Partner Violence. Domestic violence is widespread and covers a broad spectrum of behaviors. It encompasses a pattern of actual or threatened physical, sexual, or psychological abuse between family members or intimate partners and can range from intimidating behaviors to life-threatening actions.

There is no typical victim, nor is there a typical abuser. No one is immune from intimate partner violence, regardless of socioeconomic status, profession, religion, ethnicity, education, or sexual orientation. Most frequently the abuse is directed at a woman by a man. Most often, perpetrators are violent only with family members and have different public and private images. They minimize the seriousness of the violence and refuse to take responsibility for their behavior, accusing the woman of provoking them. The hallmark of their behavior is coercive control.

Although no one is immune from domestic violence, some individuals may be at increased risk of abuse: children, women who experienced abuse in childhood, adolescents, women with HIV or acquired immunodeficiency syndrome (AIDS), women with disabilities, and pregnant women. Among children living in homes where domestic violence occurs, more than half are themselves abused. Witnessing or experiencing abuse in the home is associated with higher levels of conduct problems, emotional problems, and lower levels of social functioning in childhood. Adolescent exposure is associated with anger, depression, anxiety, and posttraumatic stress. Growing up in an abusive household increases a woman's risk of abuse in adulthood.

Women between 16 and 24 years of age report the highest rates of domestic violence. Adolescents are at risk for physical and sexual abuse from two distinct groups: parents and acquaintances or dating partners. The act of screening adolescents for violence or abuse is both an effective intervention and an educational tool.

Pregnancy constitutes an increased risk for intimate partner violence. The prevalence of violence during pregnancy ranges from 1–20%, with most studies identifying rates between 4–8%. Research indicates that violence may begin or escalate during pregnancy; it may become even more prevalent in the postpartum period. Intimate partner violence is more common than other conditions for which pregnant women are routinely screened.

There may be no pathognomic signs or symptoms of domestic violence; hence, universal screening is warranted. Patients may, however, present with diagnostic clues that may include nonspecific stress-related symptoms, including depression and chronic pain, or with injuries in various stages of healing for which the explanation is inconsistent with the findings. An overly solicitous partner who answers all questions and refuses to be separated from the partner may be a batterer. A physical examination may reveal bruises, burns, and injuries, particularly on the head, neck, breasts, abdomen, and groin.

Although patients may be reluctant to bring up their abuse, they often are responsive to direct inquiry. Questions must be asked in privacy and in a nonjudgmental manner. The following three questions are easily incorporated routinely into the review of systems:

1. "Have you been hit, slapped, kicked, or otherwise physically hurt by someone?"
2. "Are you in a relationship with a person who threatens or physically hurts you?"
3. "Has anyone pressured or forced you into sexual activities when you did not want them?"

When there are injuries, it is appropriate to ask the direct question: "Did someone cause these injuries?" The patient's answer will provide directions to pursue a series of questions relating to issues of safety both for the woman and for her children, the role of friends and family, and the range of available options. If the patient will be returning to an unsafe home, safety planning should be conducted and referrals should be provided to service agencies in the community (see "Domestic or Intimate Partner Violence" in Part 4).

The clinician's role is to 1) know the signs and symptoms of intimate partner violence; 2) ask all patients about past or present exposure to violence; 3) intervene and refer as appropriate; and 4) assess the patient's risk of danger (see box). Community resources include emergency housing (usually in shelters), peer group and individual counseling, and legal and social services advocacy. Most communities have agencies and programs to help abused women and families seek viable alternatives. The clinician should reinforce that the patient has done nothing to deserve the abuse and that domestic violence is a crime. Clinicians should remember that a woman is always the best judge of her safety. Respect must be given for a decision to stay or leave her abuser. Clinicians should remind the patient that he or she remains a resource.

Child Abuse. Child abuse is generally categorized in four ways: 1) physical abuse, 2) emotional/psychologic abuse, 3) sexual abuse, and 4) neglect. In 1996, child protective services identified almost 1 million children as victims of substantiated or indicated abuse or neglect, nearly a 20% increase since 1990. It is believed that these figures significantly underestimate the extent of the problem.

The majority of child physical abuse cases involve boys; girls are sexually abused three times more often than boys. Young single mothers who were themselves abused are at risk for abusing children; they are most

The RADAR Model of the Physician's Approach to Domestic Violence

R: Remember to ask about violence and victimization.
A: Ask directly: "At any time or in the last year, have you been hit, hurt, threatened, or frightened by someone with whom you are in a relationship?"
D: Document findings in the medical records for the patient's legal protection.
A: Assess the patient's immediate safety.
R: Review options and refer (for example, crisis center, women's shelter) as appropriate.

Massachusetts Medical Society. Partner violence: how to recognize and treat victims of abuse. 3rd ed. Waltham, Massachusetts: MMS, 1999.

often involved in cases of physical abuse and neglect. Most perpetrators of child sexual assault are males, often fathers, step-fathers, or other male family members.

Child Sexual Abuse. Although specific definitions of child sexual abuse vary among states, there is widespread agreement that abusive sexual contact can include breast or genital fondling, oral and anal sex, and vaginal intercourse. Recently, definitions have expanded to include noncontact activities such as coercion to watch or perform sexual acts or participate in child pornography. The actual incidence of childhood sexual abuse in the United States is unknown. However, studies consistently find that approximately 20% of women have such a history. A recent Department of Justice/Centers for Disease Control and Prevention survey found that 18% of women surveyed had experienced an attempted or completed rape at some time in their life. Of this 18%, 22% had been younger than 12 years of age and 32% had been 12–17 years of age when they were first raped (see "Sexual Assault or Rape" in Part 4).

Although there is no single syndrome that is universally prevalent in adult survivors of childhood sexual abuse, there is a growing body of research that links such history with a wide range of long-lasting emotional and behavioral responses that represent a woman's attempt to cope with her traumatic experience. These responses may, in turn, lead to additional health care problems and are frequently associated with an overuse of health care resources.

Clinical presentations frequently include depression; anxiety; post-traumatic stress symptoms; eating disorders; alcohol, drug, and tobacco use and abuse; suicide attempts or ideation; poor self-care; and somatic disorders (eg, chronic pelvic pain, migraine, gastrointestinal disorders). Adolescents and adult women with such histories are at increased risk of STDs (including HIV and AIDS). These patients are less likely to have regular Pap tests. Adult survivors of childhood sexual abuse also may have histories that include early, unplanned pregnancy, abortions, and little or no prenatal care. Suspected child abuse must be reported to the appropriate agency.

Abuse and Neglect of the Elderly. Elder abuse refers to acts of omission or commission that result in harm or threatened harm to the health or welfare of an older adult (generally persons older than 60 years of age). The exact incidence of elder abuse is unknown. However, a 1991 report from Congress suggests that between 1.5 and 2 million older adults are abused annually in the United States. Often family members or caregivers perpetrate the abuse.

Clinicians who provide care to older women should conduct universal screening for elder abuse. The screening questions for domestic or intimate partner violence are applicable to the older female patient. When elder abuse is suspected or identified, physicians should assess mistreatment according to accepted guidelines for domestic violence. Referrals to legal and social services agencies are appropriate. Currently, state laws that define elder abuse vary considerably from one jurisdiction to another. Mandates for reporting generally apply to the incapacitated elderly individual; however, clinicians should be familiar with state laws that may require reporting cases of suspected elder abuse.

Depression

Major depressive disorders may begin at any age, with the average age of onset in the mid 20s. In one half of women the onset of depression occurs between 20 and 50 years of age. Depression can be overdiagnosed in women who have experienced grief reactions or who are undergoing situational stress. Because women often seek care from obstetrician–gynecologists for a general medical check-up rather than for a specific condition, it can be assumed that many patients treated by obstetrician–gynecologists will have a depressive illness.

The presenting symptoms of depressive disorders are frequently somatic or behavioral and sometimes can be attributed to an organic condition. In some cases, depression may be related to a condition for which a woman is receiving care, such as infertility, or perinatal loss or postpartum depression. Psychologic symptoms such as depressed mood, crying spells, loss of interest in usual activities, or suicidal thoughts are obvious, but a high index of suspicion is needed in the differential diagnosis, regardless of symptoms. Diagnostic criteria, such as that provided in the American Psychiatric Association's *Diagnostic and Statistical Manual of Mental Disorders*, can be useful.

The clinician should be alert for additional symptoms of depression, which may include but are not limited to:

- Loss of interest or pleasure in normally enjoyable activities, including sex
- Persistent physical symptoms that do not respond to treatment, such as headaches, digestive disorders, or chronic pain
- Exaggerated or prolonged depressive symptoms following common reproductive events, conditions, or procedures, such as miscarriage, stillbirth, prematurity, infertility, hysterectomy, mastectomy, childbirth, or menopause
- Multiple somatic complaints that may include dysmenorrhea, dyspareunia, and sexual dysfunction
  —Chronic, clinically unconfirmed vulvovaginitis, idiopathic vulvodynia, or chronic vaginal pain and burning
  —Chronic pelvic or genitourinary tract pain
  —Severe, incapacitating premenstrual syndrome

Patients should be screened for psychosocial stressors as described earlier in this section. The history should include previous psychologic problems, including consultations with a mental health professional, previous psychiatric illness, or contemplation of suicide. The family history should include a question concerning depression in relatives, especially first-degree relatives. When the initial screening suggests a depressive disorder, a more comprehensive history is in order.

All depressed patients should be evaluated for suicidal thinking and impulses. This is best done by direct questioning. If a woman has specific plans or significant risk for suicide, such as prior attempts or hopelessness, a mental health specialist should be consulted immediately (see "Depression" in Part 4).

Substance Abuse

Screening (with prior patient approval) is helpful in identifying patients in denial of substance abuse. The following are risk factors associated with substance abuse:

- Young age
- Biological daughter of substance-abusing parent(s)
- Spouse or partner who abuse substances
- History of recent traumatic life experience
  - —Divorce or separation
  - —Death of spouse or significant other
  - —Job loss
  - —Retirement
  - —Rape or sexual abuse
  - —Witness to a traumatic event
- Physical disability
- Health care professional
- Psychiatric disorder

When there is no suspicion of substance abuse, random checks for substance abuse without the patient's permission are unethical. However, medical circumstances occasionally arise in which consent is considered unnecessary or unobtainable (eg, the patient is unconscious, stuporous, or showing obvious signs of intoxication). These patients need to be tested to direct further medical interventions (see "Substance Use and Abuse" in Part 4).

Suggested Reading

American College of Obstetricians and Gynecologists. Adult manifestations of childhood sexual abuse. ACOG Educational Bulletin 259. Washington, DC: ACOG, 2000

American College of Obstetricians and Gynecologists. Androgen treatment of decreased libido. ACOG Committee Opinion 244. Washington, DC: ACOG, 2000

American College of Obstetricians and Gynecologists. Domestic violence. ACOG Educational Bulletin 257. Washington, DC: ACOG, 1999

American College of Obstetricians and Gynecologists. Prevention of adolescent suicide. ACOG Committee Opinion 190. Washington, DC: ACOG, 1997

American College of Obstetricians and Gynecologists. Primary and preventive health care for female adolescents. ACOG Educational Bulletin 254. Washington, DC: ACOG, 1999

American Psychiatric Association. Diagnostic and statistical manual of mental disorders: DSM-IV-TR. 4th ed. Washington, DC: APA, 2000

Association of Professors of Gynecology and Obstetrics. Cardiovascular disease in women: pathophysiology, diagnosis and treatment. APGO Educational Series on Women's Health Issues. Washington, DC: APGO, 1998

Barber HR. Perimenopausal and geriatric gynecology. New York: MacMillan, 1988

Benedet JL, Bender H, Jones H 3rd, Ngan HY, Pecorelli S. FIGO staging classifications and clinical practice guidelines in the management of gynecologic cancers. FIGO Committee on Gynecologic Oncology. Int J Gynaecol Obstet 2000;70:209–262

Byyny RL, Speroff L. A clinical guide for the care of older women: primary and preventative care. 2nd ed. Baltimore: Williams and Wilkins, 1996

Canadian Consensus Conference on Menopause and Osteoporosis: part I: consensus statement. J SOGC 1998;20:1243–1272

Centers for Disease Control and Prevention. 1998 guidelines for treatment of sexually transmitted diseases. MMWR Morb Mortal Wkly Rep 1998;47(RR-1):1–111

Clinical guidelines on the identification, evaluation, and treatment of overweight and obesity in adults: the evidence report. Bethesda, Maryland: National Heart, Lung, and Blood Institute, 1998

Coluzzi PH. Cancer pain management: newer perspectives on opioids and episodic pain. Am J Hosp Palliat Care 1998;15:13–22

Council on Resident Education in Obstetrics and Gynecology. Basic geriatric care objectives for residency training in obstetrics and gynecology. Washington, DC: CREOG, 1999

Executive Summary of the Third Report of The National Cholesterol Education Program (NCEP) Expert Panel on Detection, Evaluation, and Treatment of High Blood Cholesterol in Adults (Adult Treatment Panel III). JAMA 2001;285:2486–2497

The Expert Committee on the Diagnosis and Classification of Diabetes Mellitus. Report of the Expert Committee on the diagnosis and classification of diabetes mellitus. Diabetes Care 2000;23(suppl 1):S4–S19

Greenlee RT, Hill-Harmon MB, Murray T, Bolden S, Thun M. Cancer statistics, 2001. CA Cancer J Clin 2001;51:15–36

Institute of Medicine. Committee on Prevention and Control of Sexually Transmitted Diseases. The hidden epidemic: confronting sexually transmitted diseases. Washington, DC: National Academy Press, 1997

Iso H, Hennekens CH, Stampfer MJ, Rexrode KM, Colditz GA, Speizer FE, et al. Prospective study of aspirin use and risk of stroke in women. Stroke 1999;30:1764–1771

LCDC Expert Working Group on Canadian Guidelines for Sexually Transmitted Diseases. Canadian STD Guidelines. Ottawa, Ontario: Health Canada, 1998

National High Blood Pressure Education Program. Update on the Task Force report (1987) on high blood pressure in children and adolescents: a Working Group report from the National High Blood Pressure Education Program. Bethesda, Maryland: National Institutes of Health, National Heart, Lung, and Blood Institute, 1996: NIH publication no. 96-3790

Pignone MP, Phillips CJ, Atkins D, Teutsch SM, Mulrow CD, Lohr KN. Screening and treating adults for lipid disorders. Am J Prev Med 2001;20(3 suppl):77–89

Rich-Edwards JW, Manson JE, Hennekens CH, Buring JE. The primary prevention of coronary heart disease in women. N Engl J Med 1995;332:1758–1766

Risen CB. A guide to taking a sexual history. Psychiatr Clin North Am 1995;18:39–53

Screening adults for lipid disorders. Recommendations and rationale. U.S. Preventive Services Task Force. Am J Prev Med 2001;20(3 suppl):73–76

Sixth Report of the Joint National Committee on the prevention, detection, evaluation, and treatment of high blood pressure. Bethesda, Maryland: National Heart, Lung, and Blood Institute, 1997

Stenchever MA, ed. Care of the aging woman: a primary care resource for obstetrics and gynecology training programs. Washington, DC: Association of Professors of Gynecology and Obstetrics, 1994

U.S. Preventive Services Task Force. Guide to clinical preventive services: report of the U.S. Preventive Services Task Force. 2nd ed. Baltimore: Williams and Wilkins, 1996

AMBULATORY GYNECOLOGIC SURGERY

Many surgical procedures routinely performed by the obstetrician–gynecologist can be performed safely, efficiently, and cost-effectively in a freestanding or hospital-based ambulatory surgical center or in the office setting (see box). The availability of proper equipment and appropriately trained personnel determine the extent of surgery that can safely be performed in the office (see "Facilities and Equipment" in Part 2). Although the guidance in this section is applicable in some instances to inpatient surgery, this is not the focus.

Procedures Commonly Performed in a Physician's Office or Outpatient Surgical Facilities

- Aspiration of breast cyst
- Biopsy, aspiration, or washing of the endometrium
- Cervical polypectomy
- Cervical, vaginal, and vulvar biopsies
- Colposcopy
- Cryosurgery of the cervix, vulva, or vagina
- Culdocentesis
- Cytoscopy
- Dilation and curettage of the uterus
- Early abortion
- Evacuation of incomplete abortion (spontaneous and uncomplicated)
- Hysterosalpingography
- Hysteroscopy, diagnostic
- Incision and drainage of vulvar or perineal abscesses
- Insertion and removal of contraceptive implants
- Insertion of intrauterine contraceptive devices
- Laser vaporization and excision of the cervix, vulva, or vagina
- Loop electrosurgical excision procedures of the cervix, vulva, or vagina
- Marsupialization of cysts of the Bartholin gland
- Proctosigmoidoscopy
- Removal of skin lesions

Site and Patient Selection

Many procedures performed as inpatient procedures have been replaced by procedures that can be performed safely in ambulatory sites. Examples are endometrial sampling in place of diagnostic dilation and curettage, loop electrosurgical excision procedure in place of cone biopsy of the cervix, and diagnostic laparoscopy and hysteroscopy. Ambulatory surgical procedures should be limited to those that can be performed safely; are consistent with staff expertise, facilities, and equipment; and are in accordance with the intrinsic risk of the procedure, the patient's condition, and the need for anesthesia.

Clinicians should be aware of any state and local regulations governing surgical procedures, including office surgical procedures requiring anesthesia. They also should be aware of payers' regulations regarding sites for which professional and facility charges will be paid, because these have a bearing on where procedures may be performed.

Ambulatory Care Facilities

Procedures performed in a freestanding or hospital-based ambulatory surgical facility should be those for which there is a reasonable expectation of discharge within a short time, with traditional recovery occurring at home. Healthy patients and those with stable systemic disease whose medical condition or procedure will not necessitate an overnight stay should be considered candidates for ambulatory surgery. Patients who do not meet these criteria may still be candidates for ambulatory surgery but should first undergo a preoperative anesthesia consultation. The patient's mental or emotional suitability for ambulatory surgery and the social and environmental setting into which she will return also should be taken into consideration. The importance of a follow-up evaluation should be stressed during both the preoperative and the postoperative interviews.

Elderly patients can be expected to have reduced function in organ systems that may be specifically stressed by surgery and anesthesia. Decline in cardiac, pulmonary, and renal function are of particular importance. Similar impairment may be found in younger individuals with a history of illness involving these organ systems. Such individuals may require specific preoperative testing to determine the functional status of their heart, lungs, or kidneys. When compromise or dysfunction is identified, consultation with an appropriate specialist may be necessary. The anesthesiologist should be included in the evaluation or informed of the preoperative findings in elderly patients.

Surgical procedures at ambulatory sites may be performed under local, regional block, or general anesthesia. When any form of anesthesia is used, trained personnel and proper equipment and drugs for cardiopulmonary resuscitation should be available (see "Supporting Services" in Part 2). There should be written policies and procedures providing for prompt emergency treatment or hospitalization of patients and for obtaining blood or blood products on a timely basis in the event of an unanticipated complication. The following factors place a woman at increased risk from anesthesia and should be communicated to the anesthesia care practitioner in advance to permit formulation of a management plan:

- Marked obesity
- Severe facial and neck edema
- Extremely short stature
- Difficulty opening her mouth
- Small mandible, protuberant teeth, or both
- Arthritis of the neck
- Short neck
- Anatomic abnormalities of the face or mouth
- Large thyroid
- Asthma or other chronic pulmonary disease
- Cardiac disease
- History of problems attributable to anesthetics
- Bleeding disorders
- Other significant medical complications

On rare occasions, it may be impossible to intubate a patient after the induction of general anesthesia. Emergency percutaneous transtracheal/cricothyroid ventilation may be lifesaving in this circumstance, and the necessary equipment for performing this procedure should be immediately available whenever general anesthesia is administered.

Details on the organization of a freestanding or hospital-based ambulatory care surgical facility and on the involvement of the hospital staff in the ambulatory care facility's activities are available from JCAHO and the Accreditation Association for Ambulatory Health Care, Inc. Many states have statutes or regulations that control the structure and function of ambulatory care facilities.

Office

Simple procedures of limited invasiveness that require only local anesthesia can be accomplished safely in the office with minimum extra requirements of space, personnel, and backup equipment. When more extensive procedures using local anesthesia are performed, or when conscious intravenous sedation is to be used, a more advanced level of training of office personnel and more extensive preoperative, intraoperative, and postoperative monitoring are required. Procedures that may require major emergency laparotomy should not be performed in this setting.

It should be realized that not all patients are good candidates for office surgery. Procedures that require a level of patient cooperation, such as dilation and curettage or hysteroscopy, are not practical for certain patients. Patients in the following categories, in general, may be poor candidates for office procedures performed under local anesthesia:

- Children and adolescents who have an immature lower genital tract and cannot relax sufficiently
- Postmenopausal patients with vaginal atrophy who tolerate pelvic examinations poorly
- Patients who require maximal relaxation
- Patients who are extremely obese
- Patients who are unable to understand or cooperate with the procedure

Anesthesia

Local, regional, and general anesthesia are all used in ambulatory surgical facilities, whereas anesthesia used for office-based procedures is generally limited to local anesthesia or conscious intravenous sedation. The focus of this section is anesthesia for office-based procedures. Recommendations on regional and general anesthesia are available from the American Society of Anesthesiologists and in textbooks.

Local Anesthesia

Except for simple procedures of limited invasiveness, the following resources should be available when performing surgical procedures with local anesthesia:

- Physicians and surgical assistants certified and periodically recertified in cardiopulmonary resuscitation
- Written and readily available protocols for emergency medical services and ambulance services
- Arrangements with a backup hospital reasonably accessible to the office facility
- Oxygen with an appropriate delivery system, including oral airway, nonbreathing mask, nasal cannula, and devices able to deliver positive pressure ventilation
- Emergency medications to manage allergic reactions, anesthetic toxic effects, and vasovagal reactions. These include, but are not limited to:

  —Lidocaine

  —Atropine sulfate

  —Diphenhydramine hydrochloride

  —Epinephrine

  —Diazepam
- Intravenous solutions and appropriate intravenous cannulas
- Auxiliary light source

Procedures should be in place to maintain equipment, replace outdated or recalled medications, and maintain proper training of personnel in the use of equipment and medications. Office emergency kits with appropriate instruction manuals and reordering procedures are available commercially and can be very useful in the office setting.

Selection of Agent. For safety, minimal disturbance of physiology, and rapid recovery, local anesthetic agents are chosen for most procedures performed in the office setting. When the practitioner is properly trained in the administration of local anesthetic agents for local infiltration, pudendal block, and paracervical block, these agents are extremely effective in providing anesthesia for most office procedures. It is recommended that the practitioner limit use to a few of the agents available and become very familiar with their pharmacodynamics, anesthetic properties, toxic levels, safe dosage levels, side effects, and complications.

Most gynecologists use lidocaine in the office setting because of its safety, intermediate potency, and excellent spreading characteristics. Chloroprocaine is used by some because of its rapid hydrolysis and low toxic potential. For some surgical procedures, more potent, longer-acting amides such as bupivacaine may be used. A 1:200,000 concentration of epinephrine often is used with lidocaine to retard systemic absorption, prolong the duration of anesthesia, and allow the use of smaller concentrations of anesthetic.

Adverse systemic effects of local anesthetic agents are unlikely unless blood levels exceed 5 μg/mL. Recommended maximum safe dose levels of local anesthetics are designed to minimize toxic effects by maintaining a blood level of less than 2 μg/mL. The practitioner should be familiar with the maximum allowable doses, the signs and symptoms of high levels of anesthetic in the tissues, and the administration of appropriate treatment.

Emergency Backup and Equipment for Local Anesthesia. Specialized personnel, such as anesthesiologists and nurse–anesthetists, need not be present when local anesthesia is used in the office setting. Medications used for preoperative medication and surgical anesthesia should be chosen carefully to minimize the risk of major adverse reactions. Resuscitation devices such as endotracheal tubes, defibrillators, and medications used in advanced life-support situations are not necessary if procedures are performed with local anesthesia and if potential candidates for surgery have been evaluated carefully and those with serious cardiovascular disorders excluded. The safe and effective use of this equipment requires regular and frequent practice.

Conscious Intravenous Sedation

Analgesics and sedatives such as fentanyl, meperidine, and midazolam often are used intravenously in conjunction with office surgery. Such use is referred to as conscious intravenous sedation. If such medications are used to depress the patient's level of consciousness, the patient should still have the ability to maintain her airway independently and continuously and respond appropriately to verbal and physical stimulation. Sedation to the extent that the patient is not easily aroused to consciousness or experiences complete or partial loss of preoperative reflexes is to be avoided. Prior to performing surgery using conscious intravenous sedation, the patient should abstain from food or drink for at least 4 hours. After intravenous sedation is given and before the surgical procedure is begun, the patient's mental status and ability to maintain her airway should be determined and documented.

Selection of Agents. Selection of proper analgesics or sedatives for conscious intravenous sedation is critical. Drugs should be chosen based on their ability to prepare the patient for the planned surgical procedure and their margin of safety in the office setting. Common drugs may include:

- Midazolam
- Diazepam
- Morphine
- Meperidine
- Fentanyl citrate

Conscious intravenous sedation requires the same guidelines and resources necessary for the use of local anesthesia in addition to the following recommendations:

- Medication should be given by a qualified person who has a working knowledge of the medications, monitoring equipment, and resuscitation techniques necessary for the management of adverse drug reactions.
- Vital signs, including heart rate, blood pressure, respiratory rate, level of consciousness, and oxygen saturation (pulse oximetry) should be monitored continuously and documented prior to, during, and following the procedure.
- A qualified person whose primary responsibility is patient monitoring should be available in the procedure room.
- Narcotic and benzodiazepine reversal agents, such as naloxone and flumazenil, should be available.

Emergency Backup Equipment When Using Conscious Sedation. Emergency backup equipment must be more extensive for conscious intravenous sedation than for use of local anesthetics. Advanced life support equipment, such as a laryngoscope, endotracheal tube, defibrillator, and an emergency cart with advanced life support medications, should be available. Office personnel must be trained in the proper usage and maintenance of emergency life support equipment.

Perioperative Considerations

Preoperative Evaluations

A preoperative evaluation should be performed to determine the appropriateness of the procedure. Certain criteria should be fulfilled as a result of this evaluation. The proposed procedure must be indicated, based on targeted history and physical examination. Alternative treatments should have been considered, and it should be determined that the benefits to the patient outweigh the risks. Known contraindications and risk factors should have been ruled out or considered. Informed consent must have been obtained. The surgeon must have the necessary skills and experience, and the facility must have the equipment necessary for both the procedure and anticipated complications. The following evaluations should be completed prior to outpatient surgery, and the findings should be noted in the medical record:

- A recent general and targeted history and physical examination with specific attention to pregnancy status, preexisting or concurrent illness, medications, and adverse drug reactions that may have an effect on or contraindicate the operative procedure or anesthesia
- Laboratory data as indicated, based on the patient's needs and condition and the procedure
- Informed consent, including an informed consent form or other documentation indicating that the diagnosis, the reason for the surgery, a description of the planned procedure, the intended benefits and possible risks, the possible alternatives, if any, and the probability of a successful outcome have been explained to the patient
- Preoperative written instructions that include directions regarding restrictions on food and fluid intake (and warning that failure to heed such directions may result in cancellation of the procedure)
- A preanesthetic evaluation on the day of the surgery, including an interval history, medical record review, and heart and lung examination

Because many diagnostic and therapeutic modalities may pose a direct or indirect risk to an embryo, facilities should establish specific procedures, applicable to all services, for identifying unsuspected pregnancies in women of reproductive age. A menstrual history and physical examination can be helpful in this determination. If there is any reason to suspect pregnancy, a pregnancy test should be done in advance of any such procedure.

Laboratory testing will vary considerably with the extent of the planned surgery, the patient's age, preexisting conditions, potential complications, institutional policies, and insurance requirements. Despite these variations, the guiding principle is to determine any contraindication or risk factors that should be known and to establish baselines that may be of importance in managing the postoperative course.

Patient Preparation

The extent of preoperative counseling needed to prepare patients for ambulatory surgery using local anesthesia depends on the type of procedure being performed. Some degree of counseling is necessary for virtually all procedures to allow the patient to provide informed consent, prepare her for the level of discomfort usually associated with the procedure, and help to gain her confidence. If the patient is anxious or if the procedure is to be extensive, preoperative medication such as a mild tranquilizer may be given orally 1 hour prior to the procedure.

Preoperative tests and procedures should be individualized based on the patient's age and medical status with respect to the planned surgery. This testing should be aimed at evaluating the patient's known disease and to screen for unsuspected pathology that would warrant further preoperative evaluation or alter the surgeon's planned therapeutic approach. Other issues to be considered preoperatively include bowel preparation, prophylactic use of antibiotics, skin preparation, and prevention of venous thrombosis.

Women who have a pelvic mass suspicious for malignancy, bowel symptoms, a history of bowel resection, or suspected dense peritoneal adhesions are candidates for bowel preparation to reduce infectious complications if the bowel is entered. Appropriate prophylaxis includes a mechanical bowel preparation with or without oral antibiotics and the use of a broad-spectrum parenteral antibiotic given preoperatively.

Antibiotic prophylaxis is an option for patients who are at high risk for developing endocarditis. Antibiotic selection depends on the planned procedure and published guidelines, including those by the American Heart Association. Women undergoing surgically induced abortion are candidates for antibiotic prophylaxis; doxycycline is a cost-effective regimen.

The goal of skin preparation is to reduce bacterial counts while minimizing skin irritation. Showering with chlorhexidine the day before surgery reduces wound infection rates. Hair removal should be performed only when necessary for adequate visualization and with the least amount of skin disruption (clipping rather than shaving when possible).

Preoperative patients should be classified according to levels of risk of thrombosis to determine the benefits and risks of pharmacologic and physical methods of preventing venous thromboembolism. Factors to consider include patient age, duration of surgery, and clinical risk factors such as prior deep venous thrombosis or pulmonary embolism, varicose veins, infection, malignancy, estrogen therapy, and obesity. Low-risk patients who are undergoing gynecologic surgery do not require specific prophylaxis other than early ambulation. Alternatives for thromboprophylaxis for moderate-risk patients undergoing gynecologic surgery include compression stockings, pneumatic compression, unfractionated heparin, and low-molecular-weight heparin. Alternatives for prophylaxis for high-risk patients undergoing gynecologic surgery, especially for malignancy, include pneumatic compression, unfractionated heparin, and low-molecular-weight heparin. There are no studies to confirm definitively the clinical benefit of discontinuation of oral contraceptives or HRT preoperatively. Some studies do show a small increase in the risk of thrombosis in both oral contraceptive and HRT users. However, the benefit of stopping oral contraceptives 4–6 weeks before major surgery must be balanced against the risks of pregnancy.

Some patients are allergic or sensitive to common operating room substances such as latex, povidone-iodine, and metal used for surgical staples. Patients should be evaluated preoperatively for such allergies and sensitivities.

Intraoperative and Postoperative Care

The position of both the patient and the retractor are important to prevent nerve injury. Care should be taken to avoid excessive flexion or external rotation of the patient's hips to prevent a femoral neuropathy. This is best achieved using lateral thigh supports. Proper positioning of the foot and leg will prevent pressure on the peroneal nerve. If a laparotomy is required, improper placement of retractors can cause pressure on the psoas muscle and can cause femoral nerve injury. Shallow blades and laparotomy packs under the blades may help reduce pressure. In operative procedures, such as hysteroscopy, in which osmotically active solutions are used for visualization, careful intraoperative management of fluid balance is critical to patient well-being.

Careful attention to fluid management and pain control are important facets of postoperative care. Nasogastric tube insertion should not be used routinely as it is uncomfortable, increases the incidence of pulmonary complications, and does not reduce the incidence of wound complications. Oral feeding with a regular diet immediately postoperatively is safe for most patients who have undergone an ambulatory surgical procedure.

In elderly patients, operative management should include minimizing anesthesia doses to promote cognitive recovery, avoiding dehydration, attention to position to accommodate joint fragility, and ensuring sufficient padding of bony surfaces and cushioning to prevent ulceration. Postoperatively, early mobilization and rapid removal of restraints is important. Extra precautions should be taken to prevent falls. Delirium is a serious risk of surgery in the elderly; early investigation for medical causes is important, and treatment should be augmented with frequent auditory, visual, and somatosensory orientation.

With the exception of those specimens exempted by the governing body and JCAHO, tissue removed during surgery should be submitted to a pathologist for examination. At the appropriate time, the patient should be informed of the operative findings, including the results of tissue examination. Routine pathologic examination of tissue is not necessary following the elective surgical termination of a pregnancy in which embryonic or fetal parts can be identified with certainty. In such instances, the physician should simply record a description of the gross products of conception.

Adverse Reactions

The most common adverse reactions to gynecologic procedures performed in the office setting are vasovagal reactions. These reactions include a number of cardiovascular and autonomic or central nervous system reactions such as bradycardia, hypotension, diaphoresis, nausea, and convulsions. A vasovagal reaction usually is the result of patient anxiety but also may occur with cervical dilation, peritoneal stretching, or as a result of pain. In patients who do not have CVD, vasovagal reactions usually terminate spontaneously without the need for specific therapy.

Vasovagal reactions may be prevented by preoperative patient counseling, reassurance during the procedure, and the administration of preoperative atropine or promethazine hydrochloride. If the reaction is severe, oxygen should be used in cases of prolonged apnea. Assisted respiration is rarely necessary.

A vasovagal reaction should not be confused with the much less common allergic reactions to a local anesthetic or preoperative medications. True allergic reactions to commonly used anesthetic and preoperative medications do not occur often, but personnel should be familiar with common allergic reactions and their appropriate management. Allergic reactions such as urticaria, hives, edema, and asthma may be treated with diphenhydramine, intravenously, or epinephrine may be given intramuscularly or subcutaneously.

Latex allergy has become a common health problem (see "Latex Allergy" in Part 4). The populations most commonly affected are those with repeated exposures to latex (eg, patients with spina bifida, workers who habitually wear latex gloves, and patients who have undergone multiple surgeries). Patients with hand eczema or atopic allergies also are at higher risk for being affected. The most common manifestations of latex allergy are irritant or contact dermatitis of the hand, but contact urticaria, rhinoconjunctivitis, angioedema, asthma, and anaphylaxis also occur. Treatment is avoidance of latex materials, use of powder-free gloves to decrease airborne exposure, and supportive therapy of the sensitivity response.

Length of Stay and Discharge Issues

When local anesthetic agents are used for office surgery, minimum space and services are necessary for proper postoperative recovery. When patients are alert, oriented, have stable vital signs, are free of major pain, and are able to sit up and dress themselves, they may leave the office.

When conscious intravenous sedation is used, an area sufficient for patient recovery should be provided and staffed by personnel who continue monitoring vital signs and level of consciousness. The patient should be observed until there is a return of premedication mental status and vital signs consistent with normal ranges. The patient should be discharged by order of the clinician or by predefined practitioner-approved criteria. The patient should be discharged into the care of a responsible adult.

When procedures have been performed in an ambulatory surgical center, a physician, preferably the anesthesiologist, should be present in the facility until the patient has been discharged. This physician should oversee the postanesthetic recovery area and should share with the surgeon the responsibility for discharging patients or transferring them to the backup hospital.

During the recovery period, a member of the health care team should observe the patient closely. This person should maintain a complete record of the patient's general condition, including vital signs, blood loss, and occurrence of complications. The patient should remain in the area until recovery is sufficient to permit safe discharge according to the following criteria:

- The patient's cardiovascular physiologic variables are stable.
- The patient must be able to cough, and respiration must be unobstructed.
- Optimally, the patient should have voided after the procedure. Exceptions require documentation of plans to monitor the ability to void after discharge.
- Pain and nausea must be controllable with medication in appropriate doses.
- There should be no evidence of active bleeding or significant temperature elevation.
- The patient must be able to ambulate and be aware of her surroundings and what has occurred.

- The patient should be discharged in the company of a responsible adult licensed to drive a vehicle or able to accompany the patient home by public transportation.

The patient should be examined by a health care practitioner with appropriate clinical privileges and discharged on written order. Alternatively, other practitioners may discharge patients according to approved criteria.

On discharge, the patient and any accompanying responsible adult should be given and acknowledge verbal and written instructions about medications, follow-up care, signs and symptoms of common complications, and procedures for obtaining emergency care and advice. One method of evaluating the effectiveness of care is follow-up telephone contact to substantiate the patient's well-being the day after surgery (see also "Supporting Services" in Part 2).

SUGGESTED READING

1999 Accreditation handbook for ambulatory care. Skokie, Illinois: Accreditation Association for Ambulatory Health Care, Inc, 1999

American College of Obstetricians and Gynecologists. Antibiotic prophylaxis for gynecologic procedures. ACOG Practice Bulletin 23. Washington, DC: ACOG, 2001

American College of Obstetricians and Gynecologists. Prevention of deep vein thrombosis and pulmonary embolism. ACOG Practice Bulletin 21. Washington, DC: ACOG, 2000

American College of Surgeons. Guidelines for optimal ambulatory surgical care and office-based surgery. 3rd ed. Chicago: ACS, 2000

Dajani AS, Taubert KA, Wilson W, Bolger AF, Bayer A, Ferrieri P, et al. Prevention of bacterial endocarditis. Recommendations by the American Heart Association. Circulation 1997;96:358–366

Joint Commission on Accreditation of Healthcare Organizations. 2000–2001 comprehensive accreditation manual for ambulatory care. Oakbrook Terrace, Illinois: JCAHO, 1999

Practice guidelines for sedation and analgesia by non-anesthesiologists. A report by the American Society of Anesthesiologists Task Force on Sedation and Analgesia by Non-Anesthesiologists. Anesthesiology 1996;84:459–471

PART 4

Selected Issues in the Delivery of Women's Health Care

This section of Guidelines addresses policy and management issues for conditions that have a major impact on women's health, such as depression, endometriosis, and abnormal genital bleeding. This section contains topics that may go beyond the well-woman examination or the generalist's knowledge. This section is organized by topic and includes focused information regarding the health care impact, relevant ACOG recommendations, expertise needed, legal considerations, and resources for both the patient and the professional regarding each condition. In determining the information to be included in each entry, priority was given to new information, key areas, and information important to clinicians but not readily available in standard textbooks and references. Recommendations and legal considerations are by no means inclusive, and other requirements may apply in certain situations or jurisdictions. The resource lists include ACOG patient and professional education materials, guidelines published by other organizations, seminal articles, and contact information for organizations that focus on individual topics (see also Appendix I).

Abnormal Genital Bleeding

Health Care Impact

Abnormal genital bleeding is one of the most frequent conditions that clinicians treat and is responsible for approximately 15–20% of outpatient gynecologic complaints. Genital bleeding occurs from a wide variety of conditions, including trauma, infection, lesions, or tumors. If genital bleeding is secondary to trauma, the differential diagnosis should include rape and abuse.

The uterus is the source of most abnormal genital bleeding in adults. The condition of abnormal uterine bleeding is responsible for many hysterectomies.

The major causes of abnormal uterine bleeding are leiomyomata and dysfunctional uterine bleeding. Abnormal uterine bleeding and dysfunctional uterine bleeding often are confused, but their clinical significances are very different. Abnormal uterine bleeding is a subclassification of genital bleeding, and refers to the *site* of bleeding (the uterus) *before* any diagnosis is confirmed. Dysfunctional uterine bleeding is a definitive diagnosis that is established when all pathological causes of abnormal uterine bleeding (leiomyomata, polyps, endometrial hyperplasia or cancer, coagulopathy) have been excluded. Dysfunctional uterine bleeding is produced from hormonal imbalances in estrogen/progesterone stability of the endometrium, and usually is treated medically. It is difficult to track the epidemiologic and clinical aspects of dysfunctional uterine bleeding, because dysfunctional uterine bleeding often is included in discussion of abnormal uterine bleeding, and the term abnormal uterine bleeding also is used to describe anovulatory uterine bleeding.

Women with coagulation disorders initially may be evaluated for uterine bleeding. These disorders include defects in primary hemostasis or platelet deficiency (leukemia, idiopathic thrombocytopenia), platelet dysfunction (von Willebrand's disease), and abnormalities of secondary homeostasis (congenital factor deficiencies).

Abnormal genital bleeding affects women of all ages. Four major groupings of the differential causes of abnormal genital bleeding have been suggested:

1. Reproductive tract disease or condition (pregnancy, leiomyomata, infection, trauma, malignancy)
2. Systemic disease (coagulation defect, hypothyroidism)
3. Iatrogenic causes (hormones, drugs, chemotherapy, dialysis)
4. Anovulatory bleeding

An ordering of the differential diagnosis based on the age of the patient when symptoms occur may be more clinically relevant:

- In adolescents, abnormal genital bleeding most often occurs as a result of chronic anovulation (dysfunctional bleeding), contraceptive use, pregnancy, and coagulation disorders
- Women in the third and fourth decades of life most often develop abnormal genital bleeding from pregnancy, structural lesions (leiomyomata), anovulation, hormonal therapy, and endometrial hyperplasia
- Menopausal women most often develop bleeding from hormone therapy, endometrial atrophy, leiomyomata, or endometrial hyperplasia or malignancy

Other less common events that are associated with abnormal genital bleeding include vascular anomalies of the uterus, infection, cirrhosis, drug therapy, and thyroid dysfunction. In pediatric patients, the vagina often is the source of abnormal genital bleeding. A foreign body, vaginitis, urethral prolapse, neoplasm, trauma, or precocious puberty frequently causes this type of bleeding (see also "Pediatric Gynecology" in Part 4).

Abnormal genital bleeding is classified by the timing of the bleeding and the duration of flow. Bleeding that occurs at abnormal times of an ovarian cycle (or that occurs more frequently than every 21 days) is called metrorrhagia, and excess bleeding (≥80 mL or bleeding >7 days) during the time of expected menstrual flow is termed menorrhagia. The development of anemia as a consequence of bleeding adds urgency to treatment.

ACOG Recommendations

Once an accurate diagnosis for the cause of bleeding is established, the primary goal of management is to treat the underlying disorder to normalize the bleeding pattern. No single approach is appropriate in the management of all patients with abnormal uterine bleeding. The approach depends on the amount of bleeding and the patient's age, medical status, reproductive desires, and underlying contributory disorders. An underlying coagulopathy should be considered in all patients (particularly adolescents) with abnormal uterine bleeding, especially when bleeding is not otherwise easily explained or does not respond to medical therapy.

In adolescents, endometrial assessment should be considered, particularly for those who have a history of 2–3 years of untreated anovulatory bleeding and especially for those who are obese. Unlike in adults, such sampling may need to be performed with a dilation and curettage as opposed to office endometrial biopsy because of patient tolerance.

Based on age alone, endometrial assessment to exclude cancer is indicated in any woman older than 35 years of age who is suspected of having anovulatory uterine bleeding. Although endometrial carcinoma is rare in women younger than 35 years of age, patients between 19 and 35 years of age who do not respond to medical therapy or have prolonged periods of unopposed estrogen stimulation secondary to chronic anovulation are candidates for endometrial assessment. All women older than 40 years of age who present with suspected anovulatory uterine bleeding should be evaluated with endometrial assessment (after pregnancy has been excluded).

The treatment of choice for anovulatory uterine bleeding is medical therapy with oral contraceptives. Cyclic progestins also are effective. Women who have failed medical therapy and no longer desire future childbearing are candidates for endometrial ablation, which appears to be an efficient and cost-effective alternative treatment to hysterectomy for anovulatory uterine bleeding. However, endometrial ablation may not be the definitive therapy.

As new techniques are introduced into clinical management, it is important to separate those that represent tested and efficacious modalities from developmental or experimental approaches. Effective treatments usually are established over time after long-term outcomes have been established.

Expertise

Proper evaluation of abnormal genital bleeding may include the following services, as indicated:

- Evaluation for pregnancy
- Physical examination for lower genital tract lesions
- Evaluation of genital tract lesions (cervical cytology, biopsy, sonography, sonohysterography, and hysteroscopy)
- Evaluation for thyroid dysfunction and coagulation disorders
- Evaluation for trauma or sexual assault
- Evaluation for infection/sexually transmitted diseases

Clinicians should be familiar with any state reporting requirements regarding trauma indicative of abuse or domestic violence.

RESOURCES

Patient

American College of Obstetricians and Gynecologists. Abnormal uterine bleeding. ACOG Patient Education Pamphlet AP095. Washington, DC: ACOG, 1999

American College of Obstetricians and Gynecologists. Endometrial ablation. ACOG Patient Education Pamphlet AP134. Washington, DC: ACOG, 2000

Professional

American College of Obstetricians and Gynecologists. Management of anovulatory bleeding. ACOG Practice Bulletin 14. Washington, DC: ACOG, 2000

American College of Obstetricians and Gynecologists. Pediatric gynecologic disorders. ACOG Technical Bulletin 201. Washington, DC: ACOG, 1995

Brenner PF. Differential diagnosis of abnormal uterine bleeding. Am J Obstet Gynecol 1996;175:766–769

Brill AI. What is the role of hysteroscopy in the management of abnormal uterine bleeding? Clin Obstet Gynecol 1995;38:319–345

Jennings JC. Abnormal uterine bleeding. Med Clin North Am 1995;79:1357–1376

Royal College of Obstetricians and Gynaecologists. The initial management of menorrhagia. RCOG Evidence-Based Clinical Guidelines No. 1. London: RCOG, 1998

Royal College of Obstetricians and Gynaecologists. The management of menorrhagia in secondary care. RCOG Evidence-Based Clinical Guidelines No. 5. London: RCOG, 1999

Stewart EA, Nowak RA. Leiomyoma-related bleeding: a classic hypothesis updated for the molecular era. Hum Reprod Update 1996;2:295–306

Abnormal Cervical Cytology

Health Care Impact

Although the incidence of and death rate from cervical cancer have decreased by more than 70% since the introduction of the Pap test more than 50 years ago, there are still approximately 12,900 new cases of cervical cancer each year. Approximately 50 million cervical cytology tests are performed in the United States each year, with 3–10% of these tests being reported as ASCUS (atypical squamous cells of undetermined significance) and another 2–5% being reported as indicating more severe abnormalities. Appropriate management of patients with ASCUS test results has been the subject of considerable debate. Information from the ALTS trial (ASCUS-LSIL Triage Study), a clinical trial sponsored by the National Cancer Institute, is expected to be valuable in determining which method of management is the most appropriate.

ACOG Recommendations

In the evaluation of the cervix following an abnormal cytology report, the first objective is to exclude the presence of invasive carcinoma. Once this has been accomplished, the objectives are to determine the grade and distribution of the intraepithelial lesion. Visual inspection of the cervix and vagina and bimanual pelvic examination should be performed. In addition, repeat cytology, colposcopic examination with directed biopsies, and endocervical curettage (ECC) should be performed, as indicated.

Many colposcopists advocate routine ECC except during pregnancy. The ECC should be performed under direct colposcopic visualization. Because of potential sampling errors with ECC use, many colposcopists recommend vigorous sampling of the endocervical canal with an endocervical brush.

Diagnostic conization is indicated in the following instances:

- An intraepithelial lesion or microinvasive carcinoma is present in the endocervical canal.
- Cytologic assessment indicates a significant abnormality that is not consistent with the tissue diagnosis.
- The entire transformation zone is not visible.
- Microinvasive carcinoma is diagnosed by directed biopsy.
- Cytologic or biopsy evidence of premalignant or malignant glandular epithelium is detected.

Women with atypical glandular cells on cytology should undergo a colposcopic evaluation with a directed cervical biopsy, if indicated, an ECC, as well as an endometrial assessment.

Despite the fact that there are large numbers of cervical cytology evaluations being reported as minimally abnormal (ASCUS and low-grade squamous intraepithelial lesion [LSIL] categories), the current recommendations for management are still evolving and require some individualization. Because the prognosis of patients with an ASCUS test result can vary depending on the laboratory or cytopathologist, the clinician is encouraged to have good communication and understanding with the cytopathologist. In a high-risk patient population, which includes patients at risk for noncompliance, the safest practice is to colposcope patients after the first ASCUS test result. In a low-risk patient population, it may be sufficient to monitor the patient with repeat smears every 6 months, with colposcopy reserved for the patient who experiences a second abnormal smear.

For patients with an LSIL test result, because of the high rate of false-negative results in cervical screening, physicians should consider performing a colposcopic examination after the initial LSIL test result to determine whether a lesion is present. At a minimum, these patients should be monitored very closely with cervical smears repeated at 4–6-month intervals with immediate colposcopy if the abnormality persists. Because approximately 15% of these lesions progress to high-grade squamous intraepithelial lesions (HSIL), ablation or excision is a reasonable treatment. On the other hand, because approximately 60% of these lesions regress spontaneously over two or more years, follow-up is an appropriate form of management for a compliant patient when indicated. If follow-up and no ablation or excision is selected and the lesion persists, reevaluation and possible treatment are indicated.

Any patient with atypical glandular cells of undetermined significance or HSIL test results should undergo colposcopic examination with directed biopsies as appropriate. When a lesion is visualized and biopsy confirms HSIL, ablative or excisional therapy aimed at destruction or removal of the entire transformation zone usually should be performed. Ablation can be undertaken only if the entire lesion and limits of the transformation zone are seen and results of ECC are negative.

A variety of techniques for ablation and excision have been used in the treatment of squamous intraepithelial lesions, including surgical excision, cryosurgery, laser vaporization procedures, and more recently, loop electrosurgical excision procedure (LEEP). Loop electrosurgical excision procedure allows the clinician to combine diagnosis and treatment using a relatively simple outpatient procedure done under local anesthesia. Unlike colposcopically directed biopsies, the loop excision specimen usually includes the entire transformation zone, which potentially reduces the risk of missing invasive cancer. In most circumstances, LEEP should be reserved for cases that persist, progress, or recur after other conservative measures have been attempted and for patients thought to be unreliable for follow-up. Women with HSIL are the most appropriate candidates for LEEP.

Because all therapeutic modalities carry an inherent recurrence rate of up to 10%, cytologic follow-up at approximately 3-month intervals for

1 year is necessary. After invasive cancer has been excluded, ambulatory therapy is appropriate when the following conditions exist:

- The lesion is located on the ectocervix.
- There is no involvement of the endocervix as determined by coloscopic examination and ECC.

Some patients with HSIL may be candidates for hysterectomy after appropriate evaluation, particularly if other gynecologic disorders (eg, menorrhagia) exist. It also may be appropriate for those with recurrent HSIL or those who have lesions that cannot be treated adequately with local therapies.

Expertise

The expertise required to evaluate and manage patients with abnormal cytologic findings includes a thorough knowledge of the significance and natural history of cervical preinvasive disease. Additionally, the person responsible for evaluating the abnormal test also should be appropriately trained and experienced in colposcopy and aware of the various treatment options available for managing cervicovaginal abnormalities. Access to appropriate cytologic and histopathologic laboratory expertise also is required.

Equipment needed for evaluation of the patient with an abnormal test result includes:

- Colposcope
- Acetic acid solution, 3–5%, hemostasis solution such as Monsel's solution
- Endocervical speculum to optimize visualization of the endocervical canal
- Cervical biopsy instruments, including endocervical curettes
- Appropriate fixative solution

The Clinical Laboratory Improvement Amendments have established requirements for review of abnormal cervical cytology and follow-up of tests of identified high-risk patients (see "Compliance with Government Regulations" in Part 1). In addition, clinicians should be familiar with any state requirements in this area.

Resources

Patient

American College of Obstetricians and Gynecologists. Colposcopy. ACOG Patient Education Pamphlet AP135. Washington, DC: ACOG, 2000

American College of Obstetricians and Gynecologists. Disorders of the cervix. ACOG Education Pamphlet AP033. Washington, DC: ACOG, 1999

American College of Obstetricians and Gynecologists. The Pap test. ACOG Education Pamphlet AP085. Washington, DC: ACOG, 1999

Professional

Agency for Health Care Policy and Research. Evaluation of cervical cytology. AHCPR Evidence Report/Technology Assessment no. 5. Rockville, Maryland: AHCPR, 1999

American College of Obstetricians and Gynecologists. Role of loop electrosurgical excision procedure in the evaluation of abnormal pap test results. ACOG Committee Opinion 195. Washington, DC: ACOG, 1997

American Society for Colposcopy and Cervical Pathology
(301) 773-3640
www.asccp.org

Behavior Modification

Health Care Impact

Behavior disorders, such as drug use and abuse, eating disorders, and noncompliance with medical and exercise recommendations, complicate the lives of many women. The clinician is frequently asked for advice and may be in the position to either positively affect behavior or unintentionally reinforce suboptimal behavior through his or her approach to these conditions. The identification of patient needs, followed by an expression of concern about the behavior and a willingness to work with the patient on a behavior modification plan may increase the likelihood of the clinician having a positive influence on patient behavior change efforts (see also "Eating Disorders" and "Substance Use and Abuse" in Part 4).

ACOG Recommendations

The clinician is in the position to improve women's health through attention to compliance with medical, dietary, and exercise recommendations. In addition, the clinician has a role in substance abuse prevention and treatment. Knowledge of key risk factors, familiarity with substance abuse screening techniques, and identification of the symptoms and signs of abuse are components in the process.

Expertise

The clinician should be familiar with approaches to behavior change, especially as they relate to women, such as those based on stages of change theory, reasoned action, and social cognitive theory. Consensus on how behavior change can be effected does not exist. Regardless of approach, good communication skills are essential for eliciting accurate reports of patient behavior. Maintaining a nonjudgmental, open approach, asking the right questions, and observing and listening carefully for evidence of harmful behaviors, as well as evidence of a desire to change those behaviors, may be of assistance (see also "Primary and Preventive Care" in Part 3).

Although the role of the physician cannot be underestimated, assistance from social workers, other clinicians, and community resources may be useful. The clinician also should be familiar with other common resources to aid women in behavior modification:

- Smoking
  —Patient education pamphlet from ACOG
  —Self-help smoking cessation materials
  —Smoking cessation programs
  —Nicotine replacement therapy
  —Other pharmacologic aids
- Alcohol abuse
  —Drug rehabilitation programs
  —Alcoholics Anonymous and other sobriety programs
- Drug dependency (prescription and nonprescription)
  —Drug treatment programs
  —Narcotics Anonymous
- Eating disorders
  —Psychologists, psychiatrists, multidisciplinary programs for intervention
- Wellness programs
  —Frequently available through hospitals and employers, or freestanding

Clinicians should be familiar with state statutes requiring illicit drug use reporting.

Resources

Patient

Alcoholics Anonymous
(212) 870-3400
www.alcoholics-anonymous.org/

The American Cancer Society
The Great American Smokeout
800-ACS (227)-2345
www.cancer.org/gas/

American College of Obstetricians and Gynecologists. It's time to quit smoking. ACOG Patient Education Pamphlet AP065. Washington, DC: ACOG, 2000

American College of Obstetricians and Gynecologists. Staying healthy for women of all ages. ACOG Patient Education Pamphlet AB006. Washington, DC: ACOG, 1994

American College of Obstetricians and Gynecologists. Weight control: eating right and keeping fit. ACOG Patient Education Pamphlet AP064. Washington, DC: ACOG, 1999

American Lung Association
800-LUNG-USA (800-586-4872)
www.lungusa.org/

Narcotics Anonymous
(818) 773-9999
www.na.org/

Professional

American College of Obstetricians and Gynecologists. Smoking and women's health. ACOG Educational Bulletin 240. Washington, DC: ACOG, 1997

American College of Obstetricians and Gynecologists. Substance abuse. ACOG Technical Bulletin 194. Washington, DC: ACOG, 1994

A clinical practice guideline for treating tobacco use and dependence: A US Public Health Service report. The Tobacco Use and Dependence Clinical Practice Guideline Panel, Staff, and Consortium Representatives. JAMA 2000;283:3244–3254

BREAST DISORDERS

Health Care Impact

Concerns regarding breast disorders are commonly raised at gynecologic or obstetric visits. Ten percent of women younger than 21 years of age experience complaints related to fibrocystic conditions of the breasts. Such complaints are more common in the premenopausal period. With increasing frequency, women expect their obstetrician–gynecologists to assume responsibility for education, screening, counseling, and treatment concerning benign conditions of the breast.

ACOG Recommendations

The obstetrician–gynecologist is in a favorable position to diagnose breast disease and should have a good understanding of the natural history as well as the diagnosis and treatment of these conditions. Established screening guidelines should be followed to allow early detection of breast cancer. The final diagnosis of a breast mass rests on histologic examination. Physical examination, imaging, and cytologic evaluations all contribute information but are not definitive.

The American College of Obstetricians and Gynecologists recognizes the obstetrician–gynecologist's role in diagnosing and treating breast disease. The College has adopted the goals of assisting in educating obstetrician–gynecologists in the diagnosis and treatment of benign breast disease and in the reduction of mortality from breast cancer.

Expertise

Obstetrician–gynecologists should be able to diagnose and refer for management or refer for diagnosis and management those at risk for life-threatening breast disease (cancer) and diagnose and manage non-life-threatening breast disease, consistent with their experience and training (see also "Neoplasms" in Part 4).

The evaluation of breast disease is based on risk factors and age and is determined by history, physical examination, imaging studies, cytologic examination, and biopsy. The clinician should be able to:

- Elicit a history related to breast disorders including:
  —Duration, onset, and cyclicity of signs and symptoms
  —Menstrual and reproductive history
  —Hormone use
  —Dietary habits
  —Breast implants
- Perform a thorough physical examination of the breasts (see "Primary and Preventive Care" in Part 3)
- Educate patients on the technique of breast self-examination
- Counsel patients on the appropriate screening and diagnostic modalities for life-threatening breast disease, such as mammography and sonography, including timing and follow-up
- Diagnose and manage (consistent with training and experience) or refer for management, patients with:
  —A solid or cystic breast mass
  —A mammographic abnormality
  —Breast pain
  —Physiologic and pathologic nipple discharge
  —Mastitis
  —Fibrocystic conditions
- Counsel patients on familial risk and behavioral factors related to breast disease

The clinician should be knowledgeable regarding the indications and options for breast cancer prevention, including chemoprevention and prophylactic mastectomy. In some circumstances, and with appropriate training and experience, the obstetrician–gynecologist may diagnose by biopsy or participate in the treatment of life-threatening breast disease or both.

Obstetrician–gynecologists who provide mammography services should be in compliance with the Mammography Standards Quality Act and its regulations (see "Compliance with Government Regulations" in Part 1).

Resources

Patient

American College of Obstetricians and Gynecologists. Detecting and treating breast problems. ACOG Patient Education Pamphlet AP026. Washington, DC: ACOG, 1999

American College of Obstetricians and Gynecologists. Mammography. ACOG Patient Education Pamphlet AP076. Washington, DC: ACOG, 1999

Professional

American College of Obstetricians and Gynecologists. Role of the obstetrician–gynecologist in the diagnosis and treatment of breast disease. ACOG Committee Opinion 186. Washington, DC: ACOG, 1997

American College of Obstetricians and Gynecologists. Routine cancer screening. ACOG Committee Opinion 247. Washington, DC: ACOG, 2000

Cholesterol

Health Care Impact

Coronary heart disease (CHD) is the leading cause of death for both men and women in the United States and accounts for about 500,000 deaths each year. Clinical trials have shown that a 1% reduction in serum cholesterol levels results in a 2% reduction in CHD rates. Approximately one quarter to one third of individuals who have a first coronary event will die as a result. Although a short-term benefit from cholesterol reduction is anticipated in patients at high risk for future CHD, the near-term benefit of decreasing cholesterol is greater among those patients with established CHD. Thus, primary prevention (ie, for patients without established CHD) and secondary prevention (ie, for patients with established CHD) are both important health issues.

ACOG Recommendations

Beginning at 45 years of age, women should have their cholesterol level checked every 5 years. Earlier screening may be appropriate in women with risk factors (see "Routine Detection and Prevention of Disease" in Part 3).

Expertise

The National Cholesterol Eduation Program Expert Panel on Detection, Evaluation, and Treatment of High Blood Cholesterol in Adults (Adult Treatment Panel III) has released revised recommendations for treatment of high blood cholesterol. Research indicates that elevated low-density lipoprotein (LDL) cholesterol is a major cause of CHD. In addition, recent clinical trials show that LDL cholesterol-lowering therapy reduces the risk for CHD. For these reasons, the panel considers elevated LDL cholesterol as the primary target of cholesterol-lowering therapy.

Recommended levels of LDL cholesterol are based on risk assessment. Factors to be considered in determining a patient's level of risk include the presence or absence of CHD, diabetes mellitus, and other clinical forms of artherosclerotic disease; cigarette smoking; hypertension; low high-density lipoprotein cholesterol; family history of premature CHD; and age. The panel recommends the use of a risk assessment tool that predicts 10-year risk for developing CHD. Decisions regarding treatment are based on this risk measure.

Treatment of high LDL cholesterol can include therapeutic lifestyle changes and drug therapy, or both, depending on the risk category of the patient. Therapeutic lifestyle changes include dietary changes to reduce intake of saturated fats and cholesterol and enhance intake of plant stanols/sterols and soluble fiber, weight reduction, and increased physical activity. Drug therapy options include statins, bile acid sequestrants, and nicotinic acids. To assist clinicians in the evaluation and treatment of high blood cholesterol, the National Heart, Lung, and Blood Institute has developed a quick desk reference for clinicians based on the recommendations of the Panel (see "Resources").

The Clinical Laboratory Improvement Amendments require federal oversight for all laboratories, including physician offices, that perform tests that examine human specimens for the diagnosis, prevention, or treatment of any disease, impairment of health, or health assessment (see "Compliance with Government Regulations" in Part 1 and Appendix C).

Resources

Patient

American College of Obstetricians and Gynecologists. Cholesterol and your health. ACOG Patient Education Pamphlet AP101. Washington, DC: ACOG, 1995

American College of Obstetricians and Gynecologists. Keeping your heart healthy. ACOG Patient Education Pamphlet AP122. Washington, DC: ACOG, 1998

Professional

American College of Obstetricians and Gynecologists. Hormone replacement therapy. ACOG Educational Bulletin 247. Washington, DC: ACOG, 1998

Association of Professors of Gynecology and Obstetrics. Cardiovascular disease in women: pathophysiology, diagnosis and treatment. APGO Educational Series on Women's Health Issues. Washington, DC: APGO, 1998

Association of Professors of Gynecology and Obstetrics. Managing hyperlipidemia in women. APGO Educational Series on Women's Health Issues. Washington, DC: APGO, 1999

Executive Summary of The Third Report of The National Cholesterol Education Program (NCEP) Expert Panel on Detection, Evaluation, and Treatment of High Blood Cholesterol In Adults (Adult Treatment Panel III). JAMA 2001;285:2486–2497

Chronic Pelvic Pain

Health Care Impact

Chronic pelvic pain is defined as episodic or continuous pain for 6 months or longer that is severe enough to affect daily function. More than 10% of all gynecologic referrals are for chronic pelvic pain, and the affiliated cost to diagnose and treat this condition is estimated to exceed $2 billion each year. This condition leads to 70,000 hysterectomies annually. Endometriosis is the most common condition associated with chronic pelvic pain. See the box for a list of most of the conditions that are associated with chronic pelvic pain (see also "Endometriosis" in Part 4).

ACOG Recommendations

Evaluation of chronic pelvic pain includes history, physical examination, and laboratory testing that depends on the clinical findings. Treatment should be directed at correcting the underlying condition whenever possible. However, it is not always necessary or possible to establish a diagnosis prior to therapy, and patients in this group can be effectively treated using the general principles of pain management (see also "Pain Management" in Part 4).

Conditions Associated with Chronic Pelvic Pain

GYNECOLOGIC

- Extrauterine
  - —Adhesions
  - —Chronic ectopic pregnancy
  - —Chronic pelvic infection
  - —Endometriosis
  - —Residual ovary syndrome
- Uterine
  - —Adenomyosis
  - —Chronic endometritis
  - —Leiomyomata
  - —Intrauterine contraceptive device
  - —Pelvic congestion
  - —Pelvic support defects
  - —Endometrial polyps

UROLOGIC

- Chronic urinary tract infection
- Detrusor overactivity
- Interstitial cystitis
- Stone
- Suburethral diverticulitis
- Urethral syndrome

GASTROINTESTINAL

- Cholelithiasis
- Chronic appendicitis
- Constipation
- Diverticular disease
- Enterocolitis
- Gastric/duodenal ulcer
- Inflammatory bowel disease (Crohn's disease, ulcerative colitis)
- Irritable bowel syndrome
- Neoplasia

MUSCULOSKELETAL

- Coccydynia
- Disk problems
- Degenerative joint disease
- Fibromyositis
- Hernias
- Herpes zoster (shingles)
- Low back pain
- Levator ani syndrome (spasm of pelvic floor)
- Myofascial pain (trigger points, spasms)
- Nerve entrapment syndromes
- Osteoporosis (fractures)
- Pain posture
- Scoliosis/lordosis/kyphosis
- Strains/sprains

OTHER

- Abuse (physical or sexual, prior or current)
- Heavy metal poisoning (lead, mercury)
- Hyperparathyroidism
- Porphyria
- Psychiatric disorders (depression, bipolar disorder, inadequate personality disorder)
- Psychosocial stress (marital discord, work stress)
- Sickle cell crisis
- Sleep disturbances
- Somatoform disorders
- Substance use (especially cocaine)
- Sympathetic dystrophy
- Tabes dorsalis (third-degree syphilis)

Expertise

In general, four areas of expertise are required to evaluate and treat women with chronic pelvic pain:

1. Evaluation expertise—History, physical examination, and interpretation of the results of specialized diagnostic studies (eg, magnetic resonance imaging, sonography, barium enema, pyelography)
2. Surgical expertise—Diagnostic laparoscopy, operative laparoscopic skills, familiarity with indications for pelvic denervation procedures (sacral and presacral procedures), hysterectomy with or without salpingo-oophorectomy, and pelvic floor reconstruction
3. Pain management—Positive reinforcement and support, ability to assess psychologic factors, prompt pain treatment, consideration of multiple treatment modalities, and knowledge of indication and precautions for narcotic drug use
4. Multidisciplinary—Referral for psychotherapy, pain management, marriage and sex counseling, biofeedback, depression treatment, or physiotherapy

Clinicians should be familiar with any state requirements for reporting domestic violence.

RESOURCES

Patient

American College of Obstetricians and Gynecologists. Pelvic pain. ACOG Patient Education Pamphlet AP099. Washington, DC: ACOG, 1999

Professional

American College of Obstetricians and Gynecologists. Medical management of endometriosis. ACOG Practice Bulletin 11. Washington, DC: ACOG, 1999

Crisis Intervention

Health Care Impact

Crises, such as angry, violent, suicidal, or psychotic patients, partners, or family members, may arise during the course of patient care. Women may present acutely as victims of violence. Others may be undergoing social distress and require emergency attention. Mechanisms for dealing with security issues, psychiatric emergencies (including involuntary commitment), and urgent social needs such as shelter, safety, and transportation should be established.

ACOG Recommendations

The American College of Obstetricians and Gynecologists recommends that clinicians be able to recognize signs of abuse and mental crises and to refer patients to support services available in the community. These support services include shelters for battered women, nonresidential counseling services, community resources, and agencies that can advise women of their legal rights.

Expertise

Clinicians should identify approaches and resources for women in crisis. The clinician's ability to recognize evidence of crisis, elicit information from the patient, and work out a plan with the patient is critically important. In most cases these approaches are likely to include assistance from mental health care practitioners, such as psychiatrists, psychologists, social workers, and case managers. Some patients may have access to confidential counseling resources through employee assistance programs provided by employers.

For situations of violence or social distress, plans should include safe locations to which women can be referred to stay as problems are worked through. Clinicians should be familiar with any state requirements for reporting domestic violence. In the case of acute mental illness, this may include admission to a psychiatric care unit. Staff and clinicians also may be threatened, and mechanisms for protection and emergency response should be available and periodically reviewed (see also "Facilities and Equipment" in Part 2).

RESOURCES

Patient

American College of Obstetricians and Gynecologists. The abused woman. ACOG Patient Education Pamphlet AP083. Washington, DC: ACOG, 1998

American College of Obstetricians and Gynecologists. Depression. ACOG Patient Education Pamphlet AP106. Washington, DC: ACOG, 1999

Professional

American College of Obstetricians and Gynecologists. A guide to responding to violence against health providers. Washington, DC: ACOG, 1996

American College of Obstetricians and Gynecologists. Domestic violence. ACOG Educational Bulletin 257. Washington, DC: ACOG, 1999

Sibbald B. Physician, protect thyself. CMAJ 1998;159:987–989

DEPRESSION

Health Care Impact

Mood disorders, especially depression, are among the most common psychiatric illnesses in women. The risk of developing depression during a woman's lifetime is approximately 20%, in contrast with 10% for men, and is higher in women in their reproductive years, with a prevalence of 8–10%. The reasons for this disparity are multidimensional and may include biological, social, and economic issues that are particular to women.

The economic cost of depressive illnesses is $30–44 billion per year; the human costs cannot be estimated. The lives of 17.6 million adults and millions more family members and friends are affected. Of all people hospitalized for depression, 15% will eventually take their own lives.

ACOG Recommendations

Obstetrician–gynecologists should be able to diagnose and initiate therapy for most patients with uncomplicated depression (see also "Routine Detection and Prevention of Disease" in Part 3). As a part of patient education, it should be emphasized that depression is a medical illness and not a character defect or weakness and that in most cases it can be treated effectively. However, the risk of recurrence is significant; patients should be alert to early signs and symptoms of recurrence and seek treatment.

Expertise

Health care professionals working with women have a unique advantage to identify and diagnose depression. It is estimated that 1 in 10 U.S. adults experience depression each year, and nearly two thirds do not get the help they need. If depression is identified, it can be effectively treated in up to 85% of cases. Treatment may include medication, psychotherapy, or both. Clinicians will need to provide follow-up care for any patients that have not been referred elsewhere. The likelihood of a recurrence is 50% after a major episode of depression, and continues to increase with each occurrence.

Selection of treatment should, whenever possible, be a collaborative decision between practitioner and patient. Such shared decision making is likely to increase adherence and, therefore, treatment effectiveness. Medications should be considered for patients with moderate or severe depression, prior positive response to medication, or recurrent depression and for the patient who prefers medication to psychotherapy. The obstetrician–gynecologist should be aware of several drugs in different categories that he or she would feel comfortable prescribing. Psychotherapy alone often is effective in treating cases of mild or moderate depression, and a psychotherapy referral should be considered for relatively mild depression and when it is the patient's preference. Combined treatment with both psychotherapy and medication should be considered when the depression is more severe, there is a significant psychosocial issue that would respond to therapy, or the patient has a history of treatment noncompliance or recurrent depression.

The major categories of antidepressant medication are tricyclic agents, selective serotonin reuptake inhibitors (SSRIs), heterocyclic agents, and monoamine oxidase inhibitors. No one antidepressant is clearly more effective than another. Choices often are made on the basis of side effects. Safety of the medication and lack of significant side effects make SSRIs a first choice in antidepressants. Tricyclic agents often are used because of lower initial cost and greater experience with their use. However, several studies indicate that SSRIs are as cost-effective as tricyclic agents because they have fewer side effects, require less frequent medication changes, and have a higher rate of compliance. Either SSRIs or tricyclic agents should be considered for initial treatment by the obstetrician–gynecologist. Like the SSRIs, the heterocyclics bupropion and trazodone appear safer in cases of potential overdose. Clinicians should be aware that bupropion is marketed under a different name (Zyban) for smoking cessation. Note that monoamine oxidase inhibitors can have adverse effects and fatal interactions with other medications. Only those practitioners with significant experience with these medications should prescribe them.

All depressed patients, especially adolescents, should be evaluated for suicidal thinking and impulses. This is done by direct questioning. If a woman has specific plans or significant risk for suicide, such as prior attempts or hopelessness, a mental health specialist should be consulted immediately. Alcohol and drug abuse correlates highly with symptoms of depression. Patients who abuse substances are more difficult to treat and are at higher risk for suicide; for such patients, treatment by a mental health specialist may be preferred.

There are other conditions that one must keep in mind and distinguish from depression, including bipolar disorder, grief, substance abuse, schizophrenia, dementia, medical illness, and medication effect. Patients who report symptoms of mania have a bipolar disorder, and medical treatment will vary from treatment for depression. Antidepressant medications can induce mania and should be used with caution in a patient previously treated for mania. In such cases, referral to a psychiatrist is recommended.

Referral also is recommended for the following situations:

- Depression with suicide risk
- Bipolar disorder
- Depression with psychotic symptoms (hallucinations, delusions)
- Depression in a pediatric or adolescent patient
- Failure to respond to previous interventions
- Practitioner's lack of comfort with treating the patient

The practitioner should have referral options available, such as the following sources:

- Mental health specialists
- Employee assistance programs
- Health maintenance organizations
- Community mental health centers
- Hospital departments of psychiatry or outpatient psychiatric clinics
- Family service/social agencies
- Private clinics and facilities

RESOURCES

Patient

Agency for Health Care Policy and Research. Depression is a treatable illness: a patient's guide. AHCPR Publication No. 93-0553. Rockville, Maryland: AHCPR, 1993

American College of Obstetricians and Gynecologists. Depression. ACOG Patient Education Pamphlet AP106. Washington, DC: ACOG, 1999

Professional

Agency for Health Care Policy and Research. Treatment of depression: newer pharmacotherapies. AHCPR Evidence report/technology assessment no. 7. Rockville, Maryland: AHCPR, 1999

American Psychiatric Association. Diagnostic and statistical manual of mental disorders: DSM-IV-TR. 4th ed, text revision. Washington, DC: APA, 2000

Depression Guideline Panel. Depression in primary care: detection, diagnosis, and treatment. Quick reference guide for clinicians, No. 5. Rockville, Maryland: U.S. Department of Health and Human Services, Public Health Service, Agency for Health Care Policy and Research, 1993; AHCPR publication no. 93-0552

National Mental Health Association
1021 Prince Street
Alexandria, VA 22314-2971
800-969-NMHA (6642)
www.nmha.org

Domestic or Intimate Partner Violence

Health Care Impact

Domestic or intimate partner violence is a widespread social and public health problem that disproportionately affects women of all age, racial, educational, and socioeconomic groups. Although the true extent of domestic violence is difficult to ascertain, prevalence studies estimate that nearly 5 million adult women experience domestic violence in the United States each year. Research suggests that pregnancy may increase a woman's risk for abuse, that the pattern and severity of violence may escalate during pregnancy, and that it is prevalent in the postpartum period. According to the U.S. Department of Justice, violence by an intimate partner accounts for approximately 21% of all the violent crime experienced by women. Among female murder victims, about 30% are killed by an intimate partner.

In addition to the long-term physical harm that may be caused by violence, there is a growing body of research that links violence with a wide range of emotional and behavioral sequelae. These responses may, in turn, lead to additional health care problems and are frequently associated with over-utilization of health care resources. Economic losses related to adult domestic violence, including medical costs, other tangible losses, and quality of life losses, are estimated at $67 billion each year.

ACOG Recommendations

Because of the prevalence of violence, being female is a significant enough risk factor to warrant screening every patient at periodic intervals, such as annual examinations and new patient visits (see also "Routine Detection and Prevention of Disease" in Part 3). In the office setting, the most effective and efficient strategy for providing assistance to a woman who has disclosed abuse involves acknowledging the trauma, providing education and support, and offering referrals to community support services. The clinician must remain caring and supportive of the patient as she works through these crises, even if she chooses to remain in the relationship. Clinician responsibilities in addressing domestic violence include:

- Implement universal screening
- Acknowledge the trauma
- Assess immediate safety
- Help establish a safety plan
- Review options
- Offer educational materials
- Offer a list of community and local resources
- Provide referrals
- Document interactions
- Provide ongoing support at subsequent visits

Expertise

When a patient confides that she has been abused, it is useful to have a protocol for responding that is easily implemented and uses available resources. The physician must be prepared to discuss the abuse with the woman and establish a plan to deal with medical needs, psychosocial needs, and emergent issues. When past or ongoing victimization is identified, an important step is to acknowledge the trauma and reinforce the fact that the patient is not to blame.

Once domestic violence is identified and acknowledged, the next step is to assess immediate safety. If the violence in the woman's home has escalated to the point where she is afraid for her safety, she should be offered shelter by directly contacting or referring her to social work services, women's shelters, or community services for battered women. If the patient is not in need of immediate shelter, she should be advised that shelter is available if needed in the future. She should be provided with information on community resources and referred for continued assistance and support.

In particularly distressed women, an assessment for suicide risk may be indicated. Obviously, in acute crisis situations that involve serious risks to the life of the victim, her children, or others, crisis intervention resources should by used.

Psychologic and social assistance is best provided by services that are "trauma specific," meaning the practitioners are experienced in treating victims of intimate partner abuse. Most agencies for battered women and rape crisis centers have expertise in dealing with all forms of violence against women.

Because perpetrators often retaliate when they suspect disclosure of abuse, every effort should be made to maintain confidentiality, especially regarding telephone calls or when materials, such as bills, are sent to the patient. Office staff must be informed about the importance of confidentiality when there is any contact with the patient's home.

Laws regarding reporting obligations vary widely between states, therefore, familiarity with local laws and policies is critical. In all states, physicians are required by law to report suspected child abuse. Mandatory reporting of domestic violence is required by some states, but this remains a controversial issue especially with regard to issues of patient safety and confidentiality. Information regarding state reporting requirements are available through state medical associations, local domestic violence programs, or the state attorney general's office.

Resources

Patient

American College of Obstetricians and Gynecologists. The abused woman. ACOG Patient Education Pamphlet AP083. Washington, DC: ACOG, 1998

American College of Obstetricians and Gynecologists
Violence Against Women Home Page
www.acog.com/from_home/departments/dept_web.cfm?recno=17

National 24-hour Toll-Free Hotline Numbers:
800-799-SAFE (7233) and 800-787-3224 (TDD)

Professional

American College of Obstetricians and Gynecologists. Domestic violence. ACOG Educational Bulletin 257. Washington, DC: ACOG, 1999

American College of Obstetricians and Gynecologists. Domestic violence: the role of the physician in identification, intervention, and prevention: speaker's package. Washington, DC: ACOG, 1995

American College of Obstetricians and Gynecologists. Mandatory reporting of domestic violence. ACOG Committee Opinion 200. Washington, DC: ACOG, 1998

American College of Obstetricians and Gynecologists
Violence Against Women Home Page
www.acog.com/from_home/departments/dept_web.cfm?recno=17

American Medical Association. Diagnostic and treatment guidelines on domestic violence. Chicago: AMA, 1992

American Medical Association. Diagnostic and treatment guidelines on mental health effects of family violence. Chicago: AMA, 1995

Horan DL, Chapin J, Klein L, Schmidt LA, Schulkin J. Domestic violence screening practices of obstetrician–gynecologists. Obstet Gynecol 1998;92:785–789

Jones RF 3rd, Horan DL. The American College of Obstetricians and Gynecologists: a decade of responding to violence against women. Int J Gynaecol Obstet 1997;58:43–50

Tjaden P, Thoennes N. Prevalence, incidence, and consequences of violence against women: findings from the national violence against women survey. Research in Brief. Washington, DC: U.S. Department of Justice, Office of Justice Programs, November 1998, NCJ 172837

Early Pregnancy Complications: Spontaneous Abortion and Ectopic Pregnancy

Health Care Impact

Spontaneous abortion and ectopic pregnancy are the most common complications during the first trimester of pregnancy. The management of early pregnancy complications is within the purview of obstetrician–gynecologists and other general practitioners of women's health care. Clinicians should be aware of credentialing issues at their hospitals and with their professional liability insurance carrier as to whether this is viewed as an obstetric or gynecologic issue.

Spontaneous Abortion

Approximately 15–20% of clinical pregnancies are spontaneously lost in the first or second trimester. A mathematical derivation suggests that 50–75% of all human conceptions may ultimately be lost, with the majority of losses occurring before detection of the pregnancy. Recurrent pregnancy loss is typically defined as two or three or more consecutive pregnancy losses, and affects about 1% of couples (see "Recurrent Pregnancy Loss" in Part 4).

Overall, 30–50% of spontaneous abortions are chromosomally abnormal. Spontaneously aborted tissues with chromosomal variations most commonly contain aneuploid abnormalities, and trisomy is the leading aneuploid condition.

Ectopic Pregnancy

Based on current trends, more than 150,000 ectopic pregnancies (approximately 20/1,000 live births) will be diagnosed this year in the United States. Women with known risks for ectopic pregnancy usually will seek care early in the gestation to exclude an ectopic pregnancy. Important risks include advanced reproductive age, prior fertility treatment, pelvic infection, or previous ectopic pregnancy. Unfortunately, most women who are affected with an ectopic pregnancy are unaware of any risk and usually seek care when symptoms develop (most notably pain).

The number of deaths from ectopic pregnancy has dropped during the past decade. Approximately 25–30 women die annually in the United States as a direct result of ectopic pregnancy, making ectopic pregnancy the fourth leading cause of maternal death in this country. It has been estimated that nearly half of those who died were evaluated medically before their death.

ACOG Recommendations

The American College of Obstetricians and Gynecologists has established recommendations for the medical treatment of ectopic pregnancy. Intramuscular methotrexate is appropriate for the treatment of small, unruptured tubal pregnancies in selected patients. Successful treatment may require more than one dose of methotrexate. The expectant management of threatened abortion or the surgical management of abortive or ectopic pregnancy require consideration of the reproductive desire of the patient, as well as clinical judgment. Finally, there may be a place for expectant management of women with low levels of human chorionic gonadotropin (hCG) that are falling.

Expertise

In addition to the history of signs and symptoms, diagnosis of spontaneous abortion or ectopic pregnancy may involve:

- Interpretation of serum hCG measurements
- Interpretation of endovaginal sonography
- Interpretation of serum progesterone concentrations
- Physical diagnosis
- Surgical procedures such as dilation and curettage, culdocentesis, laparoscopy, or laparotomy

Diagnosis of ectopic pregnancy is presumed in the presence of a hemoperitoneum in the first trimester, abnormally low hCG increments over time, and an empty uterus on sonography when the hCG value is above the discriminatory zone. Ectopic pregnancy is confirmed when an ectopic pregnancy can be visualized, either laparoscopically or with endovaginal sonography.

Treatment options for ectopic pregnancy include expectant observation, medical chemotherapy (principally methotrexate), and surgery, as indicated. The choice of therapy is complex and must provide for the skill of the clinician, experience with treatment modalities, and the reproductive desire of the patient. Treatment options for spontaneous abortion may include:

- Observation
- Uterine curettage
- Review of histopathology
- Evaluation for causes of recurrent spontaneous abortion (see "Recurrent Pregnancy Loss" in Part 4)
- Grief counseling, as indicated

Clinicians should be familiar with any state requirements regarding the reporting of fetal death and disposal of fetal remains.

Resources

Patient

American College of Obstetricians and Gynecologists. Early pregnancy loss: miscarriage, ectopic pregnancy, and molar pregnancy. ACOG Patient Education Pamphlet AP090. Washington, DC: ACOG, 1998

American College of Obstetricians and Gynecologists. Grieving: a way to heal. ACOG Patient Education Pamphlet AP078. Washington, DC: ACOG, 1997

RESOLVE: The National Infertility Association
1310 Broadway
Somerville, MA 02144-1731
(617) 623-0744
www.resolve.org
E-mail: resolveinc@aol.com

RTS Perinatal Bereavement Program
Gunderson Lutheran Medical Center
1910 South Avenue
La Crosse, WI 54601
800-362-9567, ext 4747
www.gundluth.org/bereave
E-mail: berservs@gundluth.org

Professional

American Academy of Pediatrics, American College of Obstetricians and Gynecologists. Appendix E. Standard terminology for reporting of reproductive health statistics in the United States. In: Guidelines for perinatal care. 4th ed. Elk Grove Village, Illinois: AAP; Washington, DC: ACOG, 1997:311–329

American College of Obstetricians and Gynecologists. Management of recurrent early pregnancy loss. ACOG Practice Bulletin 24. Washington, DC: ACOG, 2001

American College of Obstetricians and Gynecologists. Medical management of tubal pregnancy. ACOG Practice Bulletin 3. Washington, DC: ACOG, 1998

American Society for Reproductive Medicine. Early diagnosis and management of ectopic pregnancy. ASRM Guidelines for Practice. Birmingham, Alabama: ASRM, 1992

Boklage CE. Survival probability of human conceptions from fertilization to term. Int J Fertil 1990;35:75, 79–80, 81–94

Ectopic pregnancy—United States, 1990–1992. MMWR Morb Mortal Wkly Rep 1995;44: 46–48

Royal College of Obstetricians and Gynaecologists. The management of tubal pregnancies. RCOG Guideline No 21. London: RCOG, 1999

Eating Disorders

Health Care Impact

More than 5 million Americans are affected by eating disorders each year. Anorexia nervosa, bulimia nervosa, and binge-eating disorder are characterized by severe disturbances in eating behavior. They can have life-threatening consequences. Anorexia nervosa ranks third among common chronic disorders in adolescents, surpassed only by asthma and obesity. It is a disorder of self-starvation, which manifests itself in an extreme aversion to food and can cause psychologic, physiologic, endocrine, and gynecologic problems (see box). The overwhelming majority (95%) of patients diagnosed with anorexia are female. Ages most frequently affected are 12–18, but anorexia does occur in older women and has been reported in young children. Of anorexia nervosa patients, 10–15% die.

With bulimia, there also is a negative self-image and a struggle with depression and other psychologic problems. Bulimics do not deny themselves food, but indulge in excess food consumption and then purge it out of their systems using laxatives and self-induced vomiting.

Binge eating (also called compulsive eating) involves eating large amounts of food. In this way, it is similar to bulimia. However, binge eaters do not routinely engage in purging behaviors.

ACOG Recommendations

The American College of Obstetricians and Gynecologists recommends that all women be counseled on dietary and nutritional issues, yearly or as appropriate. All adolescents should be screened annually for eating disorders and obesity by determining weight and stature, calculating body mass index, and asking about body image and eating patterns.

Test results and vital signs may help to confirm the suspicion of eating disorders and identify patients needing emergency hospitalization. The following general guidelines should be used.

Diagnostic Criteria for Anorexia Nervosa and Bulimia Nervosa

ANOREXIA NERVOSA

A. Refusal to maintain body weight at or above a minimally normal weight for age and height (eg, weight loss leading to maintenance of body weight less than 85% of that expected; or failure to make expected weight gain during period of growth, leading to body weight less than 85% of that expected).
B. Intense fear of gaining weight or becoming fat, even though underweight.
C. Disturbance in the way in which one's body weight or shape is experienced, undue influence of body weight or shape on self-evaluation, or denial of the seriousness of the current low body weight.
D. In postmenarcheal females, amenorrhea, ie, the absence of at least three consecutive menstrual cycles. (A woman is considered to have amenorrhea if her periods occur only following hormone, eg, estrogen, administration.)

SPECIFY TYPE:

Restricting Type: During the current episode of anorexia nervosa, the person has not regularly engaged in binge-eating or purging behavior (ie, self-induced vomiting or the misuse of laxatives, diuretics, or enemas)

Binge-Eating/Purging Type: During the current episode of anorexia nervosa, the person has regularly engaged in binge-eating or purging behavior (ie, self-induced vomiting or the misuse of laxatives, diuretics, or enemas)

BULIMIA NERVOSA

A. Recurrent episodes of binge eating. An episode of binge eating is characterized by both of the following:
   1. Eating, in a discrete period of time (eg, within any 2-hour period), an amount of food that is definitely larger than most people would eat during a similar period of time and under similar circumstances
   2. A sense of lack of control over eating during the episode (eg, a feeling that one cannot stop eating or control what or how much one is eating)
B. Recurrent inappropriate compensatory behavior in order to prevent weight gain, such as self-induced vomiting; misuse of laxatives, diuretics, enemas, or other medications; fasting; or excessive exercise.
C. The binge eating and inappropriate compensatory behaviors both occur, on average, at least twice a week for 3 months.
D. Self-evaluation is unduly influenced by body shape and weight.
E. The disturbance does not occur exclusively during episodes of anorexia nervosa.

(continued)

Diagnostic Criteria for Anorexia Nervosa and Bulimia Nervosa *(continued)*

Specify type:

Purging Type: During the current episode of bulimia nervosa, the person has regularly engaged in self-induced vomiting or the misuse of laxatives, diuretics, or enemas

Nonpurging Type: During the current episode of bulimia nervosa, the person has used other inappropriate compensatory behaviors, such as fasting or excessive exercise, but has not regularly engaged in self-induced vomiting or the misuse of laxatives, diuretics, or enemas

Eating Disorder Not Otherwise Specified

This category is for disorders of eating that do not meet the criteria for any specific eating disorder. Examples include:

1. For females, all of the criteria for anorexia nervosa are met except that the individual has regular menses.
2. All of the criteria for anorexia nervosa are met except that, despite significant weight loss, the individual's current weight is in the normal range.
3. All the criteria for bulimia nervosa are met except that the binge eating and inappropriate compensatory mechanisms occur at a frequency of less than twice a week or for a duration of less than 3 months.
4. The regular use of inappropriate compensatory behavior by an individual of normal body weight after eating small amounts of food (eg, self-induced vomiting after the consumption of 2 cookies).
5. Repeatedly chewing and spitting out, but not swallowing, large amounts of food.
6. Binge-eating disorder: recurrent episodes of binge eating in the absence of the regular use of inappropriate compensatory behaviors characteristic of bulimia nervosa (see Appendix B in DSM-IV for suggested research criteria).

Adapted from American Psychiatric Association. Reprinted with permission from the Diagnostic and statistical manual of mental disorders: DSM-IV-TR. 4th ed, text revision. Washington, DC: APA, 2000:589–594,

Adolescents should be assessed for organic disease, anorexia nervosa, or bulimia if any of the following conditions or behaviors are found:

- Amenorrhea or abnormal menses
- Refusal to maintain body weight at or above a normal weight for age and height

- Recurrent dieting when not overweight
- Use of self-induced emesis, laxatives, starvation, or diuretics to lose weight
- Distorted body image
- Body mass index below the 5th percentile
- Hypotension, bradycardia, cardiac arrhythmia, or hypothermia
- Excessive exercising

Expertise

Women's health care practitioners are in a unique role to be able to take a history, diagnose, and refer a patient with eating disorders. The American Psychological Association has outlined the following treatment goals:

- Solve malnutrition and other biologically mediated problems
- Address psychological, behavioral, and social deficits
- Resolve culturally mediated distortions

Treatment for anorexia nervosa and bulimia nervosa may include hospitalization, nutritional rehabilitation, psychosocial treatment, medications, the use of the addiction model, or a combination of psychosocial and medication strategies. The clinician who finds indications of an eating disorder in his or her patient should consider diagnostic studies, which may include:

- Complete blood count (usually normal, may have low white blood cell count)
- Thyroid function tests (thyroxine and triiodothyronine low in anorexia)
- Electrocardiography (cardiac abnormalities: slow heart rate, disturbances of heart rhythm)
- Electrolytes (abnormal related to purgative methods)
- Creatine phosphokinase (elevated in ipecac use)
- Reproductive hormones (low in weight loss)

Medical complications of anorexia nervosa include cardiac abnormalities, dangerously low blood pressure and body temperature, low white blood cell count, chronic constipation, osteoporosis, slowed adolescent growth or development, short stature, loss of menstrual periods, infertility, hair loss, and fingernail destruction. The medical complications of bulimia nervosa include electrolyte abnormalities that can lead to heart rhythm disturbances, dehydration, dangerously low blood pressure, menstrual cycle abnormalities, enlarged parotid glands, destruction of dental enamel, dental cavities, and bowel abnormalities.

Once a suspicion or diagnosis of an eating disorder has been made, the clinician should assess his or her ability to identify continuing problems, give the needed time and energy to the patient, and refer when needed. Supporting services may include psychiatric or eating disorder programs or facilities, if available. Clinicians should be familiar with any state regulations regarding confidentiality and parental consent for treatment.

Resources

Patient

American College of Obstetricians and Gynecologists. Eating disorders. ACOG Patient Education Pamphlet AP144. Washington, DC: ACOG, 2000

American College of Obstetricians and Gynecologists. Weight control: eating right and keeping fit. ACOG Patient Education Pamphlet AP064.Washington, DC: ACOG, 1999

Eating Disorders Awareness and Prevention
603 Stewart Street—Suite 803
Seattle, WA 98101
800-931-2337
www.edap.org
E-mail: info@edap.org

Professional

American Anorexia Bulimia Association, Inc.
165 W 46th Street—Suite 1108
New York, NY 10036
(212) 575-6200
www.aabainc.org
E-mail: amanbu@aol.com

American College of Obstetricians and Gynecologists. Primary and preventive health care for female adolescents. ACOG Educational Bulletin 254. Washington, DC: ACOG, 1999

American Psychiatric Association. Diagnostic and statistical manual of mental disorders: DSM-IV-TR. 4th ed, text revision. Washington, DC: APA, 2000

Becker AE, Grinspoon SK, Klibanski A, Herzog DB. Eating disorders. N Engl J Med 1999; 340:1092–1098

Harvard Eating Disorder Center
356 Boylston Street
Boston, MA 02116
888-236-1188
www.hedc.org/
E-mail: info@hedc.org

Lucas AR, Beard CM, O'Fallon WM, Kurland LT. 50-year trends in the incidence of anorexia nervosa in Rochester, Minn.: a population-based study. Am J Psychiatry 1991; 148:917–922

Muscari ME. Thin line: managing care for adolescents with anorexia and bulimia. MCN Am J Matern Child Nurs 1998;23:130–140; quiz 141

ENDOCRINE DISORDERS

Health Care Impact

In addition to diabetes (see "Routine Detection and Prevention of Disease" in Part 3), other important alterations of endocrine homeostasis affecting women include diseases of the thyroid, hyperandrogenism, and amenorrhea. Diseases of the thyroid affect approximately 1–4% of women, and the prevalence increases with age. Between 6% and 10% of reproductive age women have hyperandrogenic chronic anovulation (eg, polycystic ovary syndrome), and nonpregnancy-related amenorrhea during reproductive age affects an estimated 0.5% of the female population.

ACOG Recommendations

Evaluation and treatment of female endocrine disorders requires an orderly approach to laboratory testing. Underlying disorders may include life-threatening diagnoses. The goals of therapy should be correction of life-threatening disorders, avoidance of endometrial abnormalities, preservation or restoration of fertility, and reversal of cosmetically disturbing hirsutism.

Expertise

Often the evaluation and treatment of these conditions require consultation or referral to a medical or reproductive endocrinologist. Diagnosis of endocrine disorders should include:

- Review of menstrual history
- Laboratory assessments for thyroid function studies, ovarian and adrenal androgens, 17-hydroxyprogesterone, prolactin, and pituitary gonadotropins
- Endometrial assessment (biopsy or ultrasonography)
- Selected central nervous system/pituitary imaging

RESOURCES

Patient

American College of Obstetricians and Gynecologists. Evaluating infertility. ACOG Patient Education Pamphlet AP136. Washington, DC: ACOG, 2000

American College of Obstetricians and Gynecologists. Polycystic ovary syndrome. ACOG Patient Education Pamphlet AP121. Washington, DC: ACOG, 1998

American College of Obstetricians and Gynecologists. Thyroid disease. ACOG Patient Education Pamphlet AP128. Washington, DC: ACOG, 1999

American College of Obstetricians and Gynecologists. Treating infertility. ACOG Patient Education Pamphlet AP137. Washington, DC: ACOG, 2000

Professional

American Society for Reproductive Medicine. Current evaluation and treatment of amenorrhea. ASRM Guideline for Practice. Birmingham, Alabama: ASRM, 1994

American Society for Reproductive Medicine. The evaluation and treatment of androgen excess. ASRM Guideline for Practice. Birmingham, Alabama: ASRM, 2000

American Society for Reproductive Medicine. Use of insulin sensitizing agents in the treatment of polycystic ovary syndrome. ASRM Committee Opinion. Birmingham, Alabama: ASRM, 2000

ENDOMETRIOSIS

Health Care Impact

Endometriosis, defined as the presence of endometrial tissue outside the uterine cavity, is a gynecologic condition that occurs in 7–10% of women in the general population and up to 50% of premenopausal women. In the infertile population, the prevalence has been reported to be 38%. A familial predisposition toward endometriosis via a proposed polygenic/multifactorial mechanism has been documented. A female patient who has an affected first-degree relative has an approximately 10-fold increased risk for developing the disease. Cervical or vaginal atresia and müllerian fusion defects with obstructed outflow are commonly associated with pelvic endometriosis; this represents another genetic or at least congenital mechanism.

Symptoms and sequelae include:

- Adnexal mass (symptomatic or asymptomatic)
- Dysmenorrhea
- Abnormal uterine bleeding
- Chronic pelvic pain
- Dyspareunia
- Infertility
- Uterosacral ligament nodularity

Classification has been attempted by many. The classification system developed by the American Society of Reproductive Medicine (previously the American Fertility Society) is the most commonly used (Fig. 4–1). This system incorporates into the classification a means to record information on the disease morphology, clearly documenting the extent and location of disease.

Both medical and surgical modalities have been used for management. Although evidence exists to support short-term benefits on pain outcomes with either modality, there are no substantive data to indicate the

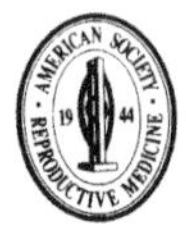

AMERICAN SOCIETY FOR REPRODUCTIVE MEDICINE
REVISED CLASSIFICATION OF ENDOMETRIOSIS

Patient's Name ________________ Date ________________

Stage I (Minimal) - 1-5
Stage II (Mild) - 6-15
Stage III (Moderate) - 16-40
Stage IV (Severe) - >40
Total ________

Laparoscopy ______ Laparotomy ______ Photography ______
Recommended Treatment ________________

Prognosis ________________

	ENDOMETRIOSIS	<1cm	1-3cm	>3cm
PERITONEUM	Superficial	1	2	4
	Deep	2	4	6
OVARY	R Superficial	1	2	4
	Deep	4	16	20
	L Superficial	1	2	4
	Deep	4	16	20

	POSTERIOR CULDESAC OBLITERATION	Partial	Complete
		4	40

	ADHESIONS	<1/3 Enclosure	1/3-2/3 Enclosure	>2/3 Enclosure
OVARY	R Filmy	1	2	4
	Dense	4	8	16
	L Filmy	1	2	4
	Dense	4	8	16
TUBE	R Filmy	1	2	4
	Dense	4*	8*	16
	L Filmy	1	2	4
	Dense	4*	8*	16

*If the fimbriated end of the fallopian tube is completely enclosed, change the point assignment to 16.

Denote appearance of superficial implant types as red [(R), red, red-pink, flamelike, vesicular blobs, clear vesicles], white [(W), opacifications, peritoneal defects, yellow-brown], or black [(B) black, hemosiderin deposits, blue]. Denote percent of total described as R___%, W___% and B___%. Total should equal 100%.

Additional Endometriosis: ________________

Associated Pathology: ________________

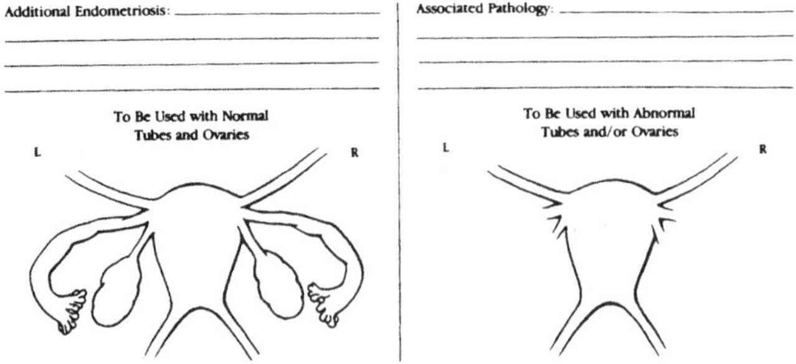

Fig. 4–1. American Society for Reproductive Medicine: Revised Classification of Endometriosis. (Reprinted by permission from the American Society for Reproductive Medicine. Revised American Society for Reproductive Medicine classification of endometriosis: 1996. Fertil Steril 1997;67:817–821)

EXAMPLES & GUIDELINES

STAGE I (MINIMAL)

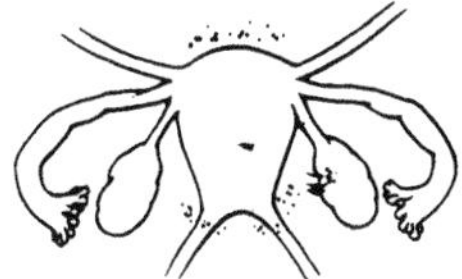

PERITONEUM			
Superficial Endo	-	1-3cm	- 2
R. OVARY			
Superficial Endo	-	< 1cm	- 1
Filmy Adhesions	-	< 1/3	- 1
TOTAL POINTS			4

STAGE II (MILD)

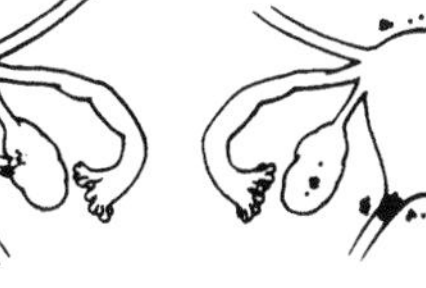

PERITONEUM			
Deep Endo	-	> 3cm	- 6
R. OVARY			
Superficial Endo	-	< 1cm	- 1
Filmy Adhesions	-	< 1/3	- 1
L. OVARY			
Superficial Endo	-	< 1cm	- 1
TOTAL POINTS			9

STAGE III (MODERATE)

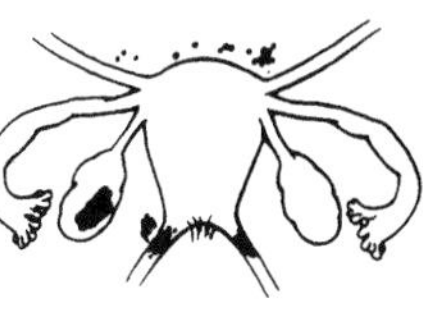

PERITONEUM			
Deep Endo	-	> 3cm	- 6
CULDESAC			
Partial Obliteration			- 4
L. OVARY			
Deep Endo	-	1-3cm	- 16
TOTAL POINTS			26

STAGE III (MODERATE)

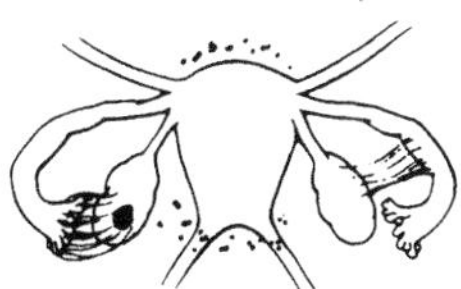

PERITONEUM			
Superficial Endo	-	> 3cm	-4
R. TUBE			
Filmy Adhesions	-	< 1/3	- 1
R. OVARY			
Filmy Adhesions	-	< 1/3	- 1
L. TUBE			
Dense Adhesions	-	< 1/3	- 16*
L. OVARY			
Deep Endo	-	< 1 cm	-4
Dense Adhesions	-	< 1/3	-4
TOTAL POINTS			30

STAGE IV (SEVERE)

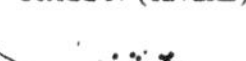

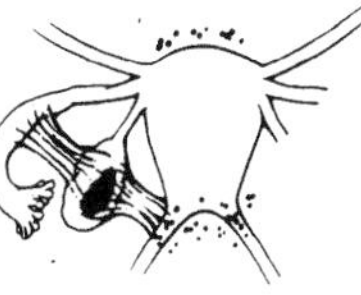

PERITONEUM			
Superficial Endo	-	> 3cm	- 4
L. OVARY			
Deep Endo	-	1-3cm	- 32**
Dense Adhesions	-	< 1/3	- 8**
L. TUBE			
Dense Adhesions	-	< 1/3	- 8**
TOTAL POINTS			52

*Point assignment changed to 16

**Point assignment doubled

STAGE IV (SEVERE)

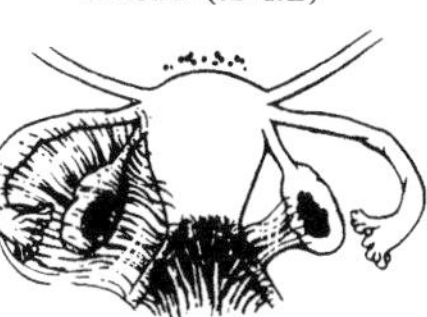

PERITONEUM			
Deep Endo	-	> 3cm	- 6
CULDESAC			
Complete Obliteration			- 40
R. OVARY			
Deep Endo	-	1-3cm	- 16
Dense Adhesions	-	< 1/3	- 4
L. TUBE			
Dense Adhesions	-	> 2/3	- 16
L. OVARY			
Deep Endo	-	1-3cm	- 16
Dense Adhesions	-	> 2/3	- 16
TOTAL POINTS			114

Determination of the stage or degree of endometrial involvement is based on a weighted point system. Distribution of points has been arbitrarily determined and may require further revision or refinement as knowledge of the disease increases.

To ensure complete evaluation, inspection of the pelvis in a clockwise or counterclockwise fashion is encouraged. Number, size and location of endometrial implants, plaques, endometriomas and/or adhesions are noted. For example, five separate 0.5cm superficial implants on the peritoneum (2.5 cm total) would be assigned 2 points. (The surface of the uterus should be considered peritoneum.) The severity of the endometriosis or adhesions should be assigned the highest score only for peritoneum, ovary, tube or culdesac. For example, a 4cm superficial and a 2cm deep implant of the peritoneum should be given a score of 6 (not 8). A 4cm deep endometrioma of the ovary associated with more than 3cm of superficial disease should be scored 20 (not 24).

In those patients with only one adenexa, points applied to disease of the remaining tube and ovary should be multipled by two. **Points assigned may be circled and totaled. Aggregation of points indicates stage of disease (minimal, mild, moderate, or severe).

The presence of endometriosis of the bowel, urinary tract, fallopian tube, vagina, cervix, skin etc., should be documented under "additional endometriosis." Other pathology such as tubal occlusion, leiomyomata, uterine anomaly, etc., should be documented under "associated pathology." All pathology should be depicted as specifically as possible on the sketch of pelvic organs, and means of observation (laparoscopy or laparotomy) should be noted.

superiority of medical versus surgical management for pain. With either method, a substantial proportion of treated women will experience a recurrence of symptoms. No data exist to indicate whether medical or surgical treatments result in the best fertility outcomes.

ACOG Recommendations

Clinicians should recognize that endometriosis is a chronic disorder. In discussing treatment options with the patient, they should plan long-term therapy based on the patient's age, reproductive desires, presenting symptoms, and severity of disease.

Expertise

Direct visualization confirmed by histologic examination, especially of lesions with nonclassical appearance, remains the standard for diagnosing endometriosis. The presence of two or more of the following histologic features is used as the threshold criteria for the diagnosis by a pathologist:

- Endometrial epithelium
- Endometrial glands
- Endometrial stroma
- Hemosiderin-laden macrophages

Nonetheless, the need for a surgical procedure to diagnose pelvic pain secondary to suspected endometriosis has been the subject of debate. Empiric therapy with a gonadotropin-releasing hormone (GnRH) agonist is an appropriate approach to the management of the woman with chronic pelvic pain, provided that a detailed initial evaluation fails to demonstrate some other cause of pelvic pain.

When medical therapy is elected for pain relief, treatment with a GnRH agonist for at least 3 months or with danazol for at least 6 months appears to be equally effective in most patients. When GnRH agonists are effective in relieving pain and continued therapy is desired, the addition of add-back estrogen therapy reduces or eliminates GnRH-induced bone mineral loss without reducing the efficacy of pain relief. For pain relief, oral contraceptives and oral or depot medroxyprogesterone acetate are effective in comparison with placebo and may be equivalent to more costly regimens. Other medical treatments for pain include the following options:

- Drug therapy
  - —Danazol
  - —Nonsteroidal antiinflammatory agents
  - —Oral contraceptives and oral or depot medroxyprogesterone acetate for pain relief
  - —Weak opioids
  - —Strong opioids
  - —Antianxiety medications
- Pain management centers
  - —Local injection of trigger points; success requires experience to detect secondary trigger points; injection alone not uniformly successful, may require addition of physical therapy and stretching exercise
- Nonpharmacologic
  - —Hypnotherapy
  - —Cognitive and relaxation techniques
  - —Massage

The efficacy of surgical therapy depends heavily on the experience and expertise of the surgeon. When surgery is elected, operative laparoscopy appears to have numerous advantages over laparotomy. However, no conservative surgical method has been shown to be superior; methods in use include:

- Excision
- Endocoagulation
- Electrocautery
- Laser vaporization

Hysterectomy, with or without bilateral oophorectomy, often is regarded as "definitive" therapy, but symptoms may recur even after hysterectomy and oophorectomy. Ovarian conservation is associated with increased likelihood of recurrent symptoms and increased likelihood of additional surgery. It has been thought that use of estrogen replacement therapy after hysterectomy may result in continued progression of endometriosis. Because there are limited data on this issue, estrogen replacement therapy is not contraindicated after hysterectomy and bilateral salpingo-oophorectomy for endometriosis.

If treatment involves modalities in which the clinician does not have expertise, referral should be considered. Supporting services include:

- Reproductive endocrinologist
- Gynecologic surgeon
- Pain management unit
- Radiographic imaging
- Alternative techniques (hypnotherapy [can identify contributing psychosocial factors], relaxation technique therapy, massage [to decrease response to pain])

RESOURCES

Patient

American College of Obstetricians and Gynecologists. Abnormal uterine bleeding. ACOG Patient Education Pamphlet AP095. Washington, DC: ACOG, 1999

American College of Obstetricians and Gynecologists. Dysmenorrhea. ACOG Patient Education Pamphlet AP046. Washington, DC: ACOG, 1999

American College of Obstetricians and Gynecologists. Evaluating infertility. ACOG Patient Education Pamphlet AP136. Washington, DC: ACOG, 2000

American College of Obstetricians and Gynecologists. Important facts about endometriosis. ACOG Patient Education Pamphlet AP013. Washington, DC: ACOG, 1998

American College of Obstetricians and Gynecologists. Pain during intercourse. ACOG Patient Education Pamphlet AP020. Washington, DC: ACOG, 1999

American College of Obstetricians and Gynecologists. Pelvic pain. ACOG Patient Education Pamphlet AP099. Washington, DC: ACOG, 1999

American College of Obstetricians and Gynecologists. Treating infertility. ACOG Patient Education Pamphlet AP137. Washington, DC: ACOG, 2000

Professional

American College of Obstetricians and Gynecologists. Medical management of endometriosis. ACOG Practice Bulletin 11. Washington, DC: ACOG, 1999

Revised American Society for Reproductive Medicine classification of endometriosis: 1996. Fertil Steril 1997;67:817–821

Female Circumcision/Female Genital Mutilation

Health Care Impact

Female circumcision/female genital mutilation (FC/FGM) is a practice based on cultural and traditional patterns dating back at least 2,000 years. According to the World Health Organization, approximately 130 million women worldwide have undergone these procedures. Although there has been increasing opposition, the practice is still widespread in parts of Africa, the Middle East, and Southeast Asia. The procedure is performed rarely in the United States, Canada, and Western Europe; however, women who have undergone the procedure often immigrate to these countries. The U.S. Department of Health and Human Services estimated that in 1990, 168,000 females in the United States had undergone or were at risk for FC/FGM. Health care practitioners should be aware of the types of FC/FGM practiced and their varying gynecologic and reproductive health effects. Clinicians should be able to deliver routine gynecologic care tailored to the special physical and psychosocial needs of circumcised women and should be able to treat complications.

The procedure of FC/FGM carries the intent of *circumcision,* the cutting of genitals based on a cultural tradition. The term *mutilation* emphasizes the degree of damage caused by this practice. It is important to recognize that most women who have undergone FC/FGM do not consider themselves to be mutilated and may be offended by such a suggestion. When talking with any woman who has undergone FC/FGM, it is important to determine how she refers to the procedure and adopt that terminology.

There are many forms of FC/FGM but the procedures performed most often have been classified by the World Health Organization as follows:

- Type I, which includes excision of the clitoral prepuce and partial or total clitoridectomy
- Type II, which includes excision of the clitoris with partial or total excision of the labia minora
- Type III, which involves removal of the clitoris and labia minora and labia majora, suturing the two surfaces together to occlude the vagina (infibulation)
- Type IV, which includes all other forms of genital cutting and manipulation. These can range from burning, cutting, or stretching to touching with cosmetics or other chemicals.

These procedures usually are performed prior to adolescence (between the ages of 1 week and 14 years) by untrained individuals without the benefit of sterile conditions or anesthesia.

The immediate physical effects of FC/FGM can include infection, tetanus, shock, hemorrhage, and even death. In addition, there are long-term physical and mental consequences, such as chronic pelvic infection, keloids, vulvar abscesses, sterility, incontinence, depression, anxiety, sexual dysfunction, and obstetric complications.

ACOG Recommendations

There is no scientific basis for the practice of FC/FGM. Physicians are reminded, however, that patients who have undergone the procedure should be treated with sensitivity and compassion. In the United States, it is a federal crime to perform any unnecessary surgery on the genitalia of a girl younger than 18 years of age. A number of states also have similar laws. The American College of Obstetricians and Gynecologists joins many other major organizations (World Health Organization, United

Nations International Children's Emergency Fund, International Federation of Gynecology and Obstetrics, American Academy of Pediatrics, and the American Medical Association) in opposing all forms of medically unnecessary surgical modification of the female genitalia. Furthermore, it is recommended that the issue be addressed by promoting awareness among the public and health care workers and by developing methods for educating physicians regarding the gynecologic and obstetric care of women who have undergone this procedure.

Expertise

It is important for clinicians to know the demographics of the local patient population to determine if FC/FGM is a medical issue that is likely to arise. Any general health care practitioner should be able to:

- Communicate effectively with circumcised patients. This requires awareness and cultural sensitivity. Practitioners may need to employ interpreters and social workers who can address the special needs of immigrants and refugees.
- Review with patients the basics of female anatomy and reproductive function and provide health education about FC/FGM and its physical and psychosexual consequences.
- Review with the patient any special gynecologic issues, including menstrual, urinary, and sexual functions; family planning; and cancer screening.
- Understand techniques for performing a pelvic examination. The routine examination may need to be altered depending on the anatomy. Use a small or narrow speculum, perform a bimanual examination with only one finger in the vagina, or use a rectal examination to assess the uterus and ovaries if unable to complete a bimanual examination. If treating bacterial vaginosis, yeast vaginitis, or atrophic vaginitis, use oral preparations whenever possible, because patients may not be comfortable with or able to insert suppositories or creams in the vagina.

The physician with special interest in pelvic/vaginal reconstructive surgery or a clinician practicing in an area of high prevalence also should:

- Be familiar with the four main classes of FC/FGM as specified by the World Health Organization, and be aware of ensuing complications including menstrual irregularities, urinary retention or incontinence, infection of the genital or urinary tracts, sexual dysfunction, and scarring or fistulas of the vagina. Obstetric complications can include difficulties of management in labor and delivery and the potential for laceration, hemorrhage, and fetal asphyxia.
- Understand surgical therapies available, including excision of cysts, introital or urethral scarring, defibulation (opening the area surgically closed), repair of fistulas, and procedures for correcting vaginal stenosis.
- Counsel the patient after surgical correction about the new appearance of her anatomy and explain changes in her urinary, menstrual, and sexual function. Clinicians may need to elicit the help of social workers and psychiatric professionals in this task.
- Communicate with policy makers, community groups, and women's groups on this issue.
- Be aware of current research on the true incidence of complications of FC/FGM and on the safest timing and techniques for repair or reconstruction.

RESOURCES

Professional

American College of Obstetricians and Gynecologists. Female circumcision/female genital mutilation: clinical management of circumcised women. Washington, DC: ACOG, 1999

Koso-Thomas O. Circumcision of women: a strategy for eradication. London: Zed Books, 1987

McCaffrey M, Jankowska A, Gordon H. Management of female genital mutilation: the Northwick Park Hospital experience. Br J Obstet Gynaecol 1995;102:787–790

Ozumba BC. Acquired gynetresia in eastern Nigeria. Int J Gynaecol Obstet 1992;37: 105–109

Toubia N. Female circumcision as a public health issue. N Engl J Med 1994;331:712–716

World Health Organization. Female genital mutilation: report of a WHO Technical Working Group, Geneva, 17–19 July 1995. Geneva: WHO, 1996

Genetics

Health Care Impact

Identification and management of genetic risk factors have the potential to affect the quality and length of a woman's life. Some estimates are that 60% of all sick individuals have diseases influenced by genetic factors. Genetic risk factors that may be identified include the more common ones of cancer and heart disease and more specific ones discovered through family history or medical history. Relatively common conditions that have or are suspected to have a genetic contribution include:

- Atherosclerotic heart disease
- Bleeding disorders (hemophilia, von Willebrand's disease)
- Cancer, including breast, ovarian, endometrial, and colon
- Clotting disorders (antithrombin III, protein C or S, factor V Leiden deficiencies)
- Cystic fibrosis
- Diabetes mellitus
- Familial hypercholesterolemia
- Fragile X
- Glaucoma
- Glucose-6-phosphate dehydrogenase deficiency
- Hemoglobinopathies (eg, sickle cell disease and thalassemias)
- Huntington disease
- Hypertension

- Marfan syndrome
- Muscular dystrophy
- Myotonic dystrophy
- Neural tube defects
- Neurofibromatosis
- Polycystic kidney disease
- Seizure disorders

Lifestyle changes, as well as medical interventions, may affect overall health as risk factors are determined.

Genetic services also may play a role in assisted reproductive techniques. Gamete donors should be screened for heritable disorders through evaluation of pedigree, counseling, and—when appropriate—testing procedures. In some circumstances it is possible to identify embryos affected by certain diseases prior to implantation. Affected embryos are then not transferred.

Concerns about the impact of information about genetic conditions on such factors as employability and insurability have been raised. Patients should be encouraged to consider the importance of relatives being made aware of genetic disorders in the family, and confidentiality issues must be considered carefully (see also "Human Resources" in Part 1).

ACOG Recommendations

A family history that may identify genetic risks should be performed. Women should be informed of genetic risks and offered appropriate counseling and testing. Testing that may have multiple medical or psychosocial consequences requires specific counseling. Both pretest and posttest counseling facilitate women's access to appropriate health care. Referral may be needed for comprehensive counseling. The patient should be informed prospectively about policies regarding use of information and legal requirements. Ordinarily, information may not be revealed without the patient's express consent. However, there may be situations in which the information may not be protected.

Expertise

Personnel capable of offering and delivering genetic services are specially trained. Most clinicians are capable of basic genetic risk identification and counseling. Personnel with more advanced training are appropriate for both basic and more unusual abnormalities. These include genetic counselors and medical geneticists.

The health care professional should be familiar with state or federal requirements regarding genetic screening, reporting, disclosure, breach of confidentiality, and discrimination based on genetic information.

RESOURCES

Patient

American College of Obstetricians and Gynecologists. Genetic disorders. ACOG Patient Education Pamphlet AP094. Washington, DC: ACOG, 1995

Professional

American College of Obstetricians and Gynecologists. Breast–ovarian cancer screening. ACOG Committee Opinion 239. Washington, DC: ACOG, 2000

American College of Obstetricians and Gynecologists. Ethical guidance for patient testing. In: Ethics in obstetrics and gynecology. Washington, DC: ACOG, 2002:32–34

American College of Obstetricians and Gynecologists. Fragile X syndrome. ACOG Committee Opinion 161. Washington, DC: ACOG, 1995

American College of Obstetricians and Gynecologists. Genetic screening for hemoglobinopathies. ACOG Committee Opinion 238. Washington, DC: ACOG, 2000

American College of Obstetricians and Gynecologists. Genetic screening for gamete donors. ACOG Committee Opinion 192. Washington, DC: ACOG, 1997

American College of Obstetricians and Gynecologists. Genetic technologies. ACOG Technical Bulletin 208. Washington, DC: ACOG, 1995

American College of Obstetricians and Gynecologists. Screening for Canavan disease. ACOG Committee Opinion 212. Washington, DC: ACOG, 1998

American College of Obstetricians and Gynecologists. Screening for Tay–Sachs disease. ACOG Committee Opinion 162. Washington, DC: ACOG, 1995

Sex selection and preimplantation genetic diagnosis. The Ethics Committee of the American Society of Reproductive Medicine. Fertil Steril 1999;72:595–598

Statement of the American Society of Clinical Oncology: genetic testing for cancer susceptibility, Adopted on February 20, 1996. J Clin Oncol 1996;14:1730–1736

GYNECOLOGIC ULTRASONOGRAPHY

Health Care Impact

Assessment of the pelvic anatomy in a woman experiencing pelvic pain, abnormal bleeding, or who has an abnormal pelvic examination, risk factors for pelvic abnormality, infertility, or early pregnancy may be aided by gynecologic ultrasonography. In addition, gynecologic ultrasonography can be of assistance when a pelvic examination provides insufficient information due to the difficulty of examination. Some management approaches to women with postmenopausal bleeding include the assessment of the thickness and characteristics of the endometrial lining, and some suggest that endometrial biopsy be reserved for those instances in which the lining is greater than 5 mm in thickness or nonhomogenous. Identification of an intrauterine or extrauterine pregnancy may be possible using gynecologic ultrasonography in the woman with pelvic pain or vaginal bleeding. Although the ultrasonography assessment increases the cost of evaluation, it may improve selection of patients for surgery and better clarify the choice of procedure.

ACOG Recommendations

Gynecologic ultrasonography should not be relied on as the sole diagnostic method but rather considered an adjunct to physical examination and other diagnostic modalities to confirm the presence or absence of a suspected problem. Results from ultrasonography examination are considered part of the medical record and should be documented and stored appropriately.

Gynecologic ultrasonography procedures should be fully explained to the patient in advance, and her involvement should be encouraged. Consideration should be given to the patient's privacy and sensitivity. Without proper preparation, the transvaginal ultrasonography examination could be construed as offensive. Because of the sensitive nature of the transvaginal examination, it may be advisable to have a chaperon present.

Expertise

Training in performance and interpretation of gynecologic ultrasonography may be acquired during residency training or from courses supplemented by supervised experience and follow-up. Ultrasound unit accreditation is available through the American Institute of Ultrasound in Medicine or the American College of Radiology.

Equipment consists of ultrasonography machines and abdominal and vaginal ultrasonography probes. The clinician should use the technique that allows for the most complete examination of the targeted organ. The vaginal probe must be covered during use (with a nonlatex covering for latex-allergic patients), and a policy for cleaning the probe between uses must be in place. Equipment should be operated only by properly trained personnel. Equipment should be well maintained and inspected at regular intervals for proper functioning and safety as specified by the manufacturer's operations manual. Personnel who can serve as chaperons should be available on clinician or patient request, especially when transvaginal ultrasonography is to be performed.

Resources

Patient

American College of Obstetricians and Gynecologists. Ultrasound exams. ACOG Patient Education Pamphlet AP025. Washington, DC: ACOG, 1998

Professional

American College of Obstetricians and Gynecologists. Medical management of tubal pregnancy. ACOG Practice Bulletin 3. Washington, DC: ACOG, 1998

American College of Radiology
Standards and Accreditation
1891 Preston White Drive
Reston, VA 20191-4397
800-227-5463
www.acr.org/f-products.html

American Institute of Ultrasound in Medicine
Ultrasound Practice Accreditation
14750 Sweitzer Lane
Suite 100
Laurel, MD 20707-5906
800-638-5352
www.aium.org/Accreditation/usp/accred.htm

HORMONE REPLACEMENT THERAPY

Health Care Impact

The median age of menopause in American women is about 51 years of age; approximately one third of the average American woman's life span occurs after menopause. Most of the important causes of morbidity and mortality in older women (eg, cardiovascular disease, osteoporosis, various cancers) appear to be influenced by female hormones. Cardiovascular disease is the leading cause of morbidity and mortality in postmenopausal women. Nearly one half of these women will develop coronary heart disease, and 30% of those who develop coronary heart disease will die as a result. An estimated 1.3 million osteoporosis-related fractures occur each year in the United States. In perspective, the lifetime risk of an osteoporotic fracture in a white woman is 16–32%, while the lifetime probability of developing endometrial or breast cancer is only about 2.6% and 10%, respectively.

Controlled trials of the clinical effects of hormone therapy are difficult to perform because of the large number of subjects and the long follow-up required. However, numerous cross-sectional, case–control, and cohort studies suggest that postmenopausal estrogen therapy has important effects on the clinical outcomes mentioned here.

There is good clinical evidence from retrospective studies and clinical trials that estrogen therapy can reduce the rate of bone loss and improve bone mineral density in postmenopausal women. An overview of 11 studies estimated that the risk of hip fracture was reduced 25% in women who had taken estrogen.

Numerous epidemiologic studies also have demonstrated a 37–44% reduction in risk of coronary heart disease in women who take estrogen. However, the Heart and Estrogen/Progestin Replacement Study trial of hormone replacement therapy in postmenopausal women with a prior cardiovascular event has raised concern over the use of estrogen in these women. In this study of women with established coronary disease, women taking conjugated equine estrogen plus medroxyprogesterone acetate showed an *increased* short-term morbidity compared with a placebo control group. However, in years 4 and 5, the morbidity for women on hormone replacement therapy was *less* than that of the controls. It is unclear what effect, if any, the progestin component in this study contributed to the negative short-term morbidity. Overall, there were no significant differences between the groups in the primary or secondary outcomes.

There are few data on which to base recommendations concerning effect on the central nervous system. Evidence is conflicting concerning the risk reduction of Alzheimer's disease, although primary and secondary studies demonstrate the potential use of hormone treatment for dementia. The Women's Health Initiative—Memory Study recently began the first long-term clinical trial to test the role of hormone replacement therapy on dementia.

Prolonged use of unopposed estrogen increases the risk of endometrial hyperplasia and endometrial cancer; this risk is elevated at all doses and increases with dose and duration of therapy. Both continuous and cyclic regimens of progestins prevent estrogen-induced endometrial hyperplasia.

Endogenous estrogens appear to be important in the etiology of breast cancer, but the effect of exogenous estrogens on breast cancer risk is uncertain. More than 40 observational studies and meta-analyses report a modest but significant increase in the risk of breast cancer among women who currently use estrogen (relative risk = 1.2 to 1.4). The dose of estrogen has no clear effect on the risk of breast cancer. A number of studies report that women who develop breast cancer during estrogen therapy have earlier disease diagnoses, lower rates of metastasis, and longer survival compared with women who had never used estrogen. There is new evidence to suggest that adding progestin therapy does moderately increase the risk of breast cancer.

A new category of drugs, selective estrogen receptor modulators, currently are indicated for treatment of osteoporosis and prevention of breast cancer. In the future, if indicated by the results of clinical trials, they may be used for hormone replacement therapy.

ACOG Recommendations

The American College of Obstetricians and Gynecologists recommends that physicians counsel all postmenopausal women about the risks and benefits of estrogen replacement and make decisions with the patient regarding hormone therapy on an individual basis. Hormone replacement therapy should always be used in a treatment plan that includes dietary control, exercise, and, when appropriate, weight reduction and behavior modification, such as cessation of smoking and reduction of alcohol intake. The American Academy of Family Physicians, the Canadian Task Force on the Periodic Health Examination, the U.S. Preventive Services Task Force, and the American College of Physicians–American Society of Internal Medicine have recommendations similar to those of the American College of Obstetricians and Gynecologists.

In women who have an intact uterus, the use of an estrogen–progestin regimen is recommended to reduce the risk of endometrial hyperplasia or endometrial cancer. For such women who do not tolerate estrogen–progestin or progestin-only regimens, estrogen-only therapy can be considered if the patient can be monitored by endometrial assessment to detect endometrial proliferation, the risk of which may approach 20% per year.

Expertise

The clinician should be able to perform a physical examination, including breast examination and pelvic examination and to identify risk based on history and physical examination. The clinician should be able to perform effective counseling regarding the benefits and risks of hormone therapy (with unopposed estrogen and estrogen–progestin combinations) and to discuss the specific regimens that are available.

The clinician should be able to perform endometrial assessment or refer as appropriate. Equipment and personnel to evaluate and manage any genital abnormalities and perform age-specific mammographic screening should be available as supporting services.

Resources

Patient

American College of Obstetricians and Gynecologists. Hormone replacement therapy. ACOG Patient Education Pamphlet AP066. Washington, DC: ACOG, 1997

American College of Obstetricians and Gynecologists. Hormone replacement therapy and your heart: what every woman should know. ACOG Patient Education Video APV04. Washington, DC: ACOG, 1998

American College of Obstetricians and Gynecologists. The menopause years. ACOG Patient Education Pamphlet AP047. Washington, DC: ACOG, 1997

American College of Obstetricians and Gynecologists. Midlife transitions: a guide to approaching menopause. ACOG Patient Education Pamphlet AB013. Washington, DC: ACOG, 1997

American College of Obstetricians and Gynecologists. Osteoporosis: what every woman should know. ACOG Patient Education Video APV01. Washington, DC: ACOG, 1998

American College of Obstetricians and Gynecologists. Preventing osteoporosis. ACOG Patient Education Pamphlet AP048. Washington, DC: ACOG, 1997

Professional

American Academy of Family Physicians. Summary of policy recommendations for periodic health examination. Kansas City, Missouri: AAFP, 2000

American College of Obstetricians and Gynecologists. Health maintenance for perimenopausal women. ACOG Educational Bulletin 210. Washington, DC: ACOG, 1995

American College of Obstetricians and Gynecologists. Hormone replacement therapy. ACOG Educational Bulletin 247. Washington, DC: ACOG, 1998

American College of Obstetricians and Gynecologists. Hormone replacement therapy in women treated for endometrial cancer. ACOG Committee Opinion 235. Washington, DC: ACOG, 2000

American College of Obstetricians and Gynecologists. Hormone replacement therapy in women with previously treated breast cancer. ACOG Committee Opinion 226. Washington, DC: ACOG, 1999

Canadian Consensus Conference on Menopause and Osteoporosis: part I: consensus statements. J SOGC 1998;20:1243–1272

Counseling postmenopausal women about preventive hormone therapy. AGS Clinical Practice Committee. J Am Geriatr Soc 1996:44;1120–1122

Guidelines for counseling postmenopausal women about preventive hormone therapy. American College of Physicians. Ann Intern Med 1992;117:1038–1041

Nawaz H, Katz DL. American College of Preventive Medicine Practice Policy Statement. Perimenopausal and postmenopausal hormone replacement therapy. Am J Prev Med 1999;17:250–254

Royal College of Obstetricians and Gynaecologists. Hormone replacement therapy and venous thromboembolism. RCOG Guideline No. 19. London: RCOG, 1999

Saver BG, Taylor TR, Woods NF, Stevens NG. Physician policies on the use of preventive hormone therapy. Am J Prev Med 1997;13:358–365

U.S. Preventive Services Task Force. Postmenopausal hormone prophylaxis. In: Guide to clinical preventive services. 2nd ed. Baltimore: Williams and Wilkins, 1996:829–843

Human Immunodeficiency Virus

Health Care Impact

In just over a decade, the proportion of all acquired immunodeficiency syndrome (AIDS) cases reported among adult and adolescent women in the U.S. more than tripled, from 7% in 1985 to 23% in 1999. It is estimated that between 120,000–160,000 adult and adolescent females are currently living with human immunodeficiency virus (HIV) infection in the United States. Approximately 6,000–7,000 women with HIV give birth each year, and perinatal transmission accounted for at least 432 AIDS cases in the United States in 1997.

ACOG Recommendations

The obstetrician–gynecologist should be prepared to educate patients about the modes of transmission of the virus, means of protection from infection, and the significance of HIV infection in pregnancy. Voluntary and confidential HIV testing should be available to any woman who wishes to be tested. Testing should be recommended to women with risk factors and offered to those who are planning a pregnancy (see "Primary and Preventive Care" in Part 3). The College also supports the Institute of Medicine recommendation for universal HIV testing with patient notification as a routine component of prenatal care. It is unethical for an obstetrician–gynecologist to refuse to accept as a patient or continue to care for persons solely because they are or are thought to be seropositive for HIV. Health care practitioners should observe standard precautions to minimize skin, mucous membrane, and percutaneous exposure to blood, secretions, and body fluids from all patients to protect against a variety of pathogens, including HIV. In making decisions about patient-care activities, a health care worker infected with HIV should adhere to the fundamental professional obligation to avoid harm to patients (see also "Human Resources" in Part 1).

Expertise

The clinician has an obligation to learn about HIV infection and its associated conditions. Necessary knowledge includes:

- Modes of transmission
- Risk groups
- Significance in pregnancy and for the newborn
- Risk reduction behaviors
- Local reporting and consent for testing requirements
- Knowledge of testing methods (screening and confirmatory)
- Pretest and posttest counseling
- Referral of HIV-positive patients for comprehensive and integrated medical and psychosocial care, and possible enrollment in research protocols
- Confidentiality issues
- Management of individuals exposed to blood or other body fluids, including postexposure prophylaxis

The health care professional should be familiar with state laws, regulations, and recommendations regarding HIV screening, reporting, disclosure, and breach of confidentiality.

RESOURCES

Patient

American College of Obstetricians and Gynecologists. HIV infection and women. ACOG Patient Education Pamphlet AP082. Washington, DC: ACOG, 1996

Professional

American Academy of Pediatrics, American College of Obstetricians and Gynecologists. Joint statement on human immunodeficiency virus screening. ACOG Statement of Policy 75. Elk Grove Village, Illinois: AAP; Washington, DC: ACOG, 1999

American College of Obstetricians and Gynecologists. Code of professional ethics of the American College of Obstetricians and Gynecologists. Washington, DC: ACOG, 2002

American College of Obstetricians and Gynecologists. Human immunodeficiency virus: ethical guidelines for obstetricians and gynecologists. In: Ethics in obstetrics and gynecology. Washington, DC: ACOG, 2002:43–47

Management of possible sexual, injecting-drug-use, or other nonoccupational exposure to HIV, including considerations related to antiretroviral therapy. Public Health Service statement. Centers for Disease Control and Prevention. MMWR Morb Mortal Wkly Rep 1998;47(RR-17):1–14

National Center for HIV, STD, and TB Prevention. Division of HIV/AIDS Prevention. www.cdc.gov/hiv/dhap.htm

The National Clinicians' Post-Exposure Hotline (PEP-Line) has been created to assist clinicians with postexposure prophylaxis issues. It is a 24-hour free service funded by the U.S. Centers for Disease Control and Prevention, Health Resources and Services Administration, and the University of California, San Francisco. The number is 888-448-4911.

Updated U.S. Public Health Service Guidelines for the Management of Occupational Exposures to HBV, HCV, and HIV and Recommendations for Postexposure Prophylaxis. MMWR Morb Mortal Wkly Rep 2001;50(RR-11):1–52

Hypertension

Health Care Impact

Hypertension affects 50 million Americans, including one of every four adults. The incidence of hypertension increases with each decade of life. Beginning soon after menopause, half of the U.S. female population is hypertensive, and the prevalence continues to increase thereafter. At every age, African-American women have a higher prevalence of hypertension than do white women.

Hypertension increases the risk of cardiovascular events, including coronary heart disease, congestive heart failure, stroke, peripheral vascular disease, and renal failure. Untreated hypertension is a major cause of mortality, with risk directly proportional to the degree of hypertension.

Most patients with hypertension have primary hypertension defined as elevated blood pressure with no demonstrable cause. High-risk groups for hypertension include African-American women, older women, women with persistently "high normal" blood pressure, women with a family history of hypertension, and women with lifestyle factors associated with hypertension (eg, obesity and excessive alcohol use).

ACOG Recommendations

Obstetrician–gynecologists can assume a pivotal role in the prevention of hypertension-related morbidity and mortality. Suggestions for modifying lifestyle can be incorporated into patient counseling to prevent the development of chronic hypertension. Treatment of mild hypertension, which comprises up to 75% of all hypertension, is within the capabilities of the obstetrician–gynecologist. More advanced stages should be referred for specialist consultation.

Expertise

Blood pressure measurement should be preceded by 5 minutes of rest in a seated position and the absence of smoking and caffeine intake for the previous 30 minutes. Blood pressure should be measured in both arms, with subsequent measures taken in the arm with the higher blood pressure level. Cuff size is important. A single measurement is insufficient for diagnosis. Classification of blood pressure for adults older than 18 years of age is shown in Table 3–10 (see also "Routine Detection and Prevention of Disease" in Part 3).

Laboratory assessments in women with hypertension include urinalysis, complete blood count, serum chemistries (eg, potassium, sodium, creatinine, fasting glucose), lipid profile, and electrocardiography. If electrocardiography indicates ventricular hypertrophy, echocardiography should be considered.

The goal of managing hypertension is to achieve a systolic blood pressure below 140 mm Hg and a diastolic blood pressure less than 90 mm Hg. Lifestyle modifications for both prevention and management of hypertension include weight loss (in overweight patients); limiting alcohol intake to less than 1 ounce of absolute alcohol daily; increasing aerobic physical activity; reducing sodium intake; ensuring adequate dietary intake of potassium, calcium, and magnesium; quitting smoking; and reducing dietary intake of saturated fat and cholesterol.

A variety of pharmacologic therapies are available for managing hypertension, including thiazide diuretics, adrenergic blockers, ACE inhibitors, and calcium channel blockers. See Fig. 4–2 for the treatment of hypertension that does not respond to lifestyle modifications.

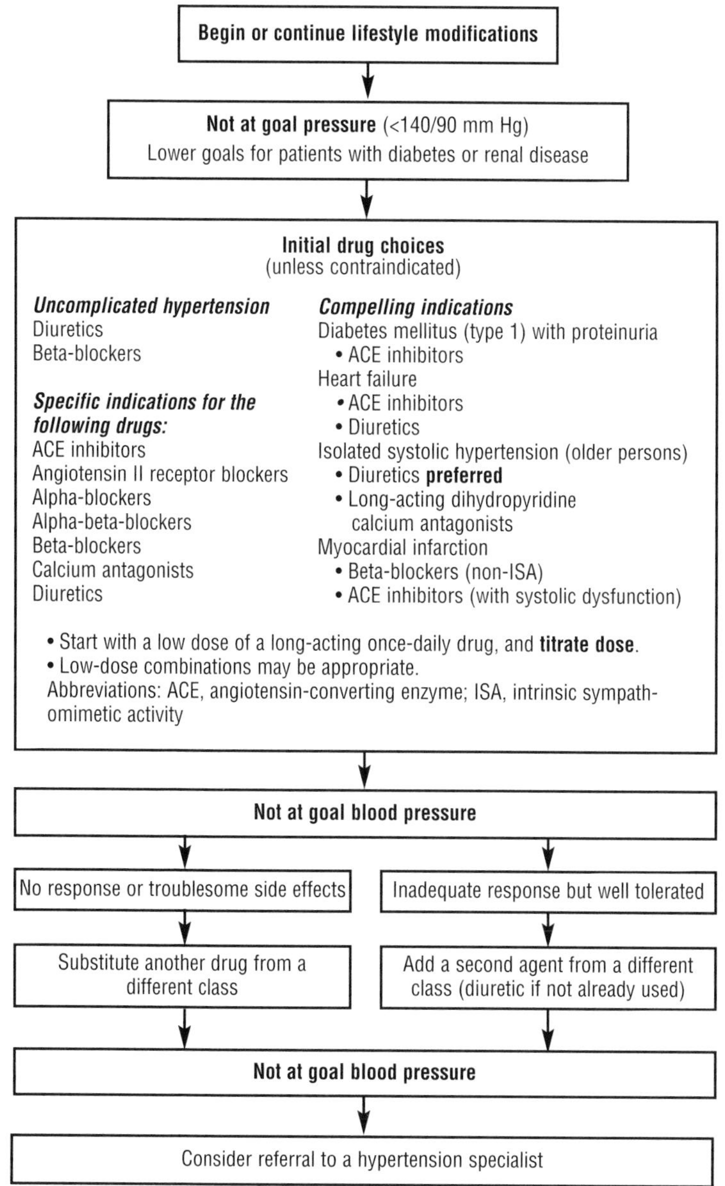

Fig. 4–2. Algorithm for the Treatment of Hypertension (Adapted from: Sixth Report of the Joint National Committee on the prevention, detection, evaluation, and treatment of high blood pressure. Bethesda, Maryland: National Heart, Lung, and Blood Institute, 1997)

RESOURCES

Patient

American College of Obstetricians and Gynecologists. Exercise and fitness: a guide for women. ACOG Patient Education Pamphlet AP045. Washington, DC: ACOG, 1998

American College of Obstetricians and Gynecologists. Healthy eating. ACOG Patient Education Pamphlet AP130. Washington, DC: ACOG, 1999

American College of Obstetricians and Gynecologists. Keeping your heart healthy. ACOG Patient Education Pamphlet AP122. Washington, DC: ACOG, 1998

American College of Obstetricians and Gynecologists. Managing high blood pressure. ACOG Patient Education Pamphlet AP123. Washington, DC: ACOG, 1998

American College of Obstetricians and Gynecologists. Staying healthy for women of all ages. ACOG Patient Education Pamphlet AB006. Washington, DC: ACOG, 1994

American College of Obstetricians and Gynecologists. Weight control: eating right and keeping fit. ACOG Patient Education Pamphlet AP064. Washington, DC: ACOG, 1999

Professional

Alliance for Aging Research, National Heart, Lung, and Blood Institute. A clinical guide: controlling high blood pressure in older women. Bethesda, Maryland: National Institutes of Health, 1998

American College of Obstetricians and Gynecologists. Health maintenance for perimenopausal women. ACOG Technical Bulletin 210. Washington, DC: ACOG, 1995

Peng TC. Hypertension. Clin Updat Womens Health Care 2002;1(1):1–56

Sixth Report of the Joint National Committee on the prevention, detection, evaluation, and treatment of high blood pressure. Bethesda, Maryland: National Heart, Lung, and Blood Institute, 1997

IMMUNIZATIONS

Health Care Impact

In the United States, vaccination programs that focus on infants and children have decreased the occurrence of many childhood, vaccine-preventable diseases. However, many adolescents and adults continue to be adversely affected by vaccine-preventable diseases (eg, influenza, varicella, hepatitis A, hepatitis B, measles, rubella, and pneumococcal pneumonia), partially because vaccine programs have not focused on improving vaccination coverage. Each year it is estimated that pneumococcal infection, influenza, and hepatitis B result in as many as 45,000 deaths in adults. Factors that have contributed to the low level of immunization in adults include (1) a general disinterest by the general public and physicians in the concept of adult immunization with the attitude that immunization is for children; (2) misconceptions about the safety and efficacy of vaccines compared with the consequences of the disease; (3) concerns about liability; and (4) a poorly developed immunization system.

Especially during their reproductive years, many women are more likely to see an obstetrician–gynecologist than other practitioners. Obstetrician–gynecologists and other clinicians who provide general health care to women therefore have multiple opportunities in which to counsel on the need for immunizations and provide vaccinations when indicated. Well-woman examinations; visits for family planning, preconception care, or hormone replacement management; and prenatal and postpartum visits are all opportunities that should be considered.

ACOG Recommendations

The American College of Obstetricians and Gynecologists recommends the following routine immunizations for women without risk factors by age group:

Age 13–18 Years:

- Tetanus–diphtheria booster (once between 11 and 16 years of age)
- Hepatitis B vaccine (one series for those not previously immunized)

Age 19–64 Years

- Tetanus–diphtheria booster every 10 years
- Influenza vaccine, annually (beginning at 50 years of age)

Age 65 and Older

- Tetanus–diphtheria booster every 10 years
- Influenza vaccine, annually
- Pneumococcal vaccine (once)

Additional or earlier immunizations are recommended for women with certain high-risk factors (see Table 3–1 in Part 3).

Expertise

Clinicians should attempt to gather a complete immunization history from each woman, including risk factors indicating the need for immunization, and attempt to obtain previous records. Clues to a woman's immunization status include the year and place of her birth, residence during childhood, previous and current occupations, military service, travel history, and lifestyle. Because serologic testing may be necessary to confirm immunization status, clinicians should have access to appropriate facilities and personnel. If there are doubts about past immunizations, it is safest to assume that a woman has not been immunized and to initiate the appropriate vaccination series.

The package insert should be read thoroughly. The storage temperature, body site for injection (usually the deltoid), route of injection (eg, intramuscular, subcutaneous, or intradermal), and length of needle are critical items in maximizing efficacy.

Severe hypersensitivity reactions following immunizations, including anaphylaxis, are rare. The reactions are almost always caused by hypersensitivity to one or more of the vaccine components (residual animal proteins, antibiotics, preservatives, or stabilizers). On rare occasions, an anaphylactic reaction will occur due to trace amounts of an antibiotic such as neomycin or streptomycin (eg, neomycin in measles–mumps–rubella vaccine). Vaccination is contraindicated in women with a previous anaphylactic reaction. Importantly, none of the current licensed vaccines contain penicillin; therefore, a history of penicillin hypersensitivity is not a contraindication to vaccination.

There are a number of misconceptions concerning contraindications to adult immunization. The following are *not* contraindications to vaccination:

- Reaction to a previous vaccination consisting of only mild to moderate local erythema or edema and fever <40.5°C (104.9°F)
- Mild upper respiratory or gastrointestinal illness with a fever <38.0°C (100.4°F)
- Current antimicrobial therapy or convalescence from a recent illness
- Pregnancy in a household contact
- Recent exposure to an infectious disease
- Breastfeeding
- Personal history of allergies
- Family history of allergies, adverse reactions to vaccination, or seizures

Federal law requires that a vaccine information statement developed by the Centers for Disease Control and Prevention be given to all patients, regardless of age, prior to administration of every dose of certain vaccines. In addition, the following information must be recorded in the patient's permanent medical record (or a permanent office log):

- The name, address, and title of the person who administered the vaccine
- The date of administration
- The vaccine manufacturer
- The lot number of the vaccine used

State health departments or the Centers for Disease Control and Prevention should be consulted to determine which vaccines are currently covered by this federal law. Vaccine information statements are available on the Internet at www.cdc.gov/nip/ or by contacting the National Immunization Information Hotline at 800-232-2522.

The federal requirement to provide relevant vaccine information statements is in addition to any applicable state laws, and no state law can negate that requirement. In addition, some states may have informed consent laws regarding immunization.

RESOURCES

Patient

American College of Obstetricians and Gynecologists. Immunizations for women. ACOG Patient Education Pamphlet AP117. Washington, DC: ACOG, 1997

National Institute of Allergy and Infectious Diseases. Understanding vaccines. Bethesda, Maryland: National Institutes of Health, 1998 January; NIH Publication no. 98-4219

Professional

American College of Physicians, Infectious Diseases Society of America. Guide for adult immunization. 3rd ed. Philadelphia: ACP; Alexandria, Virginia: IDSA, 1994

Centers for Disease Control and Prevention. Epidemiology and prevention of vaccine preventable diseases. 6th ed. Atlanta: CDC, 2000

Centers for Disease Control and Prevention. Health information for international travel 2001–2002. Atlanta: CDC, 2001

Centers for Disease Control and Prevention. International Travelers Information Line 877-394-8747 (877-FYI-TRIP)

Centers for Disease Control and Prevention
Travelers' health
www.cdc.gov/travel

Centers for Disease Control and Prevention. Vaccine information statements: what you need to know. Atlanta: CDC, 2000. Available at www.immunize.org/vis/instr00.htm. Retrieved September 26, 2000

Centers for Disease Control and Prevention National Immunization Program
www.cdc.gov/nip

General recommendations on immunization. Recommendations of the Advisory Committee on Immunization Practices (ACIP). MMWR Morb Mortal Wkly Rep 1994;43 (RR-1):1–38

Immunization Action Coalition (www.immunize.org) contains a variety of information in adult and infant immunization, including listings of state mandates (www.immunize.org/laws)

Immunization of adolescents. Recommendations of the Advisory Committee on Immunization Practices, the American Academy of Pediatrics, the American Academy of Family Physicians, and the American Medical Association. MMWR Morb Mortal Wkly Rep 1996;45(RR-13):1–16

Immunization of health-care workers: recommendations of the Advisory Committee on Immunization Practices (ACIP) and the Hospital Infection Control Practices Advisory Committee (HICPAC). MMWR Morb Mortal Wkly Rep 1997;46(RR-18):1–42

National Coalition for Adult Immunization. Resource guide for adult and adolescent immunization. 4th ed. Bethesda, Maryland: NCAI, 1999

National Network for Immunization Information
www.immunizationinfo.org

National Network for Immunization Information. Communicating with patients about immunization: resource kit. Alexandria, Virginia: NNII, 2001

Update: vaccine side effects, adverse reactions, contraindications and precautions. Recommendations of the Advisory Committee on Immunization Practices (ACIP) [published erratum appears in MMWR Morb Mortal Wkly Rep 1997 Mar 14;46(10):227]. MMWR Morb Mortal Wkly Rep 1996;45(RR-12):1–35

Vaccine Adverse Event Reporting System
www.vaers.org

INFERTILITY

Health Care Impact

Infertility affects 6.1 million people in the United states (about 10% of the population of people of reproductive age) and affects men and women equally. Sexually transmitted diseases, endometriosis, age-dependent decreasing fecundity, and population demographics (eg, the "baby boomers") are the major factors that contribute to these numbers. There is a great emphasis in modern society to have only the number of children desired at the time in a woman's reproductive life that is most convenient. Thus, many couples seek fertility services to overcome acquired diseases, enhance the naturally decreasing fertility associated with age, and accommodate their lifestyle agendas.

Infertility is established when a couple has unprotected intercourse for 12 months without conception. In general, three major potential etiologic factors are assessed to uncover the causes of infertility. Although reported infertility populations vary, on average 20% of couples will have male factor dysfunction, ovulation defects will affect 30%, and female anatomic abnormalities will be present in 25%. Other complex disorders affect about 10% of couples, and 10–15% of couples will have no explanation for their infertility.

ACOG Recommendations

It is important for health care practitioners to understand and accept the emotional and educational needs and demands of infertility patients. Physicians must honestly appraise their interests, personalities, training, and experience and be prepared to refer patients to others when appropriate. In addition, a team approach may be helpful in ensuring that patients receive an adequate workup and counseling as the need arises.

Counseling for treatment of infertility should include, among other things, information regarding the risks of multiple gestation, and the ethical issues surrounding embryo reduction should be discussed with patients before the initiation of such treatment. Physicians also have a responsibility to counsel infertility patients about adoption.

Expertise

The clinician must be able to make an assessment of the couple and refer as appropriate. Guidelines developed by the American Society for Reproductive Medicine for the provision of infertility services are outlined in the box. Supporting services may include:

- Reproductive endocrinology
- Assisted reproductive technologies, including in vitro fertilization, gamete intrafallopian transfer, zygote intrafallopian transfer; oocyte, sperm, and embryo donation; gestational and surrogate carriers; preimplantation genetic testing; and intracytoplasmic sperm injection (see Table 4–1)
- Psychologic support
- Urologic/andrology services
- Adoption agencies
- Infertility support groups
- Family counseling

Clinicians should be familiar with any state laws regarding infertility services and treatment or insurance coverage.

Resources

Patient

American College of Obstetricians and Gynecologists. Evaluating infertility. ACOG Patient Education Pamphlet AP136. Washington, DC: ACOG, 2000

American College of Obstetricians and Gynecologists. Treating infertility. ACOG Patient Education Pamphlet AP137. Washington, DC: ACOG, 2000

American Society of Reproductive Medicine. Frequently asked questions about infertility. Available at www.asrm.org/Patient/faqs.html. Retrieved September 26, 2000

RESOLVE: The National Infertility Association
1310 Broadway
Somerville, MA 02144
617-623-0744
www.resolve.org
E-mail: resolveinc.@aol.com

American Society for Reproductive Medicine Guidelines for the Provision of Infertility Services

LEVEL I CARE

- Patient Inclusion Criteria
  - —The duration of the infertility is less than 24 months
  - —The female partner is less than 30 years of age
  - —There are no risk factors for pelvic pathology or male reproductive abnormalities
  - —The couple has undergone less than 4 months of treatment without success
- Practitioner Qualifications
  - —Is prepared to consult, educate, and advise both partners
  - —Is knowledgeable about the prerequisites for successful reproduction
- Obligations
  - —Interview and physical examination
  - —Interpretation of semen analysis and confirmation of ovulation
  - —Timely referral of patients with complex disorders

LEVEL II CARE

- Patient Inclusion Criteria
  - —The duration of the infertility is less than 36 months
  - —The female partner is less than 35 years of age
  - —The couple does not qualify for Level I care
- Practitioner Qualifications
  - —Possesses the qualification for Level I care
  - —Possesses certification or documented experience in the necessary endocrinologic, gynecologic, or urologic procedures
  - —Is knowledgeable regarding the effectiveness, adverse effects, and costs of the diagnosis and treatment of infertility
- Obligations
  - —Assessment of tubal patency status
  - —Management of uncomplicated anovulation, endometriosis, and tubal disease
  - —Management of uncomplicated male infertility

(continued)

American Society for Reproductive Medicine Guidelines for the Provision of Infertility Services *(continued)*

—Access to necessary laboratory services seven days a week

—Timely referral of patients with complex disorders

Level III Care

- Patient Inclusion Criteria

—The couple does not qualify for Level I or II care

—Assisted reproductive technology (ART) is under consideration

- Practitioner Qualifications

—Possesses the qualifications for Levels I and II care

—Has certification or documented experience in assisted reproductive technology, reproductive endocrinology, or urology/andrology

—Has infertility counseling services available

- Obligations

—Management of complicated anovulation, endometriosis, and tubal disease

—Management of complicated male infertility

—The ability to provide direct access to male and female microsurgical services and ART and related services

American Society for Reproductive Medicine. Guidelines for the provision of infertility services. ASRM Committee Opinion. Birmingham, Alabama: ASRM, 1996

Table 4–1. Comparison of Reported Outcomes for Assisted Reproductive Technology Procedures*

Outcome	Standard IVF	IVF plus ICSI	GIFT	ZIFT	Donor oocyte transfer†	CPE transfer‡	CPE transfer with donor	Host uterus transfer
No. of cycles or procedures§	33,032	18,312	1,943	1,104	4,616	10,181	1,584	600
Cancellations (%)	21.7	NA	14.4	10.4	6.2	6.0	4.3	6.2
No. of retrievals	25,878	18,292	1,663	989	NA	NA	NA	563
No. of transfers	24,027	17,243	1,640	911	4,122	9,165	1,467	540
Transfers per retrieval (%)	92.8	94.3	98.6	92.1	NA	NA	NA	95.9
No. of clinical pregnancies	8,975	6,072	627	346	1,978	2,185	400	226
Pregnancy loss (%)	18.1	18.5	20.4	19.9	16.6	21.3	18.8	17.3
No. of deliveries	7,353	4,949	499	277	1,650	1,719	325	187
Deliveries per retrieval (%)	28.4	27.1	30.0	28.0	NA	NA	NA	33.2
Singleton pregnancies (%)	59.6	62.9	66.9	66.4	56.5	74.4	65.8	83.3
No. of ectopic pregnancies (EP)	220	102	16	11	21	60	10	1
EP transfer (%)	0.9	0.6	1.0	1.2	0.5	0.7	0.7	0.2
Abnormal neonates (%)	1.6	1.7	1.9	1.6	1.9	1.8	2.0	1.9

*ART, assisted reproductive technology; IVF indicates in vitro fertilization; ICSI, intracytoplasmic sperm injection; GIFT, gamete intrafallopian transfer; ZIFT, zygote intrafallopian transfer; CPE, cryopreserved embryos; CPE-DO, cryopreserved embryos from donor egg; NA, not applicable

†Includes known or anonymous but not host uterus transfer or surrogate

‡Cryopreserved embryo transfer cycles not done in combination with fresh embryo transfers and not with donor egg or embryo

§Includes all cycles regardless of maternal age and infertility diagnosis

Reprinted by permission from the American Society for Reproductive Medicine from Assisted reproductive technology in the United States: 1997 results generated from the American Society for Reproductive Medicine/Society for Assisted Reproductive Technology Registry. Fertil Steril 2000;74:641–653

Professional

American College of Obstetricians and Gynecologists. Nonselective embryo reduction: ethical guidance for the obstetrician–gynecologist. In: Ethics in obstetrics and gynecology. Washington, DC: ACOG, 2002:53–56

American College of Obstetricians and Gynecologists. Obstetrician–gynecologists' ethical responsibilities, concerns, and risks pertaining to adoption. In: Ethics in obstetrics and gynecology. Washington, DC: ACOG, 2002:57–60

American College of Obstetricians and Gynecologists. Precis, reproductive endocrinology: an update in obstetrics and gynecology. Washington, DC: ACOG, 1998

American Society for Reproductive Medicine. Guidelines for the provision of infertility services. ASRM Committee Opinion. Birmingham, Alabama: ASRM, 1996

American Society for Reproductive Medicine. Guidelines on number of embryos transferred. ASRM Committee Opinion. Birmingham, Alabama: ASRM, 1999

Collins JA, Hughes EG. Pharmacological interventions for the induction of ovulation. Drugs 1995;50:480–494

Ethical considerations of assisted reproductive technologies. By the Ethics Committee of the American Fertility Society. Fertil Steril 1994;62(Suppl 1):1S–125S

Guidelines for gamete and embryo donation. The American Society for Reproductive Medicine. Fertil Steril 1998;70(Suppl 3):1S–13S

Mosher WD, Pratt WF. Fecundity and infertility in the United States: incidence and trends [editorial]. Fertil Steril 1991;56:192–193

1997 Ethical considerations of assisted reproductive technologies. The Ethics Committee of the American Society for Reproductive Medicine. Fertil Steril 1997;67(Suppl 1):i–iii, 1–9

Posner JL, Gulianelli J. The adoption resource guide: a national directory of licensed agencies. 2nd ed. Washington, DC: Child Welfare League of America, 1990

Revised minimum standards for in vitro fertilization, gamete intrafallopian transfer, and related procedures. The American Society for Reproductive Medicine. Fertil Steril 1998;70(Suppl 2):1S–5S

The Royal College of Obstetricians and Gynaecologists. The initial investigation and management of the infertile couple. RCOG Evidence-Based Clinical Guidelines No. 2. London: RCOG, 1998

Royal College of Obstetricians and Gynaecologists. The management of infertility in secondary care. RCOG Evidence-Based Clinical Guidelines No. 3. London: RCOG, 1998

LATEX ALLERGY

Health Care Impact

Allergy to natural latex rubber is a serious health risk for many health care workers and patients. Latex products, particularly gloves, are ubiquitous in the medical setting and many consumer products (eg, condoms and diaphragms) are made of latex. Allergic reactions to latex range from mild skin reactions to systemic reactions, such as asthma and anaphylaxis, which may result in chronic illness, disability, career loss, hardship, or death.

The prevalence of latex sensitivity in the general population has been estimated to be less than 1% but may be higher. Certain high-risk groups have been identified, but it must be kept in mind that many affected people do not belong to a high-risk group. These high-risk groups include:

- Health care personnel
- Spina bifida patients and other patients who have had multiple surgeries
- Individuals subject to occupational exposure
- Individuals who have a history of atopy
- Individuals who have food allergies, especially those allergic to avocadoes, bananas, kiwi, or passion fruit

ACOG Recommendations

For patients who have latex allergy, a latex-free environment in which no latex gloves or accessories are used should be provided if feasible. Latex-allergic workers should use only nonlatex gloves, and others in the same environment should use nonlatex gloves or powder-free, low-protein gloves. Symptom reduction has been documented with the use of powder-free gloves, enabling sensitized workers to return to the workplace.

A facility-wide strategy for managing latex allergy in the health care environment should include the formation of a latex allergy task force and development of appropriate policies to deal with latex-sensitive individuals in all areas of the facility. A compendium of all latex products used at the institution should be developed, and lists of nonlatex substitutes should be made available.

Expertise

Diagnostic tools include serologic testing for antilatex immunoglobulin E, glove-use tests, patch testing, and skin tests involving pricking or scratching the skin and applying or injecting a liquid preparation containing latex allergens. The choice of testing method depends on the type of allergic reaction being evaluated (eg, contact dermatitis versus systemic symptoms) and the likelihood of a severe reaction to the allergen.

Antigen avoidance is the cardinal principle in the management of latex allergy. Immunotherapy for desensitization is not currently available. For sensitized patients undergoing procedures, pretreatment protocols using antihistamines, corticosteroids, and ephedrine, although prudent, may not afford adequate protection. Treating workers who have occupational asthma with asthma medications is not an acceptable alternative to avoidance. The prognosis for chemically induced asthma is favorable if exposure is stopped shortly after onset of symptoms.

Special warning should be given to sensitized patients regarding the use of condoms and diaphragms. Women are especially at high risk of reaction because of mucous membrane contact with these devices. Polyurethane condoms are available.

Primary prevention of sensitization to latex would require complete avoidance of latex from birth. For the general population, this is not feasible; however, in high-risk groups, measures should be taken to decrease the incidence of sensitization. Secondary prevention involves halting the acceleration of symptom severity and controlling the occurrence of potentially serious allergic reactions in those previously sensitized.

Manufacturers of medical devices are required to label products that include natural rubber latex or dry natural rubber. They may not claim that such products are hypoallergenic.

RESOURCES

Patient

Stehlin D. Latex allergies: when rubber rubs the wrong way. FDA Consum 1992;26:16–21

Professional

Hagler RM. Latex allergy. ACOG Clin Rev 1999;42:1–2,12–14

Kelly KJ. Management of the latex-allergic patient. Immunol Allergy Clin N Am 1995;15: 139–157

Latex allergy—an emerging healthcare problem. Latex Hypersensitivity Committee. Ann Allergy Asthma Immunol 1995;75:19–21

Natural rubber-containing medical devices; user labeling—FDA. Final rule. Fed Regist 1997;62:51021–51030

NIOSH alert: preventing allergic reactions to natural rubber latex in the workplace. Available at www.cdc.gov/niosh/latexalt.html. Retrieved October 6, 2000

Task Force on Allergic Reactions to Latex. American Academy of Allergy and Immunology. Committee report. J Allergy Clin Immunol 1993;92:16–18

Neoplasms

Breast Cancer

Health Care Impact

In the United States, breast cancer is the most common cancer in women, with approximately 192,200 new cases and 40,200 deaths each year. Breast cancer is the leading cause of death from cancer in women 20–59 years of age and is the second leading cause of cancer deaths overall, after lung cancer. The lifetime risk of developing breast cancer is approximately one in eight.

The most common risk factors for developing breast cancer include advancing age and female gender. Other risk factors include a personal or family history of breast cancer, nulliparity, and early menarche or late menopause. However, these and other identified risk factors, either alone or in combination, account for less than 30% of the observed risk of developing breast cancer, and all women, especially those older than 35 years of age, should be considered at risk. Mass screening with mammography is the most effective method of reducing breast cancer mortality, and attention should be given to ensuring that all eligible women are offered such screening.

ACOG Recommendations

Breast examination is an integral part of the gynecologic examination. In addition, obstetrician–gynecologists should instruct their patients in breast self-examination and inform them of the importance of periodic self-examination. The College recommends screening mammography every 1–2 years in women between 40 and 50 years of age and annually in women older than 50 years of age.

In postmenopausal women with previously treated breast cancer, the use of hormone replacement therapy may be considered, with caution exercised in all instances and in consultation with the patient's oncologist and the patient's fully informed consent. Women with breast cancer who use hormone replacement therapy must continue to be monitored for recurrent disease, and, should malignancy recur, the use of hormone replacement therapy must be reevaluated.

Genetic testing for breast–ovarian cancer should be performed only with a woman's full informed consent. Currently, such testing continues to be best performed by investigations working under research protocols approved by an institutional review board (see also "Genetics" in Part 4).

Expertise

The clinician should be able to elicit an accurate history and to document risk factors that might increase the risk of developing breast cancer (see "Primary and Preventive Care" in Part 3). The ability to perform a thorough and accurate breast examination, thus optimizing the chance of detecting breast cancer early, also is necessary. Ideally, the clinician also will have the knowledge and experience to perform cyst aspiration and fine needle aspiration as indicated by findings on examination and mammography. Otherwise, the clinician must be able to promptly refer the patient to another clinician with the expertise to appropriately evaluate any breast abnormality.

The clinician should be knowledgeable regarding the indications and options for breast cancer prevention, including prophylactic mastectomy and chemoprevention. Because a key factor to be considered is the woman's risk of breast cancer, it is important that clinicians take a thorough history to assess her risk adequately. Researchers from the National Cancer Institute and the National Surgical Adjuvant Breast and Bowel Project have developed a computer-based tool to allow clinicians to project a woman's individualized estimate of breast cancer risk. The Breast Cancer Risk Assessment Tool is a computer disk that a woman and her health care professional can use to estimate her chances of developing breast cancer based on several established risk factors. The disk is available at no charge in PC-compatible and Macintosh computer formats. To order, call the National Cancer Institute's Cancer Information Service at 800-422-6237 or visit the National Cancer Institute's cancer trials web site at http://cancertrials.nci.nih.gov/.

It is recommended that appropriate support and consideration be given to patients undergoing mastectomy, recognizing that short length of stay at the time of mastectomy is not optimal for all patients requiring such intervention.

The Cancer Rights Act of 1998 requires that insurance coverage for mastectomy include reconstructive surgery. Obstetrician–gynecologists who provide mammography services should be in compliance with the Mammography Standards Quality Act (see "Compliance with Government Regulations" in Part 1).

Cervical Cancer

Health Care Impact

Despite the fact that use of the Pap test has been associated with a 70% decline in deaths from cervical cancer during the past 50 years, there were 12,900 new cases of invasive cancer and 4,400 deaths expected in the United States in 2001. Although the median age for the occurrence of invasive carcinoma has remained constant at 44–50 years of age, this malignancy is diagnosed in women of all ages. Older women do not as often receive regular cervical cytology screening and unscreened elderly women may continue to be at high risk for the development of this malignancy.

A very large body of data has now established the fact that the human papillomavirus is a major contributor to cervical malignancy. Although the great majority of women with human papillomavirus will never develop this cancer, 95% of cervical malignancies have been associated with human papillomavirus. Certain high-risk factors have been associated with the development of cervical intraepithelial neoplasia and cervical carcinoma (see "Primary and Preventive Care" in Part 3).

ACOG Recommendations

All women who are or who have been sexually active or who have reached 18 years of age should undergo annual cervical cytology screening and pelvic examination. After a woman has had three or more consecutive, satisfactory annual examinations with normal findings, screening may be performed less frequently in a low-risk woman at the discretion of her physician.

Following treatment of preinvasive lesions of the cervix or vagina, one option is for patients to undergo cytologic evaluation at frequent intervals, every 3–4 months if feasible, for approximately 1 year and then annually thereafter. For invasive lesions, evaluation should occur every 3–4 months for approximately 2 years and then every 6 months. Close follow-up of these women is necessary because those treated for squamous cell carcinoma of the cervix are at increased risk of developing preinvasive or invasive squamous neoplasms elsewhere in the lower genital tract.

Expertise

The clinician should be able to recognize the factors that put a woman at high risk for the development of cervical neoplasia and should establish regular screening programs. Using colposcopy, the clinician also should be able to appropriately evaluate patients with an abnormal finding and accurately diagnose and appropriately treat preinvasive disease in these patients, including identifying those patients who should undergo excisional biopsy, such as cone biopsy or loop electrode excision procedure, to rule out invasive cancer (see also "Abnormal Cervical Cytology" in Part 4). These patients should be monitored carefully after treatment to rule out recurrent neoplasia. Worrisome symptoms such as postcoital bleeding and vaginal discharge should be promptly and thoroughly evaluated to rule out the presence of an early invasive cancer.

The clinician should be familiar with the options for treating women with both early and advanced cervical cancer and should facilitate referrals for this treatment. A 1999 clinical announcement from the National Cancer Institute describes that the standard of care for most patients with cervical cancer who will receive radiation therapy as either front-line or salvage therapy is to give concomitant cisplatin-based chemotherapy as a radiation sensitizer. In most cases, women diagnosed with invasive cervical cancer should be referred to a gynecologic oncologist for coordination of care, often in conjunction with a radiation therapist.

Endometrial Cancer

Health Care Impact

Carcinoma of the endometrium is the most common genital tract malignancy in the United States. The incidence of this malignancy has increased during the past 50 years as a result of the longer life expectancy of women, improved methods of diagnosis, and an increased frequency of certain predisposing conditions, such as chronic unopposed estrogen, either endogenous or exogenous. Approximately 2–3% of women in the United States will develop cancer of the endometrium at some point during their lifetime.

Adenocarcinoma of the endometrium is predominantly a disease of postmenopausal women. In the United States, white women have a 2.88% lifetime risk of developing endometrial cancer as compared with a 1.69% risk for African-American women. Risk factors for the development of endometrial cancer include excess endogenous estrogen exposure (early menarche, late menopause, obesity, chronic anovulation, estrogen-secreting tumors), unopposed exogenous estrogen exposure, tamoxifen exposure, previous pelvic radiation, hypertension, diabetes, and a personal history of breast, ovarian, or colon cancer. Factors that decrease the risk of endometrial cancer include high parity, smoking, and the use of combination oral contraceptives.

ACOG Recommendations

There are no effective screening methods to detect endometrial cancer. Endometrial cancer should be suspected in any postmenopausal woman with bleeding, and in any perimenopausal woman with increased menstrual flow, a decreased menstrual interval, or intermenstrual bleeding. Routine cervical cytology screening cannot be relied on to detect endometrial abnormalities. Although neither transvaginal nor transabdominal ultrasonography evaluation can confirm the presence or absence of cancer of the endometrium, ultrasonography can provide information to aid in diagnosis.

An endometrial biopsy, when possible, is appropriate and may eliminate the need for a formal dilation and curettage. Even though surgical staging requires pelvic and periaortic lymph node sampling, there is controversy concerning the clinical benefit of node sampling for all patients with Stage I disease. Patients with Grade 1 or 2 tumors with superficial invasion are at low risk for node metastases and may be spared the operative risks associated with node sampling. Pelvic and periaortic node sampling is recommended for all patients with suspicious nodes encountered at surgery, those with Grade 3 tumors, and those with any grade tumor with invasion into the middle third of the myometrium or cervical involvement. Postoperative therapy should be based on surgical–pathologic factors, such as depth of myometrial invasion and extrauterine extension.

Currently, there are no definitive data to support specific recommendations regarding the use of estrogen in women previously treated for endometrial cancer. At this time, the decision to use hormone replacement therapy in these women should be individualized on the basis of potential benefit and risk to the patient. Women taking tamoxifen should be monitored closely for symptoms of endometrial hyperplasia or cancer and should have a gynecologic examination at least once every year. These patients also should be encouraged to promptly report any abnormal vaginal symptoms, including bloody discharge, spotting, staining, or leukorrhea, and these symptoms should be investigated. Screening tests have not been effective in increasing the early detection of endometrial cancer in women using tamoxifen and may lead to more invasive and costly diagnostic procedures; they are not recommended. If atypical endometrial hyperplasia develops, appropriate gynecologic management should be instituted, and the use of tamoxifen should be reassessed.

Expertise

The clinician should be able to elicit an appropriate history and identify risk factors that would predispose to the development of endometrial cancer. Appropriate physical and pelvic examination should be done to determine the source of any abnormal bleeding and to rule out extrauterine etiologies. The clinician should have the appropriate expertise and equipment to perform outpatient endometrial biopsies and have the ability to obtain transvaginal ultrasound to evaluate the endometrial thickness. The clinician who plans to treat the patient with endometrial cancer must have the expertise to determine when full surgical staging is necessary and to be able to perform the required procedures, such as pelvic and periaortic node sampling. A referral to a gynecologic oncologist is appropriate.

Ovarian Cancer

Health Care Impact

Ovarian cancer is the leading cause of death from genital tract malignancy and the fifth leading cause of cancer-related death in American women. Most cases occur in women older than 50 years of age, but this disease also can affect younger women. The lifetime risk of ovarian cancer is 1.8%, with an annual incidence approaching 61.8 per 100,000 women who reach 75–79 years of age. An estimated 23,400 new cases are reported in the United States each year, with approximately 14,000 women dying from this malignancy annually. The main reason for these dismal statistics is that more than three quarters of all patients with ovarian cancer are diagnosed with Stage III and IV disease. Currently, there are no screening methods available that are appropriate for screening the general population.

The pathogenesis of ovarian carcinoma remains unclear. Pregnancy, breastfeeding, and oral contraceptive use are associated with a decreased risk of ovarian cancer. Only about 5–10% of patients with ovarian cancer have a significant family history for this malignancy. Women with *BRCA1* mutation have up to a 90% lifetime risk of developing either breast or ovarian cancer or both, compared with women without a *BRCA1* mutation.

ACOG Recommendations

During the preoperative evaluation of a woman with a pelvic mass, if there is a high probability of ovarian malignancy, the physician should consider consultation with a gynecologic oncologist. Women who have demonstrated familial ovarian or hereditary breast–ovarian cancer syndromes may benefit from screening. Genetic testing for breast–ovarian cancer should be performed only with a woman's full informed consent.

Currently, such testing continues to be best performed by investigators working under research protocols approved by an institutional review board (see also "Genetics" in Part 4).

Women who do not wish to maintain their reproductive capacity may be offered prophylactic bilateral salpingo-oophorectomy, only after a familial syndrome has been established by a full pedigree analysis by a geneticist and the patient has been counseled regarding the ethical and medical implications of this testing (see also "Genetics" in Part 4). The decision to perform prophylactic oophorectomy should not be based only on age; it should be a highly individualized decision that takes into account several patient factors and choices.

Expertise

The clinical expertise required for the evaluation of the patient with a pelvic mass includes the knowledge of common disorders, both benign and malignant, that can present as a pelvic mass. Knowledge of the appropriate preoperative evaluations required to determine the etiology of the pelvic mass is important, as is the ability to manage the perioperative patient. If an early ovarian malignancy is found, the knowledge and surgical expertise to thoroughly stage the patient is mandatory, including pelvic and periaortic lymph node sampling and omentectomy. If an advanced ovarian malignancy is encountered, the ability to use currently available tumor debulking techniques is important for the overall prognosis of the patient.

Vulvar Cancer

Health Care Impact

Vulvar cancer is fairly uncommon, accounting for approximately 5% of all gynecologic malignancies. Each year, approximately 3,600 new cases and 800 deaths occur. The great majority of malignant vulvar lesions are squamous cancers, with less common histologies including melanomas, Bartholin gland carcinomas, and a variety of sarcomas. In the recent past, the prognostic factors for vulvar cancers have been more clearly defined, and the development of more conservative surgical approaches and combination chemoradiation has contributed to improved quality of life in patients with this malignancy.

ACOG Recommendations

Because there are no macroscopic features diagnostic of vulvar cancer, biopsy should be performed promptly for any suspicious lesion, such as a confluent, wart-like mass, ulceration, thickening, or localized, unexplained itching that persists for more than one month. If a diagnosis of extensive vulvar intraepithelial neoplasia or invasive cancer is made, appropriate referral of the patient to someone with the requisite expertise to offer state-of-the-art and often multimodality therapy is required.

Expertise

To avoid significant delay in diagnosis, the clinician should have a high index of suspicion of vulvar cancer when a woman presents with vulvar symptoms or findings, especially in older women. The clinician also should be able to recognize the often subtle findings associated with preinvasive and early invasive vulvar lesions and should be able to perform appropriate diagnostic procedures, including colposcopy and vulvar biopsy, to confirm the diagnosis.

Gestational Trophoblastic Disease

Health Care Impact

Gestational trophoblastic disease (GTD) encompasses a spectrum of interrelated disease processes originating from the placenta. These histologically distinct entities include complete and partial hydatidiform moles, invasive moles, placental site trophoblastic tumors, and choriocarcinoma. With the currently available sensitive assays for human chorionic gonadotropin to monitor the disease and with effective chemotherapy regimens (both single-agent and multiagent regimens), the previously observed morbidity and mortality from these disorders have been greatly reduced. With appropriate evaluation and treatment, most women with malignant GTD can be cured and their reproductive function preserved.

Estimates of the incidence of GTD vary widely. In the United States, hydatidiform moles are observed in approximately 1 per 1,500–2,000 pregnancies. Invasive moles follow approximately 10–15% of complete hydatidiform moles. Approximately 1 of 40 moles, 1 of 5,000 ectopic pregnancies, 1 of 15,000 abortions, and 1 of 150,000 normal pregnancies result in choriocarcinoma. Approximately 3,000 cases of hydatidiform mole and 500–750 cases of malignant GTD are diagnosed in the United States each year.

ACOG Recommendations

For patients treated for a hydatidiform mole, contraception is recommended for at least 6 months to 1 year after remission. Patients with a prior partial or complete molar gestation have a 10-fold risk of a second mole in subsequent pregnancies. Therefore, all future pregnancies should be evaluated by ultrasonography early in their course. For patients treated for metastatic GTD, contraception, preferably with oral contraceptives, should be used during the first year of remission. Because of the 1–2% risk of a second molar pregnancy in subsequent pregnancies, early ultrasound examination is recommended for all future pregnancies.

Expertise

To allow for optimal treatment and outcomes, the clinician should be able to diagnose and manage women with primary molar gestations, promptly diagnose malignant GTD, and assess risk in women with malignant GTD. Once the diagnosis of malignant GTD has been made, the clinician should have access to the appropriate expertise so the patient can receive optimal therapy. Because of the increased risk of subsequent molar pregnancies, patients who become pregnant after a molar pregnancy require monitoring that may include performing an early ultrasonography to document normal gestational development, obtaining histologic evaluation of the products of conception for pregnancy loss or placenta after delivery, and documenting a quantitative human chorionic gonadotropin level at the 6-week postpartum visit.

Resources

Patient

American College of Obstetricians and Gynecologists. Cancer of the ovary. ACOG Patient Education Pamphlet AP096. Washington, DC: ACOG, 1999

American College of Obstetricians and Gynecologists. Cancer of the uterus. ACOG Patient Education Pamphlet AP097. Washington, DC: ACOG, 1999

American College of Obstetricians and Gynecologists. Colposcopy. ACOG Patient Education Pamphlet AP135. Washington, DC: ACOG, 2000

American College of Obstetricians and Gynecologists. Detecting and treating breast problems. ACOG Patient Education Pamphlet AP026. Washington, DC: ACOG, 1999

American College of Obstetricians and Gynecologists. Diseases of the vulva. ACOG Patient Education Pamphlet AP088. Washington, DC: ACOG, 2000

American College of Obstetricians and Gynecologists. Disorders of the cervix. ACOG Patient Education Pamphlet AP033. Washington, DC: ACOG, 1999

Professional

American College of Obstetricians and Gynecologists. Breast–ovarian cancer screening. ACOG Committee Opinion 239. Washington, DC: ACOG, 2000

American College of Obstetricians and Gynecologists. Concurrent chemoradiation in the treatment of cervical cancer. ACOG Committee Opinion 242. Washington, DC: ACOG, 2000

American College of Obstetricians and Gynecologists. Hormone replacement therapy in women treated for endometrial cancer. ACOG Committee Opinion 235. Washington, DC: ACOG, 2000

American College of Obstetricians and Gynecologists. Prophylactic oophorectomy. ACOG Practice Bulletin 7. Washington, DC: ACOG, 1999

American College of Obstetricians and Gynecologists. Recommendations on frequency of Pap test screening. ACOG Committee Opinion 152. Washington, DC: ACOG, 1995

American College of Obstetricians and Gynecologists. Routine cancer screening. ACOG Committee Opinion 247. Washington, DC: ACOG, 2000

American College of Obstetricians and Gynecologists. Tamoxifen and endometrial cancer. ACOG Committee Opinion 232. Washington, DC: ACOG, 2000

American College of Obstetricians and Gynecologists. Tamoxifen and the prevention of breast cancer in high-risk women. ACOG Committee Opinion 224. Washington, DC: ACOG, 1999

Benedet JL, Bender H, Jones H 3rd, Ngan HY, Pecorelli S. FIGO staging classifications and clinical practice guidelines in the management of gynecologic cancers. FIGO Committee on Gynecologic Oncology. Int J Gynaecol Obstet 2000;70:209–262

Greenlee RT, Hill-Harmon MB, Murray T, Bolden S, Thun M. Cancer statistics, 2001. CA Cancer J Clin 2001;51:15–36

Hammond CB. Gestational trophoblastic neoplasms. In Scott JR, Di Saia PJ, Hammond CB, Spellacy WN. Danforth's Obstetrics and Gynecology. 8th ed. Philadelphia: Lippincott Williams & Wilkins, 1999: 927–937

Institute of Medicine. Ensuring quality cancer care. Washington, DC: National Academy Press, 1999

Royal College of Obstetricians and Gynaecologists. The management of gestational trophoblastic disease. RCOG Guideline 18. London: RCOG, 1999

Statement of the American Society of Clinical Oncology: genetic testing for cancer susceptibility, Adopted on February 20, 1996. J Clin Oncol 1996;14:1730–1736

Winchester DP, Strom EA. Standards for diagnosis and management of ductal carcinoma in situ (DCIS) of the breast. American College of Radiology. American College of Surgeons. College of American Pathologists. Society of Surgical Oncology. CA Cancer J Clin 1998;48:108–128

OSTEOPOROSIS AND BONE DENSITOMETRY

Health Care Impact

An estimated 1.5 million osteoporosis-related fractures occur each year in the United States. Osteoporosis-related fractures commonly involve the proximal femur, vertebral body, and distal forearm. Of these sites, the proximal femur (hip) has the greatest effect on morbidity and mortality. There is a 15–20% reduction in the expected survival during the first year following a hip fracture. Hip fractures also are associated with significant pain, disability, and decreased functional independence. It has been estimated that the annual cost of osteoporosis-related fractures in the United States is nearly $14 billion in direct and indirect expenses.

The risk of postmenopausal osteoporosis is a function of both the peak bone mass acquired during adolescent growth combined with the rate of bone loss in adulthood. The principal risk factors for osteoporosis are female sex, advanced age, Caucasian race, low body weight, and bilateral oophorectomy before menopause. Smoking is a probable risk factor for hip fracture, but is a less reliable predictor than bone mass.

A number of radiologic screening tests have been proposed for both clinical and research purposes to detect low bone mass in asymptomatic persons. These include conventional skeletal radiography, computed tomography, single photon absorptiometry, dual photon absorptiometry, and dual-energy X-ray absorptiometry (DXA). Dual-energy X-ray absorptiometry is now widely used in the clinical setting and provides more reproducible measures of bone density and shorter examination times than other tests. Ultrasonography technology for assessing bone density and architecture is under development and may be of value in the future.

There is little evidence from controlled trials that women who receive bone density screening have better outcomes (improved bone density or fewer fractures) than women who are not screened. The primary argument for screening has been evidence that postmenopausal women with risk for low bone density (and risk for subsequent fractures) can be convinced to begin therapy. Women who have below-average bone density were more likely to take calcium supplements or estrogen than those with above-average values. However, the effect of bone mineral screening on long-term compliance is not known, and there are no studies determining how well perimenopausal bone density measurements will predict long-term risk of fracture.

ACOG Recommendations

The American College of Obstetricians and Gynecologists recommends that women receive counseling about the risks of osteoporosis, but does not recommend routine screening for osteoporosis. Counseling adolescents and women of reproductive age regarding exercise and calcium supplementation may be helpful in encouraging women to maximize peak bone mass. The Canadian Task Force on the Periodic Health Examination and the American College of Physicians/American Society of Internal Medicine conclude that bone density measurements "may be useful" in guiding the treatment decisions in selected postmenopausal women. The American Academy of Family Physicians recommends measuring bone mineral content in women 40–64 years of age with risk factors for osteoporosis. The U.S. Preventive Services Task Force concludes that there is insufficient evidence to recommend for or against screening in asymptomatic postmenopausal women. Instead, the U.S. Preventive Services Task Force recommends that all women should receive counseling regarding universal prevention measures related to fracture risk. Finally, the National Osteoporosis Foundation also has developed bone mineral density testing guidelines. The organization recommends bone mineral density testing to confirm the diagnosis of osteoporosis in women with fractures, for women younger than 65 years of age who have one or more risk factors for developing osteoporosis (besides menopause), and for all women 65 years of age and older, regardless of their risk for fracture.

Expertise

Several areas of expertise are required to properly evaluate and treat women at risk for osteoporosis. These areas of expertise are:

Evaluation:

- Ability to counsel all women on the risk factors for osteoporosis
- Ability to identify risk factors in patients
- Availability of bone mineral density measuring instrument (eg, DXA machine)
- Skilled technical and supporting services
- Ability to interpret the results of bone mineral density testing

Treatment:

- Advise all patients to consume adequate dietary calcium and vitamin D
- Recommend weight-bearing and strengthening exercises
- Advise all patients to avoid tobacco and minimize alcohol consumption
- Recommend pharmacologic options for osteoporosis prevention (hormone replacement therapy, alendronate, risedronate, raloxifene) and treatment (hormone replacement therapy, alendronate, risedronate, calcitonin, raloxifene)

Because the amount of emitted radiation of DXA machines is below regulated thresholds, no national standard for DXA exists. This technology is commonly regulated by local and state agencies. Check hospital, local, and state regulatory standards that apply in your area. Usually the manufacturer of the DXA equipment provides training and continuing education for technical and professional staff.

Resources

Patient

American College of Obstetricians and Gynecologists. Hormone replacement therapy. ACOG Patient Education Pamphlet AP066. Washington, DC: ACOG, 1997

American College of Obstetricians and Gynecologists. The menopause years. ACOG Patient Education Pamphlet AP047. Washington, DC: ACOG, 1997

American College of Obstetricians and Gynecologists. Midlife transitions: a guide to approaching menopause. ACOG Patient Education Pamphlet AB013. Washington, DC: ACOG, 1997

American College of Obstetricians and Gynecologists. Preventing osteoporosis. ACOG Patient Education Pamphlet AP048. Washington, DC: ACOG, 1997

Professional

American College of Obstetricians and Gynecologists. Osteoporosis. ACOG Educational Bulletin 246. Washington, DC: ACOG, 1998

Canadian Consensus Conference on Menopause and Osteoporosis: part I: consensus statements. J SOGC 1998;20:1243–1272

Gluer CC. Quantitative ultrasound techniques for the assessment of osteoporosis: expert agreement on current status. The International Quantitative Ultrasound Consensus Group. J Bone Miner Res 1997;12:1280–1288

National Osteoporosis Foundation. Physician's guide to prevention and treatment of osteoporosis. Washington, DC: NOF, 1998

Screening for postmenopausal osteoporosis. In: U.S. Preventive Services Task Force. Guide to clinical preventive services: report of U.S. Preventive Services Task Force. 2nd ed. Baltimore: Williams and Wilkins, 1996:509–516

Sturtridge W, Lentle B, Hanley DA. Prevention and management of osteoporosis: consensus statements from the Scientific Advisory Board of the Osteoporosis Society of Canada. 2. The use of bone density measurement in the diagnosis and management of osteoporosis. CMAJ 1996;155:924–929

PAIN MANAGEMENT

Health Care Impact

The heterogeneous patient population cared for by gynecologists results in a broad range of pain management challenges. The pain experienced by gynecologic patients ranges from acute pain, such as postoperative incisional pain, to chronic pain, such as that experienced by many patients with cancer. Although the treatment of patients with acute, postoperative pain is typically less challenging than the long-term management of chronic pain syndromes, studies have shown that even this acute pain often is not optimally controlled. In this setting, many patients respond adequately to the "as-needed" administration of an opioid such as morphine or meperidine, whereas other patients require a modification of the dosage or the method of administration to achieve optimal results. In general surgical patient populations, studies have documented that unrelieved postoperative pain has been reported by 25–70% of patients, and surveys of patients with chronic cancer pain have documented that approximately two thirds also suffer from acute transient pain. It is clear that even though the techniques required to provide adequate relief of pain are widely available, they often are inadequately used. The fear of regulatory scrutiny is the most common reason physicians give for failing to provide adequate treatment for chronic pain.

ACOG Recommendations

General principles of pain management are outlined in the box. Whenever possible, therapy should be directed toward resolving the underlying condition.

Expertise

The ability to optimally manage pain requires first the comprehensive assessment of pain, which includes information regarding temporal characteristics, stable versus constant course, severity, location, quality, and

Pain Management Principles

Use positive reinforcement and support.

- Placebos should not be used to assess pain.
- The placebo effect should be used to supplement other therapy through positive reinforcement.

Assess psychologic factors early in the evaluation process.

- Coexisting depression or sleep disorders should be sought.
- The diagnosis of "psychogenic pain" should not be a diagnosis of exclusion. Rather, it should be made only when there are clear indications for this diagnosis.

Treat the underlying disorder whenever possible.

- Pain receptors do not adapt and under some circumstances actually lower their thresholds causing hyperalgesia.

Treat the pain promptly and continue on a regular basis.

- Treatment that effectively suppresses pain or that is not based on the need to reexperience pain gives the best results (eg, patient-controlled analgesia for post-operative patients). Frequent, scheduled follow-ups are better than "as needed" visits.

Consider the use of multiple treatment modalities in synergy.

- Different methods of treatment work by way of different routes (eg, relaxation techniques, transcutaneous electrical nerve stimulation, physical therapy, vocational rehabilitation, and biofeedback).
- The nuances of the treatments used should be understood (eg, site of action, half-life, administration routes available, and interactions).
- Combinations of medications that increase sedation without enhancing analgesia should be avoided.

Use narcotic drugs with caution.

- Tolerance and dependence may occur with long-term use.
- Narcotics should not be withheld if other therapies are ineffective.

provocative and palliative factors. The clinician should be well versed in the various options for the management of pain.

A model approach to the selection of drug therapy, known as the "analgesic ladder," has been developed by the World Health Organization. With this approach, patients with mild to moderate pain are first treated with a nonsteroidal antiinflammatory drug, then treated with a weak opioid often with an nonsteroidal antiinflammatory drug, followed by a strong opioid as indicated to control her pain. Ideally, clinicians also should be aware of alternative approaches to the management of chronic pain, including nerve blocks, neuroaugmentive approaches such as transcutaneous electrical nerve stimulation and acupuncture, and neurosurgical approaches. Many hospitals have established comprehensive pain services, which often are directed by anesthesiologists and provide expert assessment and multimodality therapy for both acute and chronic pain. Beginning with its 2000–2001 standards manuals, the Joint Commission on the Accreditation of Health Care Organizations provides new standards for hospitals, ambulatory care facilities, and other institutions on pain assessment and treatment. Clinicians also should be aware of the option for patient-controlled analgesia.

In general, nonsteroidal antiinflammatory drugs are overused and provide minimal benefit to patients in severe pain, particularly those experiencing cancer pain. Often they are used instead of opioids with the well-intended concern that patients not become dependent. However, this class of medications generally does not control severe cancer pain, particularly at the end of life.

Guidelines for the treatment of cancer pain suggest that long-acting opioids be administered around the clock for persistent baseline pain, supplemented with short-acting oral opioids for episodes of breakthrough pain. Ninety percent of cancer pain can be controlled by relatively simple means (opioid administration via oral, rectal, or transdermal routes). Effective management requires recognition of age-related changes in drug pharmacokinetics and awareness of a drug's potential side effects.

Methods of neurostimulation, such as a transcutaneous electrical nerve stimulation unit, acupuncture, and massage, are based on the gate theory of pain control. These treatments can be useful for pain control, particularly when muscle pain is severe. Imagery, aromatherapy, and other mood modifiers can provide an atmosphere of relaxation and comfort. Finally, conduction anesthesia can be provided by continuous administration in the home or with hospice care.

Clinicians should be familiar with any relevant pain treatment legislation adopted in their state. Clinicians also should be familiar with any requirements regarding the use of controlled substances.

Resources

Patient

American College of Obstetricians and Gynecologists. Pelvic pain. ACOG Patient Education Pamphlet AP099. Washington, DC: ACOG, 1999

Professional

Agency for Healthcare Research and Quality. Management of cancer pain: summary. Evidence Report/Technology Assessment no. 35. Rockville, Maryland: AHRQ, 2001. AHRQ publication no. 01-E033. Available at www.ahcpr.gov/clinic/canpainsum.htm

The Federation of State Medical Boards of the United States, Inc. Model guidelines for the use of controlled substances for the treatment of pain. SDJ Med 1999;52:25–27

Martino AM. In search of a new ethic for treating patients with chronic pain: what can medical boards do? J Law Med Ethics 1998;26:332–349

Quality improvement guidelines for the treatment of acute pain and cancer pain. American Pain Society Quality of Care Committee. JAMA 1995;274:1874–1880

World Health Organization. Cancer pain relief and palliative care. Geneva: WHO, 1990

PEDIATRIC GYNECOLOGY

Health Care Impact

Pediatric gynecology includes the care of prepubertal and peripubertal females. A small percentage of this group will come to the attention of the health care system for problems such as vulvovaginitis, sexual differentiation abnormalities, precocious puberty, vaginal bleeding, sexual abuse, neoplasms, or other indications. Appropriate evaluation of pediatric gynecologic conditions will assist the health of the child and ensure a positive future approach to the health care system.

ACOG Recommendations

The American College of Obstetricians and Gynecologists recommends that clinicians conduct pediatric gynecologic examinations with patience and sensitivity. They also should be aware of childhood hormonal patterns and developmental stages (both psychological and physical).

Expertise

The clinician should thoroughly explain the examination and its purpose and show any instruments being used to the child. Patient positioning can be very helpful and should vary with the age of the child. A small child may be best evaluated while sitting on the parent's lap, with the child's legs separated and draped over the parent's thighs. The larger child can be positioned supine with feet in the examination table stirrups. Placement of a cooperative child in the knee-chest position causes the vagina to open, and with lateral and superior retraction of the labia majora, the upper vagina and cervix can be visualized.

Foreign bodies, often toilet paper, in the vagina are the most common cause of vaginitis. X-ray and ultrasound studies are not recommended routinely, because they fail to detect most vaginal foreign objects. Removal of the foreign body can be accomplished by lavaging the vagina with normal saline. If this is unsuccessful, the child should receive a general anesthetic and the object should be removed. Objects that have remained in the vagina for prolonged periods may become embedded in the vaginal wall or even penetrate the wall. Therefore, they should be removed with great care and examined thoroughly.

Instruments that may be useful include mirrors, hand lenses, vaginoscopes, endoscopes, hysteroscopes, or cystoscopes with irrigating capacity to obtain samples for wet mounts, forensic studies, or cultures. Plastic tubing combined with a portion of a pediatric Foley catheter also may be used to lavage the vagina for samples. Magnetic resonance imaging, computed tomography, or ultrasonography may be helpful in patients with abdominal or pelvic masses or precocious puberty, to evaluate ovaries and adrenal glands. Anesthesia may be necessary for situations that involve pain (eg, laceration repair) or inability to cooperate.

The clinician should be familiar with state statutes regarding the need for consent for examination by a parent or guardian. All states require findings in minors of signs of physical or sexual abuse to be reported to the proper state authorities.

Resources

Patient

American College of Obstetricians and Gynecologists. Growing up. ACOG Patient Education Pamphlet AP041. Washington, DC: ACOG, 1997

Professional

American College of Obstetricians and Gynecologists. Pediatric gynecologic disorders. ACOG Technical Bulletin 201. Washington, DC: ACOG, 1995

Kahn JA, Emans SJ. Gynecologic examination of the prepubertal girl. Contemp Ob Gyn 1998;43(7):71–72, 74, 77–78, 80, 83–86, 89–90

PELVIC FLOOR DYSFUNCTION

Health Care Impact

The prevalence of dysfunction of the pelvic floor increases as more women live longer. The lifetime risk of undergoing an operation for pelvic organ prolapse or urinary incontinence by 80 years of age has been estimated to be 11%. Usually women with pelvic floor dysfunction are postmenopausal and have had vaginal deliveries or chronic repetitive increases in intraabdominal pressure. Congenital weakness of the pelvic floor tissues is another cause of pelvic floor dysfunction. The urethra, bladder, rectum, or small bowel may protrude into the vaginal canal.

ACOG Recommendations

It is recommended that evaluation consist of examination of the symptomatic woman in lithotomy, sitting, and standing positions before, during, and after a maximum Valsalva effort. Treatment is determined by the age of the patient, the desire for future fertility, the desire for coital function, the severity of symptoms and degree of disability, and the presence of medical complications.

Expertise

Clinician experience with normal pelvic floor function and its variations, as well as awareness that dysfunction may respond to noninvasive as well as surgical interventions, are important in the management of pelvic floor dysfunction. In addition to medical and surgical approaches, supplementary approaches may include treatment of chronic respiratory or metabolic conditions, constipation, and intraabdominal disorders. Hormonal treatment, weight control, smoking cessation, reduction in activities that increase intraabdominal pressure, and vaginal pessaries may be of assistance. Instruction in Kegel exercises may be appropriate.

Urogynecologic investigation can be helpful if urinary incontinence or extensive bladder prolapse is present (see also “Urinary Incontinence” in

Part 4). Cystoscopy and endoscopy may be useful adjuncts to surgical repair.

Resources

Patient

American College of Obstetricians and Gynecologists. Pelvic support problems. ACOG Patient Education Pamphlet AP012. Washington, DC: ACOG, 1999

Professional

American College of Obstetricians and Gynecologists. Evaluation of cesarean delivery. Washington, DC: ACOG, 2000

Olsen AL, Smith VJ, Bergstrom JO, Colling JC, Clark AL. Epidemiology of surgically managed pelvic organ prolapse and urinary incontinence. Obstet Gynecol 1997;89:501–506

PREMENSTRUAL SYNDROME

Health Care Impact

The definition of premenstrual syndrome (PMS) is the cyclic recurrence of symptoms, which occur in the luteal phase of the menstrual cycle and cease shortly after the onset of menstruation, and are severe enough to interfere with some aspects of life. Premenstrual emotional and physical changes occur in up to 85% of women of reproductive age. It is estimated that 20–40% of these women regard these changes as difficult, and 5–10% report a significant impact on work, lifestyle, or relationships. Although the prevalence of premenstrual symptoms in the general population is high, most women do not seek care primarily for treatment of these symptoms, which include:

- Mood alterations (eg, irritability, aggression, anxiety, crying spells, depression, lethargy, sleep disorders, decreased libido, and loss of concentration)
- Breast tenderness, swelling
- Fluid retention, abdominal bloating, edema of extremities, weight gain
- Headache, migraine
- Thirst and appetite changes (food cravings)

Diagnosis of PMS depends on the exclusion of other medical and psychiatric disorders and the demonstration with a patient-completed calendar of true cyclicity of symptoms severe enough to impair the woman's life. Of those who do have severe PMS, a coexisting medical or psychiatric disorder, especially depression, may be observed. As many as 50–60% of women with a complaint of severe PMS-like symptoms have an underlying psychiatric condition, including bipolar disorder, anxiety, and personality disturbances. In many couples, marital or family problems may play a significant role in the escalation of premenstrual emotional changes. Either by structured psychometric instrument or by skilled interview, these possible problem areas should be assessed and the patient should be referred to appropriate mental health resources.

ACOG Recommendations

Women diagnosed as having PMS should meet standard diagnostic criteria and should have the timing of their symptoms confirmed using a prospective symptom calendar. As an overall clinical approach, treatments should be employed in increasing orders of complexity. Using this principle, in most cases, the therapies should be used in the following order:

Step 1: Supportive therapy, dietary complex carbohydrates, aerobic exercise, nutritional supplements (calcium, magnesium, vitamin E), spironolactone

Step 2: Selective serotonin reuptake inhibitors (fluoxetine or sertraline as the initial choice); for women who do not respond, consider an anxiolytic for specific symptoms

Step 3: Hormonal ovulation suppression (oral contraceptives or gonadotropin-releasing hormone agonists)

Expertise

Clinicians should be able to rule out pathological processes and psychiatric problems through a careful history, physical examination, and laboratory testing as needed. Access to supporting services, including mental health resources and nutritional and exercise counseling, may be helpful.

Resources

Patient

American College of Obstetricians and Gynecologists. Premenstrual syndrome. ACOG Patient Education Pamphlet AP057. Washington, DC: ACOG, 2000

Professional

American College of Obstetricians and Gynecologists. Premenstrual syndrome. ACOG Practice Bulletin 15. Washington, DC: ACOG, 2000

Lichtman R, Papera S, eds. Gynecology: well-woman care. Norwalk, Connecticut: Appleton & Lange, 1990

RECURRENT PREGNANCY LOSS

Health Care Impact

Recurrent pregnancy loss typically is defined as two or three or more consecutive pregnancy losses, and it occurs in approximately 1% of reproductive age women. Recent evidence suggests that the risk of abortion after two successive spontaneous abortions is clinically similar to the risk of recurrence among women with three or more consecutive abortions. Thus, patients with two or more consecutive spontaneous abortions are candidates for an evaluation to determine the etiology, if any, for their pregnancy losses.

Recurrent early pregnancy loss can be a difficult and frustrating problem for patients and clinicians. Factors to be considered in the evaluation of women with recurrent pregnancy loss include:

- Characteristics of prior pregnancy losses
- Exposure to toxins and drugs
- Genetic abnormalities
- Pelvic infections
- Endocrine or metabolic dysfunction
- Immunologic disorder
- Uterine abnormalities

ACOG Recommendations

It is reasonable to evaluate patients with two or more pregnancy losses for traditionally accepted causes. Couples with recurrent pregnancy loss should be tested for parental balanced chromosome abnormalities, and those affected by genetic abnormalities should be counseled regarding the risk of recurring abortion and offered prenatal genetic studies in future pregnancies. Corrective surgery for uterine defects may be reasonable, particularly in the case of a uterine septum. Women with recurrent pregnancy loss should be tested for lupus anticoagulant and anticardiolipin antibodies using standard assays. If positive for the same antibody on two consecutive occasions 6–8 weeks apart, they should be treated with heparin and low-dose aspirin in their next pregnancy attempt. Immunoglobulin and paternal leukocyte therapies are not effective in preventing recurrent pregnancy loss. The role of luteal phase defect is controversial. If a diagnosis is sought, it should be via endometrial biopsy. Luteal phase support with progesterone is of unproven efficacy.

Cultures for bacteria or viruses and tests for glucose intolerance, thyroid abnormalities, antibodies to infectious agents, antinuclear antibodies, antithyroid antibodies, paternal human leukocyte antigen status, or maternal antipaternal antibodies are not beneficial. Therefore, these are not recommended in the evaluation of otherwise normal women with recurrent pregnancy loss.

Couples with otherwise unexplained recurrent pregnancy loss should be counseled regarding the potential for successful pregnancy without treatment.

Expertise

For couples with recurrent pregnancy loss, it is reasonable to offer a basic evaluation (Table 4–2). A significant number of couples who complete this evaluation will not have an identifiable cause. Informative and supportive counseling appears to play an important role and may lead to the best pregnancy outcomes. Clinicians should be familiar with any state requirements regarding the reporting of fetal death or disposal of fetal remains.

Table 4–2. Tests Commonly Offered to Couples with Recurrent Pregnancy Loss

Tests	Potential Etiology
Luteal phase endometrial biopsy	Endocrine dysfunction
Hysterosalpingography, sonohysterography, and hysteroscopy	Uterine abnormalities
Karyotype of both partners	Genetic abnormalities
Lupus anticoagulant and anticardiolipin	Immunologic disorders

RESOURCES

Patient

American College of Obstetricians and Gynecologists. Repeated miscarriage. ACOG Patient Education Pamphlet 100. Washington, DC: ACOG, 2000

RESOLVE: The National Infertility Association
1310 Broadway
Somerville, MA 02144
(617) 623-0744
www.resolve.org
E-mail: resolveinc.@aol.com

Professional

American Academy of Pediatrics, American College of Obstetricians and Gynecologists. Appendix E. Standard terminology for reporting of reproductive health statistics in the Unites States. In: Guidelines for perinatal care. 4th ed. Elk Grove Village, Illinois: AAP; Washington, DC: ACOG, 1997:311–329

American College of Obstetricians and Gynecologists. Antiphospholipid syndrome. ACOG Educational Bulletin 244. Washington, DC: ACOG, 1998

American College of Obstetricians and Gynecologists. Management of recurrent early pregnancy loss. ACOG Practice Bulletin 24. Washington, DC: ACOG, 2001

Royal College of Obstetricians and Gynaecologists. The management of recurrent miscarriage. RCOG Guideline 17. London: RCOG, 1998

Sexual Assault or Rape

Health Care Impact

Research finds that most victims do not file police reports, making rape and sexual assault the most underreported violent crimes. Consequently, the true prevalence of rape or sexual assault is unknown. However, research estimates that more than one million rapes occur in the United States annually, and a recent U.S. Department of Justice/Centers for Disease Control and Prevention study found that 18% of the women surveyed reported experiencing attempted or completed rape at some time in their life. Most rape victims are children and adolescents. More than half of the female rape victims were younger than 18 years of age: 22% were younger than 12 years of age when they were first raped; 32% were 12–17 years of age when they were first raped. Women raped before 18 years of age are significantly more likely to be raped as adults. The overwhelming majority of rapes are perpetrated by someone known to the victim, often an intimate or family member, and acquaintances or dates in the cases of adolescents. Fewer than 25% of rapes are committed by strangers. Sexual assault frequently involves the voluntary use of alcohol, drugs, or both by both victim and offender. Alcohol is the substance most frequently associated with sexual assault. However, in the past several years, rape crisis centers increasingly have heard about other drugs being administered to a victim without her knowledge or consent. Approximately 50% of rape victims tell no one. However, most survivors experience short- and long-term consequences.

ACOG Recommendations

Clinicians should be aware that their practices will include women with a history of sexual assault and should be familiar with both the short- and long-term sequelae. All patients should be screened for a history of sexual assault (see also "Routine Detection and Prevention of Disease" in Part 3).

The physician evaluating the victim of sexual assault has a number of responsibilities, both medical and legal, and should be aware of state or local requirements regarding the reporting of the crime or that may involve the use of kits for gathering evidence. Additionally, physicians should be aware of the existence of local protocols regarding the use of specially trained Sexual Assault Forensic Examiners. Specific responsibilities are determined by the patient's needs and by state law.

Expertise

A clinician evaluating a victim of sexual assault in the acute phase should provide medical and counseling services, inform the victim of her rights, refer her to legal assistance, and help her develop prevention strategies to avoid future victimization (see box). Often, however, the victim may not make a health care visit until significant time has elapsed, and her visit may be for reasons unrelated to the assault. Physical signs of the assault may not be present, and the patient often does not initiate a discussion about her situation. Therefore, the clinician must recognize behavioral signs as well as physical health problems that often result from sexual assault.

Many jurisdictions and several clinics have developed a sexual assault assessment kit, which lists the steps necessary and the items to be obtained so that as much information as possible can be prepared for forensic purposes. Many clinics have nurses who are trained to collect needed samples and information. If these individuals are available, it is appropriate to request their assistance. Rape crisis counselors and centers also can provide valuable support.

Clinicians should be familiar with state rape and assault laws and comply with any legal requirements regarding reporting and the collection of evidence. They also must be aware that every state and the District of Columbia requires physicians to report child abuse, including sexual assault against children and adolescents. Physicians also should be familiar with any state laws requiring the reporting of statutory rape.

The Clinician's Role in Treating the Sexually Assaulted Female

- Medical
  - —Obtain informed consent from the patient
  - —Obtain an accurate gynecologic history
  - —Assess and treat physical injuries
  - —Obtain appropriate cultures and treat any existing infections
  - —Provide prophylactic antibiotic therapy and offer immunizations
  - —Provide therapy to prevent unwanted conception
  - —Offer baseline serologic tests for hepatitis B virus, human immunodeficiency virus, and syphilis
  - —Provide counseling
  - —Arrange for follow-up medical care and counseling
- Legal
  - —Provide accurate recording of events
  - —Document injuries
  - —Collect samples (pubic hair, fingernail scrapings, vaginal secretions, saliva, blood-stained clothing)
  - —Report to authorities as required
  - —Ensure chain of evidence (orderly and unbroken progress of specimens to legal authorities)

RESOURCES

Patient

American College of Obstetricians and Gynecologists. The abused woman. ACOG Patient Education Pamphlet AP083. Washington, DC: ACOG, 1998

American College of Obstetricians and Gynecologists. Stay alert! Stay safe! Washington, DC: ACOG, 1998

American College of Obstetricians and Gynecologists. Violence against women. Available at www.acog.com/from_home/departments/dept_web.cfm?recno=17

National 24-hour Toll-Free Hotline Numbers:
800-799-SAFE (7233) and 800-787-3224 (TDD)

Professional

American College of Obstetricians and Gynecologists. Adolescent victims of sexual assault. ACOG Educational Bulletin 252. Washington, DC: ACOG, 1998

American College of Obstetricians and Gynecologists. Adult manifestations of childhood sexual abuse. ACOG Educational Bulletin 259. Washington, DC: ACOG, 2000

American College of Obstetricians and Gynecologists. Sexual assault. ACOG Educational Bulletin 242. Washington, DC: ACOG, 1997

Guidelines for the evaluation of sexual abuse of children: subject review. American Academy of Pediatrics Committee on Child Abuse and Neglect. Pediatrics 1999;103:186–191 [published erratum appears in Pediatrics 1999;103:1049]

Tjaden P, Thoennes N. Prevalence, incidence, and consequences of violence against women: findings from the national violence against women survey. Research in Brief. Washington, DC: U.S. Department of Justice, Office of Justice Programs, November 1998, NCJ 172837

SEXUAL DYSFUNCTION

Health Care Impact

Although only a minority of Americans experience sexual problems, women are more often affected. An understanding of the usual pattern of sexual response (desire, arousal, orgasm, and resolution), and the variations of these responses, will assist in the identification and treatment of sexual dysfunction. An understanding of the range of sexual practices considered "normal" by different people and different cultures is necessary for appropriate counseling or referral of patients.

ACOG Recommendations

The clinician should be prepared to discuss patients' concerns about sexual function in a setting of mutual respect and trust.

Expertise

Treatment of sexual dysfunction will vary with the type of dysfunction, although many types of dysfunction are related. When medications, such as antidepressants, result in sexual dysfunction, the medication or dosage may be changed. Difficulties with prior sexual experience, insufficient foreplay, and attitudes about sexual pleasure may be discovered in careful history-taking. Behaviorally oriented, time-limited treatment programs for previously anorgasmic women have been described. Support groups of women with similar problems may be helpful. Vaginal dilation exercises may be useful with dyspareunia and vaginismus, after organic factors are excluded. Communication between partners is important in sexual health.

Although androgen therapy has been prescribed for sexual dysfunction for many years, data regarding its safety and efficacy are incomplete and physiologic androgen replacement therapy has not been shown to consistently affect the libido. Measurement of free or total testosterone levels for diagnosis or monitoring is not clinically useful. Patients most likely to benefit from androgen therapy are young women who have undergone oophorectomy. Although it is possible that other women experiencing decreased libido may benefit from a trial of androgen therapy, the lack of definitive data should lead to a cautious approach. In general, lower doses of oral preparations are preferred. Appropriate monitoring for side effects, including lipoprotein alteration, should be undertaken.

Some treatments for sexual dysfunction may be within the scope of the obstetrician–gynecologist. If not, referrals may be appropriate to psychologists, marriage or relationship counselors, or sex therapists.

Resources

Patient

American College of Obstetricians and Gynecologists. Sexuality and sexual problems. ACOG Patient Education Pamphlet AP072. Washington, DC: ACOG, 2000

Professional

American Association of Marriage and Family Therapy
1133 15th Street NW, Suite 300
Washington, DC 20005-2710
(202) 452-0109
Fax: (202) 223-2329
www.aamft.org

American Association of Sex Educators, Counselors, and Therapists
PO Box 238
Mt. Vernon, IA 52314
Fax: (319) 895-6203
www.aasect.org
E-mail: AASECT@worldnet.att.net

American College of Obstetricians and Gynecologists. Androgen treatment of decreased libido. ACOG Committee Opinion 244. Washington, DC: ACOG, 2000

The Society for Sex Therapy and Research (SSTAR)
409 12th Street, SW
Washington, DC 20024-2188
(202) 863-1646
Fax: (202) 554-0453

SEXUALLY TRANSMITTED DISEASES

Health Care Impact

The U.S. Centers for Disease Control and Prevention (CDC) reports that in excess of 90% of the common infectious diseases in women in the United States are sexually transmitted. An estimated 650,000 cases of gonorrhea and 3 million cases of chlamydia occur in the United States each year. Approximately 45 million adolescent and adult Americans have been infected with genital herpes, and the CDC estimates that 20 million carry human papillomavirus infections of some kind. Approximately 5% of the population has been infected with hepatitis B with approximately 120,000 of the 200,000 new infections each year acquired through sexual transmission. Human immunodeficiency virus (HIV) in women is a significant sexually transmitted disease (STD), with most women (40%) with acquired immunodeficiency syndrome (AIDS) infected through heterosexual contact. Syphilis remains a major concern with 70,000 new cases annually. Sexually transmitted diseases are directly related to death, cancer, and impaired fertility.

ACOG Recommendations

The American College of Obstetricians and Gynecologists recommends strategies for the prevention, diagnosis, and treatment of STDs. The

American College of Obstetricians and Gynecologists also recognizes the important role played by practitioners of women's health care.

Expertise

The clinician should provide the following care:

- Effective counseling in strategies to prevent infection
- Diagnosis and treatment of STDs in patient and partner(s)
- Adherence to local regulations regarding STD screening, reporting, partner notification, and follow-up
- Adherence to CDC guidelines for the treatment of STDs

The difficult issue of partner treatment is addressed in the CDC's *1998 Sexually Transmitted Disease Guidelines.* This document states that: "Health care practitioners should advise patients who have an STD to notify sex partners, including those without symptoms, of their exposure and encourage these partners to seek clinical evaluation…interrupting the transmission of infection is crucial to STD control." Treatment of male sexual partners is a keystone in the prevention of, transmission of, and reinfection with certain STDs. Clinicians may be asked to provide a prescription for the patient's partner without having performed an examination of the partner. There is no clear policy concerning the appropriateness of such action. In most cases, such a prescription will result in treatment without complication. An adverse reaction to the medication is uncommon but may result in a significant health hazard to the partner. Each clinician must decide whether providing such prescriptions is appropriate. Clinicians should be familiar with any federal, state, or local requirements for the screening, follow-up, and reporting of STDs.

Resources

Patient

American College of Obstetricians and Gynecologists. Genital herpes. ACOG Patient Education Pamphlet AP054. Washington, DC: ACOG, 1999

American College of Obstetricians and Gynecologists. Gonorrhea and chlamydia. ACOG Patient Education Pamphlet AP071. Washington, DC: ACOG, 2000

American College of Obstetricians and Gynecologists. HIV infection and women. ACOG Patient Education Pamphlet AP082. Washington, DC: ACOG, 2000

American College of Obstetricians and Gynecologists. How to prevent sexually transmitted diseases. ACOG Patient Education Pamphlet AP009. Washington, DC: ACOG, 1999

American College of Obstetricians and Gynecologists. Human papillomavirus infection. ACOG Patient Education Pamphlet AP073. Washington, DC: ACOG, 1999

Professional

American College of Obstetricians and Gynecologists. Hepatitis virus infections in obstetrician–gynecologists. ACOG Committee Opinion 203. Washington, DC: ACOG, 1998

American College of Obstetricians and Gynecologists. Human immunodeficiency virus: ethical guidelines for obstetricians and gynecologists. In: Ethics in obstetrics and gynecology. Washington, DC: ACOG, 2002:43–47

American College of Obstetricians and gynecologists. Management of herpes in pregnancy. ACOG Practice Bulletin 8. Washington, DC: ACOG, 1999

Institute of Medicine. The hidden epidemic: confronting sexually transmitted diseases. Washington, DC: National Academy Press, 1997

LCDC Expert Working Group on Canadian Guidelines for Sexually Transmitted Diseases. Highlights: 1998 edition of the Canadian STD guidelines. Ottawa, Ontario: Health Canada, 1998

1998 guidelines for treatment of sexually transmitted diseases. Centers for Disease Control and Prevention. MMWR Morb Mortal Wkly Rep 1998;47(RR-1):1–111

Substance Use and Abuse: Tobacco, Alcohol, and Illegal Drugs

Health Care Impact

Use of tobacco, alcohol, and illegal drugs constitutes a significant national health problem. In the United States, more than two thirds (68%) of women report ever having smoked and four fifths (80%) of women report any lifetime alcohol use. More than one fourth (27%) of U.S. women report any lifetime marijuana use, and about one third (30%) report ever having used any illegal drug. Although the prevalence of tobacco, alcohol, and illegal drug use varies, it is present in all socioeconomic, cultural, and ethnic groups.

Approximately 22 million (23%) women in the United States are current smokers. Women 18–44 years of age report the highest prevalence of smoking. More than 3 million adolescents in the United States smoke cigarettes, and the prevalence of cigarette smoking among adolescents has been increasing since 1992. Prevalence is inversely associated with education level, and is highest among women who started but did not complete high school. Among racial/ethnic groups, smoking prevalence is highest for American Indians/Alaskan Natives and lowest for Asian/Pacific Islanders. Non-Hispanic white women report a higher rate of smoking than non-Hispanic black women.

Cigarette smoking is the largest preventable cause of death and disability among women in the United States. Smoking contributes to deaths from cancer, cardiovascular diseases, and respiratory diseases. Women who smoke increase their risk for painful menstruation, secondary amenorrhea, and menstrual irregularity. Women smokers also have natural menopause at a younger age than do nonsmokers and are at increased risk for hip fracture and poorer reproductive outcomes.

About 60% of adult American women have consumed alcohol in the past year, with half of these women drinking at least once weekly and

2.6% reporting heavy use in the past month. Heavy alcohol use (five or more drinks per occasion on 5 or more days in the last month) is associated with the following factors:

- Young age (18–25)
- Less than a high school education
- Some indicators of poverty
- Major depression, generalized anxiety disorder, agoraphobia, and panic attacks

Excessive alcohol consumption contributes to more than 100,000 deaths in the United States each year. In addition to motor vehicle accidents, suicide, and homicide, heavy drinking contributes to deaths from heart disease, cancer, and stroke. Half of all cirrhosis deaths are linked with alcohol. Menstrual disorders, early menopause, and osteoporosis are among the gynecologic consequences of alcohol abuse. The effect of alcohol on the fetus (eg, fetal alcohol syndrome) is well known.

About 8% of women report any illegal drug use in the last month. About 5% of women are reported to be problem drug users or in need of drug treatment, which is associated with the following factors:

- Initiation of alcohol or drug use at younger than 19 years of age
- Unemployment
- Less than a high school education

Frequent use or dependency involving more than one substance is common; the effects of multidrug use may be synergistic.

Illegal drug abuse causes major effects in reproductive function and health, as well as in other organ systems. Malnutrition, liver disease, stroke and other cerebrovascular diseases, an increase in certain malignancies, and behavior that results in the acquisition of serious infections (human immunodeficiency virus [HIV], hepatitis, sexually transmitted diseases) are some of the consequences noted in women. In 1997, almost 16,000 deaths (both male and female) in the United States were directly related to illegal drugs. This excludes accidents, homicides, and those deaths related to infections (eg, HIV/acquired immunodeficiency syndrome [AIDS]).

ACOG Recommendations

Women's health care practitioners have important roles in the prevention, identification, and treatment of tobacco, alcohol, and substance abuse. Key areas in which clinicians can make an impact are encouraging healthy behaviors by providing appropriate information and education, screening, providing counseling and brief interventions for tobacco use, and referring patients who are abusing drugs or alcohol for assessment and intervention from those trained in substance abuse treatment.

When prescribing potentially addictive substances, the clinician should carefully assess the risks of drug treatment and consider nonpharmacologic treatments or nonaddicting medications whenever possible. Potentially addictive drugs should be initially prescribed at a dose adequate to relieve symptoms and then be reduced gradually to the smallest effective dose.

Expertise

Evaluation of a patient for tobacco, alcohol, or other substance abuse requires appreciation of the high prevalence and wide distribution among the population of such disorders, along with the ability to take a thorough history. Direct questioning of patients about their use of tobacco, alcohol, or other drugs is preferable to vague inquiry.

There are five major steps to intervention in tobacco use (see box). Placing tobacco use stickers (indicating current, former, or never user) on the patient chart or expanding the vital signs measured at each visit to include asking about tobacco use have been found to be helpful reminders.

The CAGE Questionnaire (see box) has been widely used for the detection of alcohol abuse and has been found to be 91% sensitive and 77% specific for the detection of problem drinking. Other questionnaires to detect problem drinking include the T-ACE, MAST (Michigan Alcohol Screening Test), and AUDIT (Alcohol Use Disorders Identification). Although all of these screening questionnaires were initially developed for use in detecting alcohol use, it is possible to use them for detecting other

The Five A's for Brief Tobacco Intervention

Ask about tobacco use	Identify and document tobacco use status for every patient at every visit
Advise to quit	In a clear, strong and personalized manner urge every tobacco user to quit
Assess willingness to make a quit attempt	Is the tobacco user willing to make a quit attempt at this time?
Assist in quit attempt	For the patient willing to make a quit attempt, use counseling and pharmacotherapy to help her quit
Arrange follow-up	Schedule follow-up contact, preferably within the first week after the quit date

Fiore MC, Bailey WC, Cohen SJ, Dorfman SF, Goldstein MG, Gritz ER, et al. Treating tobacco use and dependence. Clinical practice guideline. Rockville, MD: US Department of Health and Human Services. Public Health Service, 2000. ARHC Publication 00-0032

The CAGE Questionnaire To Detect Problem Drinking

CAGE QUESTIONNAIRE

C Have you ever felt you ought to **C**ut down on your drinking?

A Have people **A**nnoyed you by criticizing your drinking?

G Have you ever felt bad or **G**uilty about your drinking?

E Have you ever had a drink first thing in the morning to steady your nerves or get rid of a hangover (**E**ye opener)?

One positive response indicates reason for concern; two positive responses indicate that a problem is likely.

Ewing J. Detecting alcoholism. The CAGE questionnaire. JAMA 1984;252:1905–1907. Copyrighted 1984, American Medical Association.

drug use by adding the term drugs or a specific list of drugs of concern to the screening instrument.

Women may not disclose tobacco, alcohol, or other substance use for a variety of reasons. Most women who smoke, however, report that they would like to quit. Fears regarding disclosure can include that of intervention by government agencies when reporting can result in punishment, incarceration, or loss of child custody. "Enabling" behavior is another barrier to both disclosure and management. Clinicians can enable further substance use by misunderstanding symptoms and signs or ignoring other evidence of substance abuse.

A variety of signs and symptoms can be found in patients engaged in substance abuse. A careful search for physical findings and close attention to the psychologic manifestations may increase the likelihood of identifying patients with substance abuse problems. However, patients may not exhibit any symptoms.

There are few laboratory studies helpful in the screening and diagnosis of patients with alcohol abuse. A blood alcohol level is of limited value, because ethanol is eliminated quite rapidly; thus, it cannot predict actual drinking behaviors. Liver function studies can be of some value. A complete blood count may reflect macrocytosis due to the direct effect of ethanol or associated folate deficiency. Anemia may reflect folate deficiency, gastrointestinal bleeding, or bone marrow suppression.

Toxicologic screening can be used to detect use of various nonalcohol substances. Immunoassay procedures are generally used, but confirmatory testing will reduce false-positive results. Many laboratories perform multiple tests as a "drug panel" aimed at commonly used illegal drugs. Patient consent should be obtained prior to any toxicologic screening, and clinicians should be familiar with any state reporting requirements regarding the use or abuse of substances during pregnancy.

Treatment for tobacco, alcohol, and other substance abuse has been shown to be effective. Treatments for tobacco use have been well established and are outlined in the U.S. Public Health Service's Clinical Practice Guideline for Treating Tobacco Use and Dependence (see "Resources"). As is true of other addictions, tobacco use must be treated as a chronic disease; most former smokers report two to three quit attempts before they are successful. Brief counseling interventions, self-help materials, and referrals to support groups can increase cessation rates. Pharmacotherapy with either nicotine replacement or bupropion should be recommended for all smokers except pregnant or breastfeeding women, those with medical contraindications, those smoking fewer than 10 cigarettes a day, and adolescents.

For alcohol and illegal drug abusers, no single treatment is appropriate for all individuals. Recovery from substance abuse is a long-term process. Better outcome is seen in individualized programs that provide a greater range, frequency, and intensity of services.

Treatment programs for women should look beyond simple abstinence from further substance abuse and take into account the total health of the individual. Support services (eg, transportation, childcare services) can affect substance abuse treatment. Social service departments in many hospitals are an invaluable source of assistance and referral of patients with substance abuse problems. Many additional community and clinical resources are available (see "Resources").

RESOURCES

Patient

Alcoholics Anonymous
www.alcoholics-anonymous.org
(212) 870-3400

American College of Obstetricians and Gynecologists. Alcohol and women. ACOG Education Pamphlet AP068. Washington, DC: ACOG, 2000

American College of Obstetricians and Gynecologists. It's time to quit smoking. ACOG Patient Education Pamphlet AP065. Washington, DC: ACOG, 2000

Center for Substance Abuse Treatment referral helpline
800-662-HELP

Narcotics Anonymous
na.org/index.htm
(818) 773-9999

Professional

American College of Obstetricians and Gynecologists. Smoking and women's health. ACOG Educational Bulletin 240. Washington, DC: ACOG, 1997

American College of Obstetricians and Gynecologists. Substance abuse. ACOG Technical Bulletin 194. Washington, DC: ACOG, 1994

American Society of Addiction Medicine
(301) 656-3920
www.asam.org

Fiore MC, Bailey WC, Cohen SJ, Dorfman SF, Goldstein MG, Gritz ER, et al. Treating tobacco use and dependence. Clinical practice guideline. Rockville, MD: US Department of Health and Human Services. Public Health Service, 2000. ARHQ Publication 00-0032

Hartmann, KE. Clear and concise intervention for smoking cessation. Hosp Physician 2000; 36(8): 19-27

National Council on Alcoholism and Drug Dependence, Inc.
(212) 206-6770
Hope Line: 800-NCA-CALL
www.ncadd.org

Robert Wood Johnson Foundation. Substance abuse: the nation's number one health problem. Princeton, New Jersey: RWJF, 2001

Substance Abuse and Mental Health Services Administration. A guide to substance abuse services for primary care clinicians. Treatment Improvement Protocol (TIP) Series; no. 24. Rockville, Maryland: SAMHSA, 1997

Substance Abuse and Mental Health Services Administration National Clearinghouse for Alcohol and Drug Information
www.health.org
800-487-4890

Women and smoking: a report of the Surgeon General. Atlanta: Centers for Disease Control and Prevention, 2001. Available at www.cdc.gov/tobacco/sgr_forwomen.htm

TERMINATION OF PREGNANCY

Health Care Impact

According to data compiled by the U.S. Centers for Disease Control and Prevention, nearly 1.2 million legal induced abortions were performed in 1997, a 3% decrease from the 1996 total. There were nearly 4 million live births that same year. Women who obtained legal induced abortions were predominantly white and unmarried. Approximately 20% of women who obtained legal abortions in 1996 were 19 years of age or younger; 32% were 20–24 years of age. Curettage (suction and sharp) remained the primary abortion procedure (99% of all procedures). More than half (55%) were performed during the first 8 weeks of gestation, and approximately 88% of all abortions were performed during the first 12 weeks of pregnancy. A 1996 Alan Guttmacher Institute study found that 86% of all U.S. counties lacked an abortion practitioner, and these counties were home to 32% of all 15–44-year-old women.

ACOG Recommendations

Termination of pregnancy before viability is a medical matter between the patient and the physician, subject to the physician's clinical judgment, the patient's informed consent, relevant state laws, and the availability of appropriate facilities. The American College of Obstetricians and Gynecologists supports access to care for all individuals, irrespective of financial status, and supports the availability of all reproductive options. The American College of Obstetricians and Gynecologists opposes unnecessary laws or regulations that limit or delay access to care. If abortion is to be performed, it should be performed safely and as early as possible.

A woman has the right to choose to have an abortion and should be unencumbered by obstacles such as:

- Bans on public funding for abortion facilities and services
- Bans on specific procedures
- Stricter facility regulations for abortion than for other surgical procedures of similar risk

- Harassment of and violence against practitioners and recipients of services
- Lack of availability of practitioners
- Biased informed consent provisions
- Mandatory waiting periods
- Parental notification or consent

The College continues to affirm the legal right of a woman to obtain an abortion prior to fetal viability. The American College of Obstetricians and Gynecologists is opposed to abortion of the healthy fetus that has attained viability in a healthy woman. Viability is the capacity of the fetus to survive outside the mother's uterus. Whether or not this capacity exists is a medical determination, may vary with each pregnancy, and is a matter for the judgment of the responsible attending physician.

Clinicians are not required to perform abortions. However, they should be prepared to counsel patients fully on their options and manage complications of induced abortions as needed.

Expertise

Before an abortion, the patient should be counseled on her options for the management of the unwanted pregnancy. The patient should be fully informed in a balanced manner about all options, including raising the child herself, placing the child for adoption, and abortion. The information conveyed should be appropriate to the duration of the pregnancy. The health care professional should make every effort to avoid introducing personal bias.

An evaluation of the patient's available social support and referral to appropriate counseling or other supportive services also should be offered. Contraceptive counseling is important. The following evaluation should be completed:

- Careful history, physical examination, testing, and ultrasonography, as indicated, to diagnose pregnancy and accurately establish gestational age
- Rh factor determination

- Complete blood count, as indicated
- Vaginitis/sexually transmitted disease screening, as indicated
- Prophylactic antibiotics, as indicated

Clinicians who perform abortions in their offices should provide for prompt emergency treatment in the event that a complication occurs. Clinics and freestanding ambulatory care facilities should have an established mechanism for transferring patients who require emergency treatment.

Routine pathologic examination of tissue is not necessary following the elective surgical termination of pregnancy in which embryonic or fetal parts can be identified with certainty. In such instances, a description of the gross products of conception should be recorded. The following post-procedure care should be provided:

- Immunoprophylaxis with Rh immune globulin for Rh-negative women
- Counseling on signs of hemorrhage, uterine perforation, retained tissue, infection, subinvolution, Asherman syndrome, and missed pregnancy, as appropriate
- Psychologic or other support service consult, as indicated

Clinicians should be aware of any limitations on abortion services in their jurisdiction. The United States has no national system for the mandatory reporting of induced termination of pregnancy. However, state health departments vary greatly in approaches to the compilation of these data and clinicians should be aware of any such reporting requirements.

RESOURCES

Patient

American College of Obstetricians and Gynecologists. Induced abortion: important medical facts. ACOG Patient Education Pamphlet AP043. Washington, DC: ACOG, 1994

American College of Obstetricians and Gynecologists. Pregnancy choices: raising the baby, adoption, and abortion. ACOG Patient Education Pamphlet AP102. Washington, DC: ACOG, 1999

Planned Parenthood Federation of America
810 Seventh Avenue
New York, NY 10019
800-230-PLAN
www.plannedparenthood.org

Professional

Abortion surveillance: preliminary analysis—United States, 1997. MMWR Morb Mortal Wkly Rep 2000;48:1171–1174, 1191 [published erratum appears in MMWR Morb Mortal Wkly Rep 2000;49:23]

American College of Obstetricians and gynecologists. Abortion policy. ACOG Statement of Policy 69. Washington, DC: ACOG, 2000

American College of Obstetricians and Gynecologists. Antibiotic prophylaxis for gynecologic surgery. ACOG Practice Bulletin 23. Washington, DC: ACOG, 2000

American College of Obstetricians and Gynecologists. Medical management of abortion. ACOG Practice Bulletin 26. Washington, DC: ACOG, 2001

American College of Obstetricians and Gynecologists. Mifepristone for medical pregnancy termination. ACOG Committee Opinion 245. Washington, DC: ACOG, 2000

The National Abortion Federation
1755 Massachusetts Ave. NW, Suite 600
Washington, DC 20036
800-772-9100
www.prochoice.org

Paul M, Lichtenberg ES, Borgatta L, Grimes DA, Stubblefield PG. A clinician's guide to medical and surgical abortion. New York: Churchill Livingstone, 1999

URINARY INCONTINENCE

Health Care Impact

Urinary incontinence has been reported to affect 10–25% of women younger than 65 years of age, 15–30% of noninstitutionalized women older than 60 years of age, and more than 50% of nursing home residents. A recent estimate of the direct costs of caring for persons of all ages with incontinence is more than $15 billion annually. Urinary incontinence has been shown to affect women's social, clinical, and psychological well-being. It is estimated that less than one half of all incontinent women seek medical care, even though urinary incontinence often can be treated.

ACOG Recommendations

The obstetrician–gynecologist should recognize the factors which contribute to the development of urinary incontinence and pelvic organ prolapse. Obstetrician–gynecologists who have training, experience, and demonstrated competence in urogynecologic techniques, including cystoscopy, should be credentialed accordingly.

Expertise

The health care practitioner should be able to perform or ensure the patient has access to a practitioner who can perform the following care:

- Clarify the patient's symptoms
- Demonstrate the loss of urine objectively
- Determine the etiology of the incontinence using clinical testing
- Identify women who require more sophisticated urodynamic or imaging studies
- Identify and treat reversible causative conditions
- Discuss treatment options
- Implement a management plan consistent with the patient's condition and goals

A basic physical evaluation for urinary incontinence includes:

- Abdominal examination
- Pelvic examination
- Rectal examination
- Neurologic examination of the lower thoracic, lumbar, and sacral nerves
- Direct observation of urine loss (eg, cough, pad test)
- Postvoid residual test

Laboratory evaluation includes urinalysis and urine culture. Supplementary evaluation may include:

- Blood testing (blood urea nitrogen, creatinine, glucose, calcium)
- Urodynamic testing (water or carbon dioxide cystometry, multichannel urodynamics)
- Cystourethroscopy
- Imaging tests (eg, radiographic, ultrasonographic)

Pretest screening for bacteriuria or urinary tract infection by urine culture or urinalysis, or both, is recommended in women undergoing urodynamic testing. Those with positive results should be given antibiotic treatment.

Resources

Patient

American College of Obstetricians and Gynecologists. Urinary incontinence. ACOG Patient Education Pamphlet AP081.Washington, DC: ACOG, 2000

UTERINE LEIOMYOMATA

Health Care Impact

Uterine leiomyomata (commonly known as myomas or fibroids) are the most common solid pelvic tumors in women and the leading indication for hysterectomy. Uterine leiomyomata are clinically apparent in 25–50% of women, although studies in which careful pathologic examination of the uterus is carried out suggest the prevalence may be as high as 80%. These tumors originate from proliferation of a single myometrial cell. Factors responsible for the genesis of leiomyomata are unknown, but family history, ethnicity, and diet may play a role. Major symptoms produced by leiomyomata include abnormal genital bleeding, pelvic pain, and pregnancy loss. Size and symptoms may regress following menopause.

Uterine leiomyomata are the indication for nearly half of the 600,000 hysterectomies performed each year in the United States, and most hysterectomies for leiomyomata are performed abdominally. Subsequent consequences of hysterectomy include a postoperative recovery that requires about 4–6 weeks, infectious complications (10%), and major injuries to the bowel, bladder, ovaries, or ureter (1%).

Many women seek an alternative to hysterectomy because they wish to retain their uterus to preserve childbearing or for a variety of other reasons even if they have completed childbearing. As alternatives to hysterectomy become increasingly available, the efficacies of these treatments and the risk of potential problems are important to delineate.

ACOG Recommendations

As benign neoplasms, uterine leiomyomata usually require treatment only when they cause symptoms. The two most common symptoms for which women seek treatment are abnormal uterine bleeding and pelvic pressure or pain. However, not all bleeding is caused by leiomyomata; therefore, other causes of abnormal bleeding in the presence of leiomyomata should be ruled out.

In women with symptomatic leiomyomata, hysterectomy provides a definitive cure. Abdominal myomectomy is a safe and effective option for women who wish to retain their uterus. If this option is selected, women should be counseled preoperatively about the relatively high risk of reoperation. The clinical diagnosis of rapidly growing leiomyomata has not been shown to predict uterine sarcoma and thus should not be used as the sole indication for myomectomy or hysterectomy.

Use of gonadotropin-releasing hormone agonists preoperatively is beneficial, especially when improvement of hematologic status and uterine shrinkage are important goals. Benefits of the use of gonadotropin-releasing hormone agonists should be weighed against their cost and side-effects for individual patients.

Leiomyomata may be a factor in infertility for some patients. The issues are complex, and myomectomy for an infertility indication should not be performed without first completing a comprehensive fertility evaluation.

Postmenopausal women with leiomyomata may have more bleeding problems and some increase in leiomyoma size while taking hormone replacement therapy. However, there appears to be no reason to withhold this treatment option from women who desire or need such therapy.

Expertise

The clinician should be able to evaluate symptoms related to pelvic pain, abnormal genital bleeding, pelvic mass, and infertility. The clinician also should be able to evaluate imaging studies of the pelvis such as magnetic resonance imaging, computerized tomography, sonography, hysteroscopy, and hysterosalpingography. Treatment options for consideration include hysterectomy, myomectomy, gonadotropin-releasing hormone agonists, and hysteroscopic resection.

Resources

Patient

American College of Obstetricians and Gynecologists. Uterine fibroids. ACOG Patient Education Pamphlet AP074. Washington, DC: ACOG, 1994

Professional

Agency for Healthcare Research and Quality. Management of uterine fibroids: summary. Evidence Report/Technology Assessment no. 34. Rockville, Maryland: AHRQ, 2001. AHRQ publication no. 01-E051. Available at www.ahcpr.gov/clinic/utersumm.htm

American College of Obstetricians and Gynecologists. Surgical alternatives to hysterectomy in the management of leiomyomas. ACOG Practice Bulletin 16. Washington, DC: ACOG, 2000

American Society for Reproductive Medicine. Myomas and reproductive dysfunction. Guideline for Practice. Birmingham, Alabama: ASRM, 1992

Gehlbach DL, Sousa RC, Carpenter SE, Rock JA. Abdominal myomectomy in the treatment of infertility. Int J Gynaecol Obstet 1993;40:45–50

Lepine LA, Hillis SD, Marchbanks PA, Koonin LM, Morrow B, Kieke BA, et al. Hysterectomy surveillance–United States, 1980–1993. Mor Mortal Wkly Rep CDC Surveill Summ 1997;46:1–15

Women with Disabilities

Health Care Impact

Women with disabilities number more than 28 million in the United States. The World Health Organization defines disability as "any restriction or lack resulting from an impairment of ability to perform an activity in the manner or within the range considered normal for a human being." Health care practitioners need to take into account both a patient's disabilities and gynecologic issues. Medical treatment approaches commonly applied to all women may need to be modified to take into account the special physical and physiologic differences resulting from disabling conditions or chronic disease states. There are a variety of disabling conditions with varying impact on health. Therefore, the level of modification to a clinician's practice will vary depending on individual patient need.

ACOG Recommendations

Health care practitioners have a societal and professional ethical responsibility to accommodate and individualize the care of women with special needs. Clinicians should review the following recommendations and adopt those that will enable them to accept this responsibility:

- Assess the environment of their medical practice site and activities, and make appropriate modifications in layout, equipment, and staff training to enhance services.
- Support models of care that increase personal power of women with disabilities.
- Acquire additional knowledge and skills through continuing medical education and other resources.

Expertise

Health care practitioners need to communicate effectively with women with disabilities to learn how their condition affects reproductive functions so that the clinician can incorporate existing treatment protocols and tailor health care delivery to individual patients. The health care practitioner should be able to communicate effectively with patients with all types of disabilities, including those with visual, auditory, and cognitive impairments. The clinician should have an open exchange of information with the patient on a level and in a format where this can be clearly interpreted and understood. In some disabling conditions, this may require modified approaches. For example, sharing information with visually impaired patients will best be accomplished with audiotapes, videotapes with audio descriptions, and with clear descriptive explanations of all procedures and recommended therapies. When communicating with a deaf patient, sign language interpreters and comprehensive and clear written information will facilitate the sharing of pertinent medical knowledge between clinician and patient. When treating cognitively impaired women, it is essential to communicate in simple language with the addition of visual tools, such as models and pictures. These cognitive impairments may be significant and compromise the patient's ability to comprehend what is being told to her. All attempts should be made to simplify issues surrounding care decisions. If adequate communication is not possible, the individual or agency legally responsible for the woman's health maintenance must provide signed documentation that the examination or treatment has been preapproved.

The clinician should review with the woman all of her gynecologic issues, including sexual activity, menstrual cycles, contraception needs, gynecologic cancer screening, interest in conception, and concerns about menopause and osteoporosis. Involuntary sterilization of women with disabilities is commonplace in developing countries and is not entirely unheard of in the United States. It is important to acknowledge the woman's right to reproductive choice, whether this be contraception, conception, or sterilization, without making any assumptions about what she would or would not be able to manage. When women have cognitive impairments that leave them unable to consent to sterilization, consent typically must be obtained through a legal proceeding. An effort should be made to conform to the woman's expressed values and beliefs.

Clinicians should provide accessible examination tables or have adequate staff available to ensure the patient's safe transfer from wheelchair to table. Health care practitioners also should familiarize themselves with the woman's disability or chronic disease, as these conditions may result in urinary dysfunction, bowel dysfunction, excess muscle spasms, weakness, chronic pain, or other medical conditions. An understanding of the medications used for disabling conditions, possible interactions, and their effects on gynecologic issues (eg, anticonvulsants' impact on contraceptive efficacy, corticosteroids' association with osteoporosis) also is important.

As with other patients, clinicians should obtain the patient's dietary and exercise history. Many women with disabilities are in excellent health, but the requirements to maintain this status may differ from those applying to nondisabled women. For example, these women may engage in wheelchair sports and have good stamina, but may still be at increased risk for the development of early-onset osteoporosis because of lack of weight-bearing activities. Frequently, dairy foods are avoided by women with disabilities because of concern for increased risk of nephrolithiasis. Although this may be an issue for some women, there is no definite prohibition against calcium supplementation and use of dairy products in women with disabilities. These issues may be clarified during individual consultations with a urologist.

Depending on a woman's disability or chronic condition, her optimal functional status may vary with the extent of her limitations. For example, it would not be realistic to have women with multiple sclerosis or polio engage in rigorous physical exercise, as this may compromise energy levels. Instead, basic maintenance of physical activity may be preferable as such women may be at a higher risk for weight gain and obesity. Blood pressure control and cholesterol monitoring are essential. Many women with disabilities have limited access to healthy food choices and frequently eat high-fat, high-sodium, processed foods because of ease of preparation. It may be helpful to have a dietitian realistically review choices to facilitate improved dietary selection.

Abuse of women with disabilities is extremely common. Their vulnerability, whether perceived or actual, can make them targets for physical, sexual, and emotional abuse perpetrated by caregivers, spouses, family members, or others. Accessible shelters are few; thus women may be trapped in a seemingly hopeless situation. It is critical for the clinician to be observant and pick up subtle signs of abuse and neglect and assist the woman in identifying protective services and viable escape options (see also "Domestic or Intimate Partner Violence" in Part 4).

Title III of the Americans with Disabilities Act requires that a public accommodation operated by a private entity, including professional offices of health care practitioners, take steps to ensure that no individual with a disability is discriminated against on the basis of the disabling limitation (see Appendix E). The Americans with Disabilities Act requires the reduction of environmental barriers through both modifications of physical access and provision of auxiliary aids and services to persons with disabilities. The Americans with Disabilities Act does not require massive reconstruction of existing facilities, nor does it require provision of aids and services if doing so would be unduly burdensome.

Services provided to women with cognitive impairments may be subject to widely differing federal, state, and local laws and regulations. For example, federal funds may not be used for the sterilization of "mentally impaired" or "institutionalized" persons. Clinicians should be familiar with laws and regulations that have a bearing on the consent of women with cognitive disabilities and the delivery of services to them.

RESOURCES

Professional

American College of Obstetricians and Gynecologists. Access to health care for women with physical disabilities. ACOG Committee Opinion 202. Washington, DC: ACOG, 1998

American College of Obstetricians and Gynecologists. Routine cancer screening. ACOG Committee Opinion 247. Washington, DC: ACOG, 2000

American College of Obstetricians and Gynecologists. Sterilization of women, including those with mental disabilities. In: Ethics in obstetrics and gynecology. Washington, DC: ACOG, 2002:92–95

Kirschner KL, Gill CJ, Reis JP, Welner S. Health issues for women with disabilities. In: DeLisa JA, Gans BM, eds. Rehabilitation medicine: principles and practice. 3rd ed. Philadelphia: Lippincott-Raven, 1998:1695–1716

McNeil JM. Americans with disabilities: 1994–1995. Current Population Reports. 1997; Series P70-61:1–8

U.S. Department of Justice. Americans with Disabilities Act. ADA Home Page. ADA Information Line 800-514-0301 or 800-514-0383 (TDD) www.usdoj.gov/crt/ada/adahom1.htm

Welner SL. Screening issues in gynecologic malignancies for women with disabilities: critical considerations. J Womens Health 1998;7:281–285

Welner SL, Foley CC, Nosek MA, Holmes A. Practical considerations in the performance of physical examinations on women with disabilities. Obstet Gynecol Surv 1999:54:457–462

APPENDIX A

CODE OF PROFESSIONAL ETHICS OF THE AMERICAN COLLEGE OF OBSTETRICIANS AND GYNECOLOGISTS

Obstetrician–gynecologists, as members of the medical profession, have ethical responsibilities not only to patients, but also to society, to other health professionals, and to themselves. The following ethical foundations for professional activities in the field of obstetrics and gynecology are the supporting structures for the Code of Conduct. The Code implements many of these foundations in the form of rules of ethical conduct. Certain documents of the American College of Obstetricians and Gynecologists, including Committee Opinions and *Ethics in Obstetrics and Gynecology*, also provide additional ethical rules. Selections relevant to specific points are set forth in the Code of Conduct, and those particular documents are incorporated into the Code by reference. Noncompliance with the Code, including referenced documents, may affect an individual's initial or continuing Fellowship in the American College of Obstetricians and Gynecologists. These documents may be revised or replaced periodically, and Fellows should be knowledgeable about current information.

Ethical Foundations

I. The patient–physician relationship: The welfare of the patient (*beneficence*) is central to all considerations in the patient–physician relationship. Included in this relationship is the obligation of physicians to respect the rights of patients, colleagues, and other health professionals. The respect for the right of individual patients to make their own choices about their health care (*autonomy*) is fundamental. The principle of justice requires strict avoidance of discrimination on the basis of race, color, religion, national origin, or any other basis that would constitute illegal discrimination (*justice*).

II. Physician conduct and practice: The obstetrician–gynecologist should deal honestly with patients and colleagues (*veracity*). This includes not misrepresenting himself or herself through any form of communication in an untruthful, misleading, or deceptive manner. Furthermore, maintenance of medical competence through study, application, and enhancement of medical knowledge and skills is an obligation of practicing physicians. Any behavior that diminishes a physician's capability to practice, such as substance abuse, must be immediately addressed and rehabilitative services instituted. The physician should modify his or her practice until the diminished capacity has been restored to an acceptable standard to avoid harm to patients (*nonmaleficence*). All physicians are obligated to respond to evidence of questionable conduct or unethical behavior by other physicians through appropriate procedures established by the relevant organization.

III. Avoiding conflicts of interest: Potential conflicts of interest are inherent in the practice of medicine. Physicians are expected to recognize such situations and deal with them through public disclosure. Conflicts of interest should be resolved in accordance with the best interest of the patient, respecting a woman's autonomy to make health care decisions. The physician should be an advocate for the patient through public disclosure of conflicts of interest raised by health payor policies (managed care or others) or hospital policies.

IV. Professional relations: The obstetrician–gynecologist should respect and cooperate with other physicians, nurses, and other health care professionals.

V. Societal responsibilities: The obstetrician–gynecologist has a continuing responsibility to society as a whole and should support and participate in activities that enhance the community. As a member of society, the obstetrician–gynecologist must respect the laws of that society. As professionals and members of medical societies, physicians are required to uphold the dignity and honor of the profession.

Code of Conduct

I. Patient–Physician Relationship

1. The patient–physician relationship is the central focus of all ethical concerns, and the welfare of the patient should form the basis of all medical judgments.
2. The obstetrician–gynecologist should serve as the patient's advocate and exercise all reasonable means to ensure that the most appropriate care is provided to the patient.
3. The patient–physician relationship has an ethical basis and is built on confidentiality, trust, and honesty. If no patient–physician relationship exists, a physician may refuse to provide care, except in emergencies. Both the patient and the obstetrician–gynecologist are free to establish or discontinue the patient–physician relationship. The obstetrician–gynecologist must adhere to all applicable legal or contractual constraints in dissolving the patient–physician relationship.
4. Sexual misconduct on the part of the obstetrician–gynecologist is an abuse of professional power and a violation of patient trust. Sexual contact or a romantic relationship between a physician and a current patient is always unethical (1).
5. The obstetrician–gynecologist has an obligation to obtain the informed consent of each patient (2). In obtaining informed consent for any course of medical or surgical treatment, the obstetrician–gynecologist should present to the patient, or to the person legally responsible for the patient, in understandable terms, pertinent medical facts and recommendations consistent with good

medical practice. Such information should include alternate modes of treatment and the objectives, risks, benefits, possible complications, and anticipated results of such treatment.

6. It is unethical to prescribe, provide, or seek compensation for therapies that are of no benefit to the patient.
7. The obstetrician–gynecologist should respect the rights of patients, colleagues, and others and safeguard patient information and confidences within the limits of the law. If during the process of providing information for consent it is known that results of a particular test or other information must be given to governmental authorities or other third parties, that should be explained to the patient (3).
8. The obstetrician–gynecologist should not discriminate against patients based on race, color, national origin, religion, or on any other basis that would constitute illegal discrimination.

II. Physician Conduct and Practice

1. The obstetrician–gynecologist should recognize the boundaries of his or her particular competencies and expertise, and provide only those services and use only those techniques for which he or she is qualified by education, training, or experience.
2. The obstetrician–gynecologist should participate in continuing medical education activities to maintain current scientific and professional knowledge relevant to the medical services he or she renders. The obstetrician–gynecologist should provide medical care involving new therapies or techniques only after undertaking appropriate training and study.
3. In emerging areas of medical treatment where recognized medical guidelines do not exist, the obstetrician–gynecologist should exercise careful judgment and take appropriate precautions to protect patient welfare.
4. The obstetrician–gynecologist should not publicize or represent himself or herself in any untruthful, misleading, or deceptive man-

ner to patients, colleagues, other health care professionals, or the public.

5. The obstetrician–gynecologist who has reason to believe that he or she is infected with the human immunodeficiency virus or other serious infectious agents that might be communicated to patients should voluntarily be tested for the protection of his or her patients. In making decisions about patient-care activities, a physician infected with such an agent should adhere to the fundamental professional obligation to avoid harm to patients (4).
6. The obstetrician–gynecologist should not practice medicine while impaired by alcohol, drugs, or physical or mental disability. The obstetrician–gynecologist who experiences substance abuse problems or who is physically or emotionally impaired should seek appropriate assistance to address these problems and limit his or her practice until the impairment no longer affects the quality of patient care.

III. Conflicts of Interest

1. Potential conflicts of interest are inherent in the practice of medicine. Conflicts of interest should be resolved in accordance with the best interest of the patient, respecting a woman's autonomy to make health care decisions. If there is concern about a possibly significant conflict of interest, the physician should disclose his or her concerns to the patient. If a conflict of interest cannot be resolved, the obstetrician–gynecologist should take steps to withdraw from the care of the patient. If conflicts of interest are unresolved, the physician should seek consultation with colleagues or an institutional ethics committee.
2. Commercial promotions of medical products and services may generate bias unrelated to product merit, creating, or appearing to create, inappropriate undue influence. The obstetrician–gynecologist should be aware of this potential conflict of interest and offer medical advice that is as accurate, balanced, complete, and devoid of bias as possible (5, 6).

3. The obstetrician–gynecologist should prescribe drugs, devices, and other treatments based solely upon medical considerations and patient needs, regardless of any direct or indirect interests in or benefit from a pharmaceutical firm or other supplier.
4. When the obstetrician–gynecologist receives anything of substantial value, including royalties, from companies in the health care industry, such as a manufacturer of pharmaceuticals and medical devices, this fact should be disclosed to patients and colleagues when material.
5. Financial and administrative constraints imposed by managed care may create disincentives to treatment otherwise recommended by the obstetrician–gynecologist as in the patient's best interest. Any pertinent constraints should be disclosed to the patient (7).

IV. Professional Relations

1. The obstetrician–gynecologist's relationships with other physicians, nurses, and health care professionals should reflect fairness, honesty, and integrity, sharing a mutual respect and concern for the patient.
2. The obstetrician–gynecologist should consult, refer, or cooperate with other physicians, health care professionals, and institutions to the extent necessary to serve the best interests of their patients.
3. The obstetrician–gynecologist should respect all laws, uphold the dignity and honor of the profession, and accept the profession's self-imposed discipline. The professional competence and conduct of obstetrician–gynecologists are best examined by professional associations, hospital peer-review committees, and state medical and/or licensing boards. These groups deserve the full participation and cooperation of the obstetrician–gynecologist.
4. The obstetrician–gynecologist should strive to address through the appropriate procedures the status of those physicians who demonstrate questionable competence, impairment, or unethical or illegal

behavior. In addition, the obstetrician–gynecologist should cooperate with appropriate authorities to prevent the continuation of such behavior.

V. Societal Responsibilities

1. The obstetrician–gynecologist should support and participate in those health care programs, practices, and activities that contribute positively, in a meaningful and cost-effective way, to the welfare of individual patients, the health care system, or the public good.
2. Obstetrician–gynecologists who provide expert medical testimony in courts of law recognize their duty to testify truthfully. The obstetrician–gynecologist should not testify concerning matters about which he or she is not knowledgeable (8). The obstetrician–gynecologist should be prepared to have testimony, given in any judicial proceeding, subjected to peer review by an institution or professional organization to which he or she belongs. It is unethical for a physician to accept compensation that is contingent on the outcome of litigation.

References

1. American College of Obstetricians and Gynecologists. Sexual misconduct in the practice of obstetrics and gynecology: ethical considerations. In: Ethics in obstetrics and gynecology. Washington, DC: ACOG, 2002:89–91
2. American College of Obstetricians and Gynecologists. Ethical dimensions of informed consent. In: Ethics in obstetrics and gynecology. Washington, DC: ACOG, 2002:19–27
3. American College of Obstetricians and Gynecologists. Ethical guidance for patient testing. In: Ethics in obstetrics and gynecology. Washington, DC: ACOG, 2002:32–34
4. American College of Obstetricians and Gynecologists. Human immunodeficiency virus: ethical guidelines for obstetricians and gynecologists. In: Ethics in obstetrics and gynecology. Washington, DC: ACOG, 2002:43–47
5. American College of Obstetricians and Gynecologists. Guidelines for relationships with industry. In: Ethics in obstetrics and gynecology. Washington, DC: ACOG, 2002:40–42

6. American College of Obstetricians and Gynecologists. Commercial enterprises in medical practice: selling and promoting products. In: Ethics in obstetrics and gynecology. Washington, DC: ACOG, 2002:7–9

7. American College of Obstetricians and Gynecologists. Physician responsibility under managed care: patient advocacy in a changing health care environment. In: Ethics in obstetrics and gynecology. Washington, DC: ACOG, 2002:64–68

8. American College of Obstetricians and Gynecologists. Ethical issues related to expert testimony by obstetricians and gynecologists. In: Ethics in obstetrics and gynecology. Washington, DC: ACOG, 2002:38–39

APPENDIX B

Occupational Safety and Health Administration Regulations on Occupational Exposure to Bloodborne Pathogens*

In 1970, the U.S. Congress enacted the Occupational Safety and Health Act to protect workers from unsafe and unhealthy conditions in the workplace. To oversee this effort, the law also created the Occupational Safety and Health Administration (OSHA) within the U.S. Department of Labor. The Occupational Safety and Health Administration has the responsibility for developing and implementing job safety and health standards and regulations. Its standards and regulations apply to all employers and employees. To promote and ensure compliance with its standards, OSHA has the authority to conduct unannounced workplace inspections. It also maintains a reporting and record-keeping system to monitor job-related injuries and illnesses. Failure to comply with OSHA standards may result in the assessment of civil or criminal penalties.

In December 1991, OSHA issued new regulations on occupational exposure to bloodborne pathogens that are designed to minimize the transmission of human immunodeficiency virus (HIV), hepatitis B virus (HBV), and other potentially infectious materials in the workplace. The regulations cover all employees in physician offices, hospitals, medical laboratories, and other health care facilities where workers could be "rea-

*Adapted from Kaminetzky HA, Rutledge P. OSHA regulations and medical practice. Prim Care Update Ob/Gyns. 1995;2:143–149

sonably anticipated" as a result of performing their job duties to come into contact with blood and other potentially infectious materials. The regulations were revised, effective April 2001, to comply with the Needlestick Safety and Prevention Act of 2000.

Approved State Plans

Under the federal law that created OSHA, states are encouraged to develop and operate—under OSHA guidance—state job safety and health plans. Currently, 23 states and 2 other jurisdictions have OSHA-approved plans, which require them to provide standards and enforcement programs that are at least as effective as the federal standards. They are:

- Alaska
- Arizona
- California
- Connecticut†
- Hawaii
- Indiana
- Iowa
- Kentucky
- Maryland
- Michigan
- Minnesota
- Nevada
- New Mexico
- New York†
- North Carolina
- Oregon
- Puerto Rico
- South Carolina
- Tennessee
- Utah
- Vermont
- Virgin Islands
- Virginia
- Washington
- Wyoming

A list of these state OSHA offices is available on the OSHA website at http://www.osha.gov/oshdir/states.html; call the number listed to receive a copy of the state's standards on occupational exposure to blood-borne pathogens. In Connecticut and New York, the state plans cover state and local government employees only; the private sector is covered by the federal OSHA standard. In addition, states with an OSHA-approved state plan must comply with the federal OSHA standard.

Complying with the Regulations

Exposure Control Plan

In order to comply with the regulations, health care employers are required to prepare a written "Exposure Control Plan" designed to elimi-

†The state OSHA plan covers state and local government employees only.

nate or minimize employee exposure to bloodborne pathogens. This plan must list all job classifications in which employees are likely to be exposed to infectious materials and the relevant tasks and procedures performed by these employees. Infectious materials include blood, semen, vaginal secretions, peritoneal fluid, amniotic fluid, any body fluid visibly contaminated with blood, all body fluids in which it is impossible to differentiate between the body fluids, any unfixed human tissue or organ (living or dead), as well as HIV-containing cell or tissue cultures, organ cultures, and HIV- or HBV-containing culture medium or other solutions.

Under the plan, employers are required to adopt universal precautions, engineering and work practice controls, and personal protective equipment requirements. Employers must also establish a schedule for implementing the following controls:

- Housekeeping requirements
- Employee training and record-keeping requirements
- Hepatitis B virus vaccination for employees and postexposure evaluation and follow-up procedures
- Communication of hazards

A detailed discussion of each of these requirements follows. The plan must be accessible to employees and made available to OSHA upon request. The Exposure Control Plan must be reviewed annually and updated to reflect changes in technology that eliminate or reduce exposure to bloodborne pathogens. The employer must document this annual consideration and use of appropriate effective safer medical procedures and devices that are commercially available. In designing and reviewing the Exposure Compliance Plan, the employer must solicit input from non-managerial employees who are potentially exposed to injuries from contaminated sharps. Employers must document, in the Exposure Control Plan, how they received input from employees.

Mandatory Universal Precautions

The regulations require that universal precautions must be used to prevent contact with blood or other potentially infectious materials. It is

OSHA's intention to follow the Centers for Disease Control and Prevention's guidelines on universal precautions. As defined by the Centers for Disease Control and Prevention, the concept of universal precautions requires the employer and employee to assume that blood and other body fluids are infectious and must be handled accordingly.

Engineering and Work Practice Controls

Specific engineering and work practice controls for the workplace must be implemented and examined for effectiveness on a regular schedule. These include the following controls:

1. Employers are required to provide hand-washing facilities that are readily accessible to employees; when this is not feasible, employees must be provided with an antiseptic hand cleanser with clean cloth/paper towels or antiseptic towelettes. It is the employer's responsibility to ensure that employees wash their hands immediately after gloves and other protective garments are removed.
2. Contaminated needles and other contaminated sharp objects shall not be bent, recapped, or removed unless the employer can demonstrate that no alternative is feasible or that a specific medical procedure requires such action. Shearing or breaking of contaminated needles is prohibited. Recapping or needle removal must be accomplished by a mechanical device or a one-handed technique. Contaminated reusable sharp objects shall be placed in appropriate containers until properly reprocessed; these containers must be puncture resistant, leakproof, and labeled or color coded in accordance with the regulations for easy identification.
3. Eating, drinking, smoking, applying cosmetics or lip balm, and handling contact lenses are prohibited in work areas where there is a reasonable likelihood of exposure to potentially infectious materials.
4. Food and drink must not be kept in refrigerators, freezers, shelves, cabinets, or on countertops where blood or other potentially infectious materials are present.
5. All procedures involving blood or other infectious materials shall be performed in a manner to minimize splashing, spraying, spattering,

and creating droplets; mouth pipetting/suctioning of blood or other potentially infectious materials is prohibited.

6. Specimens of blood or other potentially infectious materials must be placed in closed containers that prevent leakage during collection, handling, processing, storage, transport, or shipping; containers must be labeled or color coded in accordance with the regulations for easy identification. However, when a facility uses universal precautions in the handling of all specimens, the required labeling or color coding of specimens is not necessary as long as containers are recognizable as containing specimens; this exemption applies only while the specimens and containers remain in the facility. If outside contamination of the primary container occurs, it must be placed within a second container that is leakproof, puncture resistant, and labeled or color coded accordingly.
7. Equipment that could be contaminated with blood or other infectious materials must be examined prior to servicing or shipping and shall be decontaminated as necessary, unless the employer can demonstrate that decontamination of the equipment or parts of the equipment is not feasible. A label must be attached to the equipment stating which parts remain contaminated. The employer must ensure that this information is conveyed to all affected employees, the servicing representative, and/or the manufacturer prior to handling, servicing, or shipping so that the necessary precautions will be taken.

Personal Protective Equipment

The regulations also stress the importance of appropriate personal protective equipment that employers are required to provide at no cost to employees whose job duties expose them to blood and other infectious materials. Appropriate personal protective equipment includes but is not limited to gloves, gowns, laboratory coats, face shields or masks, eye protection, mouthpieces, resuscitation bags, pocket masks, or other ventilation devices. As defined by OSHA, personal protective equipment is considered "appropriate" if it prevents blood or other potentially infectious materials from reaching an employee's work clothes and skin, eyes, mouth, or other mucous membranes under normal conditions of use.

Employers must ensure that the employee uses appropriate personal protective equipment unless the employer can demonstrate that the employee temporarily declined to use the equipment, when under rare and extraordinary circumstances, it was the employee's professional judgment that use of personal protective equipment would have prevented the delivery of health care services or would have posed an increased hazard to the safety of the worker or co-worker. When an employee makes this judgment, the circumstances shall be investigated and documented in order to determine whether changes can be made to prevent such situations in the future.

Personal protective equipment in the appropriate sizes must be accessible at the worksite or issued to employees. The employer shall provide for laundering and disposal of personal protective equipment, as well as repair and replace this equipment when necessary to maintain its effectiveness, at no cost to the employee. If a garment(s) is penetrated by blood or other infectious materials, it must be removed immediately or as soon as feasible. All personal protective equipment must be removed before leaving the work area, whereupon it shall be placed in a designated area or storage container for washing or disposal.

Gloves must be worn when it can reasonably be anticipated that the employee may have hand contact with blood, other potentially infectious materials, mucous membranes, and nonintact skin; when performing vascular access procedures; and when handling or touching contaminated surfaces. Disposable gloves shall be replaced as soon as practical when contaminated or when torn or punctured; they shall not be washed or decontaminated for reuse. Utility gloves may be decontaminated for reuse but must be discarded if a glove is cracked, peeling, torn, punctured, or shows other signs of deterioration.

Masks in combination with goggles or protective eye shields must be worn whenever splashes, spray, spatter, or droplets of blood may be created and eye, nose, or mouth contamination can reasonably be anticipated. Gowns and other protective body clothing such as, but not limited to, gowns, aprons, lab coats, clinic jackets, or similar outer garments, shall be worn in occupational exposure situations. The type and characteristics will depend upon the task and degree of exposure anticipated. Surgical caps or hoods and/or shoe covers must be worn in situations in which "gross contamination" can reasonably be anticipated (eg, autopsies, orthopedic surgery).

Housekeeping

Employers must ensure that the worksite is maintained in a clean and sanitary condition and shall develop and implement a written schedule for cleaning and method of decontamination based upon the location within the facility, type of surface to be cleaned, type of soil present, and tasks or procedures being performed in the area. All equipment and working surfaces shall be cleaned and decontaminated after contact with blood or other potentially infectious materials.

Contaminated work surfaces shall be decontaminated with an appropriate disinfectant after tasks and procedures are completed; immediately or as soon as feasible when surfaces are contaminated or after any spill of blood or other potentially infectious materials; and at the end of the work shift if the surface may have become contaminated since the last cleaning. Protective covering (eg, plastic wrap, aluminum foil, or imperviously backed absorbent paper used to cover equipment and environmental surfaces) must be removed and replaced as soon as feasible upon contamination or at the end of the work shift if they may have become contaminated during the shift. All bins, pails, cans, and similar containers intended for reuse shall be inspected and decontaminated on a regularly scheduled basis and cleaned immediately or as soon as feasible upon visible contamination.

Broken glassware that may be contaminated must not be picked up directly with the hands; it must be cleaned up using a brush and dustpan, tongs, or forceps. Contaminated reusable sharp objects must not be stored or processed in a manner that requires employees to reach by hand into the containers in which these sharp objects have been placed. Containers for contaminated sharp objects must be closable, puncture resistant, leakproof on the sides and bottom, and labeled or color coded in accordance with the regulations. During use, containers for contaminated sharp objects shall be easily accessible to personnel and located as close as possible to the immediate area where sharp objects are used. Additionally, these containers must be maintained upright throughout use, replaced routinely, and not be allowed to be overfilled. Reusable containers shall not be opened, emptied, or cleaned manually or in any other manner which would expose employees to the risk of percutaneous injury. Containers of contaminated disposable sharp objects and personal protective equipment are defined as regulated waste; such containers must prevent the spillage or protrusion of contents during handling, storage, transport, or shipping.

Contaminated laundry shall be handled as little as possible and must be placed in bags or containers at the location where it was used; it must not be sorted or rinsed in the location of use. Contaminated laundry shall be transported in clearly labeled or color-coded bags or containers in accordance with the regulations. Employers shall ensure that employees who have contact with contaminated laundry wear protective gloves and other appropriate personal protective equipment. When a facility ships contaminated laundry offsite to a second facility that does not use universal precautions in handling all laundry, the facility generating the contaminated laundry must clearly mark or color code the bags or containers with appropriate biohazard labels.

Hepatitis B Vaccination

Employers are required to provide the vaccination for HBV free of charge to all employees who are at risk for occupational exposure. The vaccine must be provided within 10 days of an employee's initial assignment, except in the following cases:

- The employee has previously received the complete HBV vaccination series.
- Antibody testing has revealed that the employee is immune.
- The vaccine is contraindicated for medical reasons.

The regulations prohibit employers from making employees participate in a prescreening program as a prerequisite for receiving the vaccination. Employees who refuse the vaccination must sign a "Hepatitis B Vaccine Declination" form stating that they have declined the vaccine. If the U.S. Public Health Service ever recommends booster doses of HBV vaccine they must also be provided to employees free of charge. The employee, however, is allowed to change his or her mind and elect to receive the vaccine at any time at the employer's expense.

Postexposure Evaluation and Follow-up

Following a report of an employee exposure incident, the employer must make immediately available to the exposed employee a confidential medical evaluation and follow-up, including at least the following information and follow-up care:

1. Documentation of the route(s) of exposure and the circumstances under which the exposure occurred
2. Identification and documentation of the individual who is the source of the blood or potentially infectious material, unless the employer can establish that such identification is not feasible or is prohibited by state or local law. The source individual's blood shall be tested as soon as possible and after consent is obtained, in order to determine HBV or HIV infectivity. If consent is not obtained, the employer must document that legally required consent cannot be obtained. If the source individual's consent is not required by law, the source individual's blood if available shall be tested and the results documented. However, when the source individual is already known to be infected with HBV or HIV, blood testing for HBV or HIV is not required. Results of the source individual's blood test shall be made available to the exposed employee, and the employee shall be informed of all applicable laws concerning the disclosure of the source individual's identity and infectious status.
3. Collection and testing of the exposed employee's blood for HBV and HIV serologic status as soon as feasible after the employee gives consent. If the employee consents to baseline blood collection but does not give consent at that time for HIV serologic testing, the sample shall be preserved for 90 days. Testing of the blood shall take place within the 90 days if the employee decides to do so.

4. Postexposure prophylaxis when medically indicated, as recommended by the U.S. Public Health Service
5. Counseling
6. Evaluation of reported illnesses

The employer must ensure that the health professional responsible for the employee's HBV vaccination is provided a copy of the OSHA regulation on bloodborne pathogens. In the case of a health professional evaluating an exposed employee, the employer shall ensure that the health professional is provided the following information:

- A copy of the OSHA bloodborne pathogens regulations
- A description of the exposed employee's duties as they relate to the exposure incident
- Documentation of the routes of exposure and circumstances under which exposure occurred
- Results of the source individual's blood testing, if available
- All medical records relevant to the appropriate treatment of the exposed employee, including vaccination status, which is the employer's responsibility to maintain

The employer must obtain and provide the employee with a copy of the evaluating health professional's written opinion within 15 days of completion. The health professional's written opinion for HBV vaccination shall be limited to whether HBV vaccination is indicated for the employee and if the employee has received such vaccination. The health professional's written opinion for postexposure evaluation and follow-up shall be limited to the following information:

- The employee has been informed of the results of the evaluation.
- The employee has been told about any medical conditions resulting from exposure to blood or other potentially infectious materials which require further evaluation or treatment.

All other findings or diagnoses must remain confidential and shall not be included in the written report.

Communications of Hazards to Employees

Warning Labels and Signs. The regulations require warning labels on containers of regulated waste and refrigerators and freezers containing blood or other potentially infectious materials. Warning labels must also be affixed to containers used to store, transport, or ship blood or other potentially infectious materials. The warnings must be fluorescent orange or orange-red; however, red bags or red containers may be substituted for labels.

Employee Training. Employers must ensure that all employees at risk for occupational exposure participate in a training program at no cost to employees and during working hours. Training shall take place at the time of an employee's initial assignment to tasks that risk exposure and at least annually thereafter. Annual training for employees shall be provided within 1 year of their previous training. Additional training must be provided when changes such as modifications of tasks or procedures or introduction of new tasks and procedures affect the worker's exposure risk. The training must be conducted by a person knowledgeable about the subject matter, and the material shall be presented at an educational level appropriate to the employees. The training program at a minimum must include the following information:

1. A copy of the bloodborne pathogens regulations and an explanation of their contents
2. A general explanation of the epidemiology and symptoms of bloodborne diseases
3. An explanation of the modes of transmission of bloodborne diseases
4. An explanation of the employer's Exposure Control Plan and information on how the employee can obtain a copy of the plan
5. An explanation of the appropriate methods for identifying tasks and other activities that may involve exposure
6. An explanation of the methods that will prevent or reduce exposure (including appropriate engineering controls, work practices, and personal protective equipment)

7. Information on the types, proper use, location, removal, handling, decontamination, and disposal of personal protective equipment
8. An explanation of the basis for selection of personal protective equipment
9. Information on the HBV vaccine (efficacy, safety, method of administration, benefits of being vaccinated, and that the vaccine will be offered free of charge)
10. Information on the appropriate actions to take and persons to contact in an emergency involving blood or other infectious materials
11. An explanation of the procedure for follow-up if an exposure incident occurs (including the method for reporting incident and the medical follow-up that may be available)
12. Information on the postexposure evaluation and follow-up that the employer is required to provide for the employee
13. An explanation of the signs and labels and/or color-coding requirements
14. An opportunity for interactive questions and answers with the person conducting the training session

Record-Keeping Requirements

The employer shall maintain an accurate record for each employee at risk for occupational exposure that includes the following information:

- The name and social security number of employee
- The employee's HBV vaccination status (dates and any medical information relative to the employee's ability to receive the vaccination)
- The results of examinations, medical testing, and follow-up procedures
- The employer's copy of the health professional's written evaluation as required following an exposure incident

- A copy of the information provided to the health professional as required following an exposure incident

The employer shall ensure the confidentiality of employee records; information shall not be disclosed without the employee's written consent. The employer is required to maintain records for the duration of employment plus 30 years. The employer must also maintain records of the training sessions that include the dates, the names and qualifications of persons who conducted training sessions, and the names and job titles of employees who attended sessions. These records shall be maintained for 3 years from the date the training session occurred.

All records shall be made available to the assistant secretary of OSHA for examination and copying, including employee medical records, for which the employee's consent is not needed. In the event of an employer going out of business, these records must be transferred to the new owner or must be offered to the National Institute for Occupational Safety and Health.

Sharps Injury Log

An employer with more than 10 employees shall maintain a "sharps injury log" to record percutaneous injuries from contaminated sharps. The information in the log shall be kept in a way to protect the confidentiality of the injured employee. The log must contain:

- The type and brand of device involved in the incident
- The department or work area where the exposure incident occurred
- An explanation of how the incident occurred

The bloodborne pathogens regulations are just one of the OSHA standards that physician offices must follow to be in compliance. Other OSHA regulations include standards on the hazards of chemicals in the workplace, compressed gases, office equipment, and an action plan in case of fire. An emergency hotline number has been established by OSHA to report emergencies: 800-321-OSHA.

APPENDIX C

Clinical Laboratory Improvement Amendments of 1988

The Clinical Laboratory Improvement Amendments of 1988 (CLIA) require federal oversight for all laboratories, including physician offices, that perform tests that examine human specimens for the diagnosis, prevention, or treatment of any disease, impairment of health, or health assessment. All physician offices that conduct any such tests must register their laboratory with the Centers for Medicare and Medicaid Services (CMS) (formerly known as the Health Care Financing Administration) and obtain an appropriate certificate. The Centers for Medicare and Medicaid Services also maintains a registry of laboratories that it has determined to not be in conformance with CLIA regulations.

The majority of obstetrician–gynecologists' offices have either certificates of waiver or certificates for provider-performed microscopy (PPM) procedures. This appendix provides more information on these two types of certificates.

Certificates of Waiver

Physician offices performing only waived tests must obtain a certificate of waiver from CMS in order to perform these tests. No additional complex tests may be performed by the laboratory without prior authorization from CMS. Currently, an extensive list of waived tests exists and can be obtained on the CMS website at http://www.hcfa.gov/medicaid/clia/waivetbl.htm. This list is revised periodically, and physicians should check with CMS to obtain the current list.

Offices performing only waived tests are exempt from the bulk of CLIA regulatory requirements, including proficiency testing, patient test management, quality control, personnel, quality assurance, and routine inspections. However, physician offices must follow manufacturer's instructions for performing the test. Physician offices also are subject to random announced or unannounced inspections to determine whether only waived tests are being performed and to collect information about waived tests. Complaints filed against an office also will be investigated through an inspection.

Certificates of waiver are issued for 2 years and cost $150. Renewal applications for certificates of waiver must be submitted to the U.S. Department of Health and Human Services no less than 9 months and no more than 12 months prior to the expiration of the certificate.

Certificate for Provider-Performed Microscopy Procedure

A certificate for PPM procedures is issued to a laboratory that conducts tests that fall under the PPM category. The procedures that are now defined as PPM are as follows:

- Wet mounts, including preparations of vaginal, cervical, or skin specimens
- All potassium hydroxide preparations
- Pinworm examinations
- Fern test
- Postcoital direct, qualitative examinations of vaginal or cervical mucus
- Urinalysis; microscopic only
- Urinalysis, by dipstick or tablet reagent for bilirubin, glucose, hemoglobin, ketones, leukocytes, nitrite, pH, protein, specific gravity, urobilinogen, any number of these constituents; nonautomated, with microscopy
- Urinalysis, by dipstick or tablet reagent for bilirubin, glucose, hemoglobin, ketones, leukocytes, nitrite, pH, protein, specific gravity, uro-

bilinogen, any number of these constituents; automated, with microscopy (NOTE: May only be used when the laboratory is using an automated dipstick urinalysis instrument approved as waived.)

- Urinalysis; two or three glass test (CWF effective date 7/14/97)
- Fecal leukocyte examination
- Semen analysis; presence and/or motility of sperm excluding Huhner
- Nasal smears for eosinophils

A PPM certificate also permits laboratories to perform waived tests but not other tests of moderate or high complexity. Prior to performing any other tests in the waived or PPM lists, a laboratory must obtain a registration certificate to cover the additional tests of greater complexity.

A laboratory with a PPM certificate also must have a laboratory director, and, if required by state law, the director must possess a state laboratory director license. The laboratory director must be a physician or a midlevel practitioner authorized to practice independently in the state where the laboratory is located. A midlevel practitioner is defined as a nurse–midwife, nurse practitioner, or physician assistant licensed by the state within which the individual practices, if such licensing is required in the state in which the laboratory is located.

The regulations also require that the microscopic tests be personally performed by a physician, a midlevel practitioner under a physician's supervision, or a midlevel practitioner in independent practice, if authorized by the state. To qualify under the PPM category, the procedure also must occur during the patient's visit on a specimen obtained from the practitioner's own patient or from a patient of the group medical practice, clinic, or other health care practitioner where the physician or midlevel practitioner is a member or an employee.

Laboratories with a PPM certificate do receive significant relief from two of the CLIA regulatory requirements. They are not subject to routine inspections, and the cost of the certificates, $200, is significantly less than the cost of a certificate for a laboratory performing tests of greater complexity. Announced or unannounced inspections may be conducted, however, to determine laboratory compliance in performing only the PPM or waived procedures listed, to evaluate complaints, and to collect data on microscopy procedures.

Other CLIA Requirements

Laboratories with a PPM certificate also must comply with the proficiency testing, patient test management, quality control, and quality assurance requirements of the CLIA for laboratories performing tests of moderate complexity:

- Generally, the regulations prescribe that as of January 1994 each laboratory must enroll in a proficiency testing (PT) program. At this time, none of the tests in the PPM category are required to fulfill the PT requirements. Laboratories with PPM certificates are still required, however, to meet the CLIA quality assurance requirements. Basically this requires a laboratory to verify the accuracy, at least twice a year, of any test not subject to PT. This can be accomplished in a number of ways, including splitting specimens with a reference laboratory, evaluating the patient's clinical picture, or enrolling in a non-CLIA-approved PT program that does PT for PPM procedures.
- Patient test management requirements state that each laboratory must have available and follow written policy and procedures for specimen submission and handling. A written procedure manual also must be available and followed by office personnel for quality control purposes.

Certificates for PPM are valid for up to 2 years. To renew a PPM certificate, the appropriate renewal paperwork must be returned to the U.S. Department of Health and Human Services 9–12 months prior to the expiration of the certificate.

Information about CLIA is available at the CMS web site: www.hcfa.gov. Information on how to apply for a CLIA certificate is available from local state survey agencies. A listing of state survey agency contacts is available on the CMS web site.

APPENDIX D

Federal Requirements for Patient Screening and Transfer

In 1986, Congress first enacted legal requirements specifying how Medicare-participating hospitals with emergency services must handle individuals with emergency medical conditions or women who are in labor. Since then, the patient screening and transfer law has undergone numerous refinements and revisions. The most recent regulations, promulgated by the Health Care Financing Administration (HCFA) (currently known as the Centers for Medicare and Medicaid Services), became effective July 22, 1994. Physicians should expect that this law will continue to evolve and that there will be additional modifications to it in the future.

Requirements for an Appropriate Medical Screening Examination

Federal law requires that all Medicare-participating hospitals with emergency services must provide an "appropriate medical screening examination" for any individual who comes to the emergency department for medical treatment or examination to determine whether the patient has an emergency medical condition. This examination must be made within the capability of the hospital's emergency department, including ancillary services routinely available to the emergency department. For example, "[i]f a hospital has a department of obstetrics and gynecology, the hospital is responsible for adopting procedures under which the staff and resources of that department are available to treat a woman in labor who comes to its emergency department."

Medical screening examinations also must "...be conducted by individuals determined qualified by hospital by-laws or rules and regulations."

Thus, it is up to a hospital to designate who is a "qualified medical person" to provide an appropriate medical screening examination. The law does not require that physicians perform all screening examinations. Therefore, a hospital can determine under what circumstances a physician is required to provide medical screening and when screening can be done by a nonphysician.

Determining Whether a Patient Has an Emergency Medical Condition

The legal definition of "emergency medical condition" is not the same as the medical one. Under the law, it is defined as follows:

> A medical condition manifesting itself by acute symptoms of sufficient severity (including severe pain, psychiatric disturbances and/or symptoms of substance abuse) such that the absence of immediate attention could reasonably be expected to result in
>
> (A) Placing the health of the individual (or, with respect to a pregnant woman, the health of the woman or her unborn child) in serious jeopardy;
>
> (B) Serious impairment to bodily functions; or
>
> (C) Serious dysfunction of any bodily organ or part.

It is important to note that with pregnant women who present to a hospital emergency room, the health of the fetus also must be considered in determining whether an "emergency medical condition" exists.

Special Determination of Emergency Medical Condition for Pregnant Women

The definition of emergency medical condition also makes specific reference to a pregnant woman having contractions. It provides that an emergency medical condition exists if a pregnant woman is having contractions and "...there is inadequate time to effect a safe transfer to another hospital before delivery; or that transfer may pose a threat to the health or safety of the woman or the unborn child." An emergency medical condition does not exist even when a woman is having contractions as long as there is adequate time to effect a safe transfer before delivery and the transfer will not pose a threat to the health or safety of the mother or fetus.

In its 1998 state operations manual, HCFA interpreted the definition of labor to mean "...the process of childbirth beginning with the latent phase of labor or early phase of labor and continuing through delivery of the placenta. A woman experiencing contractions is in true labor unless a physician or qualified individual certifies that after a reasonable time of observation the woman is in false labor." The addition of the phrase "or qualified individual" is a recent clarification by HCFA of the requirements.

Patients with Emergency Medical Conditions

Once a patient comes to an emergency room, is appropriately screened, and is determined to have an emergency medical condition the physician has two choices as to how to proceed. The physician may:

1. Treat the patient and stabilize her condition
2. Transfer the patient to another medical facility in accordance with specific procedures outlined below

In situations in which the woman is experiencing contractions and meets the other criteria outlined above for an emergency medical condition, the only way to stabilize the patient is to deliver the child and the placenta.

Patients Can Refuse to Consent to Treatment

If a patient refuses to consent to treatment, the hospital has fulfilled its obligations under the law. If a patient refuses to consent to treatment, however, the following steps must be taken:

1. The patient must be informed of the risks and benefits of the examination and treatment, or both.
2. The medical record must contain a description of the examination and treatment that was refused by the patient.

3. The hospital must take all reasonable steps to secure the patient's written informed refusal. The written document must indicate that the person has been informed of the risks and benefits of the examination or treatment, or both.

Procedures to Follow for Transferring a Patient to Another Medical Facility

In general, a patient who meets the criteria of an emergency medical condition may not be transferred until the patient is stabilized. There are, however, some exceptions to this prohibition.

The patient may request a transfer, in writing, after being informed of the hospital's obligations under the law and the risks of transfer. The unstabilized patient's written request for transfer must indicate the reasons for the request and that the patient is aware of the risks and benefits of transfer.

An unstabilized patient also may be transferred if a physician signs a written certification that:

> *based upon the information available at the time of transfer, the medical benefits reasonably expected from the provision of appropriate medical treatment at another medical facility outweigh the increased risks to the individual or, in the case of a woman in labor, to the woman or the unborn child, from being transferred.*

The certification must contain a summary or the risks and benefits of transfer.

If a physician is not physically present in the emergency department at the time of the transfer of a patient, a qualified medical person can sign the certification described above after consulting with a physician who authorizes the transfer. The physician must countersign the certification later.

Patients Can Refuse to Consent to Transfer

If the hospital offers to transfer a patient, in accordance with the appropriate procedures, and the patient refuses to consent to transfer, the hospital also has fulfilled its obligations under the law. When a patient refuses to consent to the transfer, the hospital must take the following steps:

1. The patient must be informed of the risks and benefits of the transfer.
2. The medical record must contain a description of the proposed transfer that was refused by the patient.
3. The hospital must take all reasonable steps to secure the patient's written informed refusal. The written document must indicate that the person has been informed of the risks and benefits of the transfer and the reasons for the patient's refusal.

Additional Requirements of the Transferring and Receiving Hospitals

The transferring hospital must comply with the following requirements to ensure the transfer was appropriate:

1. The receiving hospital must have space and qualified personnel to treat the patient and must have agreed to accept the transfer. A hospital with specialized capabilities such as a neonatal intensive care unit may not refuse to accept patients if space is available.
2. The transferring hospital must minimize the risks to the patient's health, and the transfer must be executed through the use of qualified personnel and transportation equipment.
3. The transferring hospital must send to the receiving hospital all medical records related to the emergency condition available at the time of transfer. These records include available history, records related to the emergency medical condition, observations of signs or symptoms, preliminary diagnosis, results of diagnostic studies or telephone reports of the studies, treatment provided, results of any test and the informed written consent or certification, and the name of any on-call physician who has refused or failed to appear within a reasonable time to provide necessary stabilizing treatment. Other records not yet available must be sent as soon as practical.

General Requirements

1. Medical records related to transfers must be retained by both the transferring and receiving hospitals for 5 years from the date of the transfer.
2. Hospitals are required to report to the Centers for Medicare and Medicaid Services or the state survey agency within 72 hours from the time of the transfer any time it has reason to believe it may have received a patient who was transferred in an unstable medical condition.
3. Hospitals are required to post signs in areas, such as entrances, admitting areas, reception area, emergency departments, with respect to their obligations under the patient screening and transfer law.
4. Hospitals also are required to post signs stating whether the hospital participates in the Medicaid program under a state-approved plan. This requirement applies to all hospitals, not only the ones that participate in Medicare.
5. Hospitals must keep a list of physicians who are on call after the initial examination to provide treatment to stabilize a patient with an emergency medical condition.
6. Hospitals must keep a central log of all individuals who come to the emergency department seeking assistance and the result of each individual's visit.
7. A hospital may not delay providing appropriate medical screening to inquire about payment method or insurance status.

Enforcement and Penalties

Physicians and hospitals violating these federal requirements for patient screening and transfer are subject to civil monetary penalties of up to $50,000 for each violation and to termination from the Medicare program. Hospitals are prohibited from penalizing physicians who report violations of the law or refuse to transfer an individual with an unstabilized emergency medical condition.

APPENDIX E

THE AMERICANS WITH DISABILITIES ACT

In July 1990, the Americans with Disabilities Act (ADA) was signed into law. It is an ambitious federal measure that safeguards the civil rights of individuals with disabilities.

Who Is Protected by the Americans with Disabilities Act?

The ADA protects individuals with disabilities against discrimination in certain critical areas of daily living. These areas include protections for health services, employment, communication, public accommodations, education, and transportation. Disability is defined broadly to include both physical and mental impairments that substantially limit one or more major life activities of an individual. A person who has a record of either a physical or a mental impairment or a person who is regarded as having such an impairment also is considered as having a disability.

Although it is impossible to enumerate all of the impairments that are covered by the ADA, the list includes the following: visual, speech, and hearing impairments as well as epilepsy, muscular dystrophy, heart disease, cancer, human immunodeficiency virus infection (symptomatic or asymptomatic), tuberculosis, mental retardation, cosmetic disfigurement, anatomical loss, alcoholism, or emotional or mental illness. There also are a number of conditions that are specifically defined as not disabilities under the ADA. These include current use of illegal drugs, compulsive gambling, kleptomania, pyromania, and sexual behavioral disorders.

Employment Obligations

The antidiscrimination employment provisions of the ADA apply to all employers who have 15 or more employees on staff. To summarize, employers are prohibited from discriminating against a job applicant or an employee currently on staff who is a "qualified individual with a disability." All aspects of employment practices are covered by the law, including job application procedures, hiring, job advancement, compensation, benefits, and discharge. The ADA specifically prohibits pre-employment questions about a disability or the nature or severity of a disability.

Who Is a "Qualified Individual with a Disability?"

A qualified individual with a disability is defined as "an individual who, with or without reasonable accommodation, can perform the essential functions of the employment position that such individual holds or desires." In essence, an employer cannot deny a qualified individual with a disability a job or discharge such an employee based on the individual's disability.

An employer also is prohibited from discriminating against an individual because the person is known to have a relationship with a person with a disability. For instance, an employer cannot reject a potential employee solely on the basis that the applicant's spouse has cancer and the employer fears that the applicant may not be able to devote full attention to the position.

What Is a Reasonable Accommodation?

An employer also must make reasonable accommodations to assist an individual with a disability in performing a job, unless such accommodations would impose an undue hardship on the business. What comprises a reasonable accommodation varies with the circumstances. A reasonable accommodation could mean that an employer would have to make the office readily accessible and usable by individuals with disabilities. An employer also may be required to restructure an employee's assignments or modify the employee's work schedule as a reasonable accommodation.

The ADA does not require employers to hire unqualified individuals with disabilities. It permits businesses to use selection criteria or standards that screen out or tend to screen out an individual with a disability as long as the criteria are shown to be job related for the position, are consistent with business necessity, and the job functions cannot be accomplished by reasonable accommodations.

Public Accommodations

A place of "public accommodation" is defined broadly by the ADA as a privately operated entity that owns, operates, or leases a place of public accommodation. Places of public accommodation include physician offices, hospitals, grocery stores, golf courses, libraries, and day care centers, to name a few. Public accommodations, regardless of the size of the business or the number of people employed, also are prohibited from discriminating against individuals with a disability.

Are Physicians Required to Treat All Patients?

Antidiscrimination protections in the ADA prohibit a business that fits the definition of public accommodations from establishing criteria that would screen out or tend to screen out an individual with a disability. The ADA also requires businesses to make reasonable modifications for individuals with disabilities. This makes it discriminatory for physicians to deny care to an individual based solely on the individual's disability. For example, an obstetrician–gynecologist would be in violation of the ADA if the physician established a rule denying care to obstetric patients with human immunodeficiency virus. If, however, this same physician no longer practiced obstetrics and referred all pregnant women to other physicians, the physician would be under no obligation to care for this patient. A physician is not required to treat a patient with a condition outside the physician's area of practice or expertise.

A physician also is not required to provide services to an individual with a disability if the individual poses a direct threat to the health or safety of others. A "direct threat" is a significant risk to the health or safety of others that cannot be eliminated by a modification of policies, practices, or procedures or the provision or auxiliary aids and services. Physicians have to be careful, however, that a decision not to provide care is based on objective criteria relying on current medical evidence rather than stereotypes or generalizations about the effects of a particular disability.

Auxiliary Aids

Physicians also are required to provide and pay for auxiliary aids and services to communicate effectively with patients who have disabilities affecting hearing, vision, or speech, unless such accommodations create an undue burden. This is a flexible requirement, and physicians should consider the patient's needs and consult with the patient before determining what form of auxiliary aids to provide.

Other Provisions

Businesses are required to make readily achievable structural changes to their facilities to make them more accessible to the individuals with a disability. New construction also must be in compliance with the ADA. There are federal tax deductions for some expenses associated with removal of barriers and tax credits for eligible small businesses that make certain accommodations required by the ADA.

Americans with Disabilities Act Resources

For more information about or assistance with the ADA contact:

U.S. Department of Justice
ADA Information Line
800-514-0301 (voice)
800-514-0383 (TDY)
www.usdoj.gov/crt/ada/adahom1.htm

Equal Employment Opportunity Commission

Employment—questions
800-669-4000 (voice)
800-669-6820 (TDY)

Employment—documents
800-669-3362 (voice)
800-800-3302 (TDY)
www.eeoc.gov

Federal Communications Commission
TTY Help Desk–(202) 418-0124
TTY Directory–(202) 418-0370
www.fcc.gov/cib/dro

Architectural and Transportation Barriers Compliance Board
Documents and questions
800-872-2253 (voice)
800-993-2822 (TDY)
www.access-board.gov/

Department of Education
Disability and Business Technical Assistance Centers
800-949-4232 (voice/TDY)
www.adata.org

President's Committee on Employment of People with Disabilities

Employment questions
(202) 376-6200 (voice)
(202) 376-6205 (TDY)
www.50pcepd.gov/pcepd/

Job Accommodation Network
800-526-7234 (voice/TDY)
janweb.icdi.wvu.edu/

APPENDIX F

STATEMENT ON SCOPE OF PRACTICE OF OBSTETRICS AND GYNECOLOGY

ACOG Operational Mission Statement

The American College of Obstetricians and Gynecologists (ACOG) is a membership organization of obstetrician–gynecologists dedicated to the advancement of women's health through education, advocacy, practice and research.

Vision Statement

Obstetrics and gynecology is a discipline dedicated to the broad, integrated medical and surgical care of women's health throughout their lifespan. The combined discipline of obstetrics and gynecology requires extensive study and understanding of reproductive physiology, including the physiologic, social, cultural, environmental and genetic factors that influence disease in women.

Primary and preventive counseling and education are essential and integral parts of the practice of an obstetrician–gynecologist as they advance the individual and community-based health of women of all ages.

Obstetricians and gynecologists may choose a wide or more focused scope of practice from primary ambulatory health to concentration in a particular area of specialization. This study and understanding of the reproductive physiology of women gives obstetricians and gynecologists a unique perspective in addressing gender-specific health care issues.

Approved by the Executive Board of the American College of Obstetricians and Gynecologists, May 25, 2000

APPENDIX G

ACOG Woman's Health Record

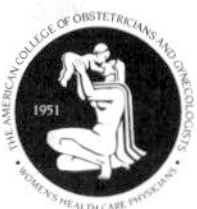

ACOG WOMAN'S HEALTH RECORD

HOW TO USE THE ACOG WOMAN'S HEALTH RECORD

The ACOG Woman's Health Record is intended to serve as a complete record for a woman's gynecologic care. It allows documentation of both preventive services and services directed to a chief complaint. This record has been specifically designed to aid in documentation and correct coding of women's health services.

The ACOG Woman's Health Record includes six sections:

1. Physician History
2. Physical Examination
3. Medical Decision Making
4. Patient Intake History
5. Problem List/Immunization Record
6. Routine and High-Risk Laboratory Records

Physician History: The Physician History can be used to record the history for every type of outpatient encounter, including consultations. A new Physician History should be completed by the physician at each visit when clinically indicated.

Physical Examination: The Physical Examination section should be completed by the physician each time a physical examination is provided. The form offers prompts to aid in documenting the services that are provided. This form is based on the 1997 HCFA guidelines for the female genitourinary system examination and can be used to document any level of examination.

Medical Decision Making: The Medical Decision Making section provides space to document minutes counseled, total encounter time, and other services needed to determine the correct level of medical decision making.

Patient Intake History: This optional form gives practices the flexibility to have patients complete their own history at or before the visit. It uses language that a patient is likely to understand and includes ample space for physician notes. Space at the end of the form allows physicians to review the history and sign off for 4 years. At year 5, the patient should be asked to complete a new Patient Intake History.

Problem List and Immunization Record: The Problem List captures problems, allergies, family history, and current medication use. The Immunization Record lists immunization services recommended by ACOG for either routine use or in high-risk patients, as defined in the enclosed table of high-risk factors. Ample space for listing problems and immunization services allows the same form to be used for years.

Routine and High-Risk Laboratory Records: The Routine and High-Risk Laboratory Records provide ample space to document laboratory services provided. The Routine Laboratory Record includes those laboratory tests recommended by ACOG for routine use and provides reminders for recommended frequency of services. The High-Risk Laboratory Record includes those laboratory tests recommended by ACOG on the basis of the risk factors defined in the enclosed table of high-risk factors.

The ACOG Woman's Health Record also includes helpful reference information (one each per package):

Coding Tips: This sheet includes all the reminders a physician needs to code correctly the history, physical examination, and medical decision making provided during the visit. Once these elements have been coded correctly, the summary tables can be used to select the appropriate code for the visit.

Table of High-Risk Factors: The table (see back of this card) lists in one place the risk factors that should prompt recommended interventions, laboratory tests, and immunizations. It is to be used in completing the Immunization Record and the Routine and High-Risk Laboratory Records.

PHYSICIAN HISTORY

PATIENT NAME:	BIRTH DATE: / /	ID NO.:	DATE: / /
☐ NEW PATIENT ☐ ESTABLISHED PATIENT	☐ CONSULTATION ☐ REPORT SENT: / /		
PRIMARY CARE PHYSICIAN:	WHO SENT PATIENT:		
OTHER PHYSICIAN(S):			
CHIEF COMPLAINT (CC) (REQUIRED FOR ALL VISITS):	CURRENT MEDICATIONS: ☐ NONE		
LAST MENSTRUAL PERIOD: / /	ALLERGIES (DESCRIBE REACTION): ☐ NONE		
LAST PAP TEST: / /			
LAST MAMMOGRAM: / /			
LAST COLORECTAL SCREENING: / /			

PAST HISTORY (PH)

☐ NONCONTRIBUTORY ☐ NO INTERVAL CHANGE SINCE: / /

SURGERIES:

ILLNESSES:

INJURIES:

IMMUNIZATIONS/TUBERCULOSIS TEST:

FAMILY HISTORY (FH)

☐ NONCONTRIBUTORY ☐ NO INTERVAL CHANGE SINCE: / /

MOTHER: ☐ LIVING ☐ DECEASED—CAUSE: AGE:	FATHER: ☐ LIVING ☐ DECEASED—CAUSE: AGE:

SIBLINGS: NUMBER LIVING: NUMBER DECEASED: CAUSE(S)/AGE(S):

CHILDREN: NUMBER LIVING: NUMBER DECEASED: CAUSE(S)/AGE(S):

☐ DIABETES	☐ HEART DISEASE	☐ HYPERLIPIDEMIA
☐ CANCER	☐ HYPERTENSION	☐ DEEP VENOUS THROMBOEMBOLISM/PULMONARY EMBOLISM
☐ OTHER		

American College of Obstetricians and Gynecologists ■ 409 12th Street, SW ■ PO Box 96920 ■ Washington, DC ■ 20090-6920

PHYSICIAN HISTORY *(Continued)*

PATIENT NAME:	BIRTH DATE: / /	ID NO.:	DATE: / /

SOCIAL HISTORY (SH)

☐ NONCONTRIBUTORY ☐ NO INTERVAL CHANGE SINCE: / /

	YES	NO	NOTES
TOBACCO USE	☐	☐	
ALCOHOL/DRUG USE	☐	☐	
DOMESTIC VIOLENCE	☐	☐	
HEALTH HAZARDS AT HOME/WORK	☐	☐	
SEAT BELT USE	☐	☐	
DIET DISCUSSED	☐	☐	
FOLIC ACID INTAKE	☐	☐	
CALCIUM INTAKE	☐	☐	
REGULAR EXERCISE	☐	☐	
CAFFEINE INTAKE	☐	☐	
OTHER			

☐ NO CHANGES SINCE: / /

REVIEW OF SYSTEMS (ROS)

1. CONSTITUTIONAL	☐ NEGATIVE ☐ WEIGHT LOSS ☐ WEIGHT GAIN ☐ FEVER ☐ FATIGUE ☐ OTHER TALLEST HEIGHT ______
2. EYES	☐ NEGATIVE ☐ VISION CHANGE ☐ GLASSES/CONTACTS ☐ OTHER
3. EAR, NOSE, AND THROAT	☐ NEGATIVE ☐ ULCERS ☐ SINUSITIS ☐ HEADACHE ☐ HEARING LOSS ☐ OTHER
4. CARDIOVASCULAR	☐ NEGATIVE ☐ ORTHOPNEA ☐ CHEST PAIN ☐ DIFFICULTY BREATHING ON EXERTION ☐ EDEMA ☐ PALPITATION ☐ OTHER
5. RESPIRATORY	☐ NEGATIVE ☐ WHEEZING ☐ HEMOPTYSIS ☐ SHORTNESS OF BREATH ☐ COUGH ☐ OTHER
6. GASTROINTESTINAL	☐ NEGATIVE ☐ DIARRHEA ☐ BLOODY STOOL ☐ NAUSEA/VOMITING/INDIGESTION ☐ CONSTIPATION ☐ FLATULENCE ☐ PAIN ☐ FECAL INCONTINENCE ☐ OTHER
7. GENITOURINARY	☐ NEGATIVE ☐ HEMATURIA ☐ DYSURIA ☐ URGENCY ☐ FREQUENCY ☐ INCOMPLETE EMPTYING ☐ INCONTINENCE ☐ DYSPAREUNIA ☐ ABNORMAL OR PAINFUL PERIODS ☐ PMS ☐ ABNORMAL VAGINAL BLEEDING ☐ ABNORMAL VAGINAL DISCHARGE ☐ OTHER
8. MUSCULOSKELETAL	☐ NEGATIVE ☐ MUSCLE WEAKNESS ☐ MUSCLE OR JOINT PAIN ☐ OTHER
9a. SKIN	☐ NEGATIVE ☐ RASH ☐ ULCERS ☐ DRY SKIN ☐ PIGMENTED LESIONS ☐ OTHER
9b. BREAST	☐ NEGATIVE ☐ MASTALGIA ☐ DISCHARGE ☐ MASSES ☐ OTHER
10. NEUROLOGIC	☐ NEGATIVE ☐ SYNCOPE ☐ SEIZURES ☐ NUMBNESS ☐ TROUBLE WALKING ☐ SEVERE MEMORY PROBLEMS ☐ OTHER
11. PSYCHIATRIC	☐ NEGATIVE ☐ DEPRESSION ☐ CRYING ☐ SEVERE ANXIETY ☐ OTHER
12. ENDOCRINE	☐ NEGATIVE ☐ DIABETES ☐ HYPOTHYROID ☐ HYPERTHYROID ☐ HOT FLASHES ☐ HAIR LOSS ☐ HEAT/COLD INTOLERANCE ☐ OTHER
13. HEMATOLOGIC/LYMPHATIC	☐ NEGATIVE ☐ BRUISES ☐ BLEEDING ☐ ADENOPATHY ☐ OTHER
14. ALLERGIC/IMMUNOLOGIC	(SEE FIRST PAGE)

PHYSICAL EXAMINATION

PATIENT NAME: | BIRTH DATE: / / | ID NO.: | DATE: / /

CONSTITUTIONAL

• VITAL SIGNS (RECORD ≥ 3 VITAL SIGNS):

HEIGHT: ______ WEIGHT: ______ BMI: ______ BLOOD PRESSURE (SITTING): ______ TEMPERATURE: ______ PULSE: ______ RESPIRATION: ______

• GENERAL APPEARANCE (NOTE ALL THAT APPLY):

☐ WELL-DEVELOPED ☐ OTHER ☐ NO DEFORMITIES ☐ OTHER

☐ WELL-NOURISHED ☐ OTHER ☐ WELL-GROOMED ☐ OTHER

☐ NORMAL HABITUS ☐ OBESE ☐ OTHER

NECK

• NECK ☐ NORMAL ☐ ABNORMAL ______

• THYROID ☐ NORMAL ☐ ABNORMAL ______

RESPIRATORY

• RESPIRATORY EFFORT ☐ NORMAL ☐ ABNORMAL ______

• AUSCULTATED LUNGS ☐ NORMAL ☐ ABNORMAL ______

CARDIOVASCULAR

• AUSCULTATED HEART

SOUNDS ☐ NORMAL ☐ ABNORMAL ______

MURMURS ☐ NORMAL ☐ ABNORMAL ______

• PERIPHERAL VASCULAR ☐ NORMAL ☐ ABNORMAL ______

GASTROINTESTINAL

• ABDOMEN ☐ NORMAL ☐ ABNORMAL ______

• HERNIA ☐ NONE ☐ PRESENT ______

• LIVER/SPLEEN

LIVER ☐ NORMAL ☐ ABNORMAL ______

SPLEEN ☐ NORMAL ☐ ABNORMAL ______

• STOOL GUAIAC, IF INDICATED

LYMPHATIC

• PALPATION OF NODES (CHOOSE ALL THAT ARE APPLICABLE)

NECK ☐ NORMAL ☐ ABNORMAL ______

AXILLA ☐ NORMAL ☐ ABNORMAL ______

GROIN ☐ NORMAL ☐ ABNORMAL ______

OTHER SITE ☐ NORMAL ☐ ABNORMAL ______

SKIN

• INSPECTED/PALPATED ☐ NORMAL ☐ ABNORMAL

NEUROLOGIC/PSYCHIATRIC

• ORIENTATION ☐ TIME ☐ PLACE ☐ PERSON ☐ COMMENTS

• MOOD AND AFFECT ☐ NORMAL ☐ DEPRESSED ☐ ANXIOUS ☐ AGITATED ☐ OTHER

GYNECOLOGIC (AT LEAST 7)

• BREASTS ☐ NORMAL ☐ ABNORMAL ______

• EXTERNAL GENITALIA ☐ NORMAL ☐ ABNORMAL ______

• URETHRAL MEATUS ☐ NORMAL ☐ ABNORMAL ______

• URETHRA ☐ NORMAL ☐ ABNORMAL ______

• BLADDER ☐ NORMAL ☐ ABNORMAL ______

• VAGINA/PELVIC SUPPORT ☐ NORMAL ☐ ABNORMAL ______

• CERVIX ☐ NORMAL ☐ ABNORMAL ______

• UTERUS ☐ NORMAL ☐ ABNORMAL ______

• ADNEXA/PARAMETRIA ☐ NORMAL ☐ ABNORMAL ______

• ANUS/PERINEUM ☐ NORMAL ☐ ABNORMAL ______

• RECTAL ☐ NORMAL ☐ ABNORMAL ______

• TOTAL NUMBER OF BULLET (•) ELEMENTS EXAMINED:

American College of Obstetricians and Gynecologists ■ 409 12th Street, SW ■ PO Box 96920 ■ Washington, DC ■ 20090-6920

MEDICAL DECISION MAKING

PATIENT NAME:	BIRTH DATE: / /	ID NO.:	DATE: / /

AMOUNT AND COMPLEXITY OF DATA REVIEWED:

TEST(S) ORDERED:

☐ LABORATORY

—PAP TEST

—WET MOUNT

—OTHER: __________

☐ RADIOLOGY/ULTRASOUND

—MAMMOGRAM

—OTHER: __________

REVIEW OF RECORDS:

☐ PREVIOUS TEST RESULTS: __________

☐ DISCUSSION OF TEST RESULTS WITH PERFORMING PHYSICIAN: __________

☐ OLD RECORDS REVIEWED AND SUMMARIZED: __________

☐ HISTORY OBTAINED FROM OTHER SOURCE: __________

☐ INDEPENDENT REVIEW OF IMAGE/SPECIMEN: __________

DIAGNOSES/MANAGEMENT OPTIONS

☐ ESTABLISHED PROBLEM ☐ NEW PROBLEM

ASSESSMENT AND PLAN:

PATIENT COUNSELED ABOUT:

MINUTES COUNSELED:	TOTAL ENCOUNTER TIME:
SIGNATURE:	DATE: / /

American College of Obstetricians and Gynecologists ■ 409 12th Street, SW ■ PO Box 96920 ■ Washington, DC ■ 20090-6920

FOR OFFICE USE ONLY
☐ NEW PATIENT
☐ ESTABLISHED PATIENT
☐ CONSULTATION
☐ REPORT SENT: / /

PATIENT INTAKE HISTORY

PATIENT NAME:	BIRTH DATE: / /	ID NO.:	DATE: / /
ADDRESS:			
CITY:	STATE/ZIP:		
HOME TELEPHONE: ( )	WORK TELEPHONE: ( )		
EMPLOYER:	INSURANCE:		
NAME YOU WOULD LIKE US TO USE:			
NAME OF SPOUSE/PARTNER:	EMERGENCY CONTACT:		
	RELATIONSHIP:		
	HOME TELEPHONE: ( )	WORK TELEPHONE: ( )	
REFERRED BY:			
WHY HAVE YOU COME TO THE OFFICE TODAY?			
IF YOU ARE HERE FOR AN ANNUAL EXAMINATION IS THIS A ☐ PRIMARY CARE VISIT OR ☐ GYNECOLOGY ONLY			
IS THIS A NEW PROBLEM?			
PLEASE DESCRIBE YOUR PROBLEM, INCLUDING WHERE IT IS, HOW SEVERE IT IS, AND HOW LONG IT'S LASTED.			

If you are uncomfortable answering any questions, leave them blank; you can discuss them with your doctor or nurse.

GYNECOLOGIC HISTORY

	PHYSICIAN'S NOTES
LAST NORMAL MENSTRUAL PERIOD (FIRST DAY): / /	
AGE PERIODS BEGAN:	
LENGTH OF PERIODS (NUMBER OF DAYS OF BLEEDING):	
NUMBER OF DAYS BETWEEN PERIODS:	
ANY RECENT CHANGES IN PERIODS?	
ARE YOU CURRENTLY SEXUALLY ACTIVE?	
HAVE YOU EVER HAD SEX?	
NUMBER OF SEXUAL PARTNERS (LIFETIME):	
SEXUAL PARTNERS ARE ☐ MEN ☐ WOMEN ☐ BOTH	
PRESENT METHOD OF BIRTH CONTROL:	
HAVE YOU EVER USED AN INTRAUTERINE DEVICE (IUD) OR BIRTH CONTROL PILLS?	
IF YES, FOR HOW LONG?	
WHEN WAS YOUR LAST PAP TEST?	
WHAT WAS THE RESULT?	
HAVE YOU EVER HAD AN ABNORMAL PAP TEST?	
DO YOU DO REGULAR BREAST SELF-EXAMINATIONS?	

American College of Obstetricians and Gynecologists ■ 409 12th Street, SW ■ PO Box 96920 ■ Washington, DC ■ 20090-6920

PATIENT INTAKE HISTORY *(Continued)*

PATIENT NAME:	BIRTH DATE: / /	ID NO.:	DATE: / /

OBSTETRIC HISTORY

	NUMBER		NUMBER		NUMBER
PREGNANCIES		ABORTIONS		MISCARRIAGES	
PREMATURE BIRTHS (<37 WEEKS)		LIVE BIRTHS		LIVING CHILDREN	

NO.	BIRTH DATE	WEIGHT AT BIRTH	BABY'S SEX	WEEKS PREGNANT	TYPE OF DELIVERY (VAGINAL, CESAREAN, ETC.)	COMPLICATIONS?
1.						
2.						
3.						
4.						

PHYSICIAN'S NOTES ON OBSTETRIC HISTORY:

CURRENT MEDICATIONS
(Including hormones, vitamins, herbs, nonprescription medications)

DRUG NAME	DOSAGE	WHO PRESCRIBED	DRUG NAME	DOSAGE	WHO PRESCRIBED

FAMILY HISTORY

MOTHER: ☐ LIVING ☐ DECEASED—CAUSE: AGE:	FATHER: ☐ LIVING ☐ DECEASED—CAUSE: AGE:
SIBLINGS: NUMBER LIVING: NUMBER DECEASED: CAUSE(S)/AGE(S):	
CHILDREN: NUMBER LIVING: NUMBER DECEASED: CAUSE(S)/AGE(S):	

ILLNESS	YES	WHICH RELATIVE(S) AND AGE OF ONSET	PHYSICIAN'S NOTES
DIABETES	☐		
STROKE	☐		
HEART DISEASE	☐		
BLOOD CLOTS IN LUNGS OR LEGS	☐		
HIGH BLOOD PRESSURE	☐		
HIGH CHOLESTEROL	☐		
OSTEOPOROSIS (WEAK BONES)	☐		
HEPATITIS	☐		
HIV/AIDS	☐		
TUBERCULOSIS	☐		
BIRTH DEFECTS	☐		
DRINKING OR DRUG PROBLEMS	☐		
BREAST CANCER	☐		
COLON CANCER	☐		
OVARIAN CANCER	☐		
UTERINE CANCER	☐		
MENTAL ILLNESS/DEPRESSION	☐		
ALZHEIMER'S DISEASE	☐		
OTHER	☐		

American College of Obstetricians and Gynecologists ■ 409 12th Street, SW ■ PO Box 96920 ■ Washington, DC ■ 20090-6920

PATIENT INTAKE HISTORY *(Continued)*

PATIENT NAME:	BIRTH DATE: / /	ID NO.:	DATE: / /

SOCIAL HISTORY

	YES	NO	PHYSICIAN'S NOTES
EVER SMOKED? CURRENT SMOKING: PACKS PER DAY: YEARS:	☐	☐	
ALCOHOL: DRINKS PER DAY: DRINKS PER WEEK:	☐	☐	
RECREATIONAL DRUG USE	☐	☐	
SEAT BELT USE	☐	☐	
REGULAR EXERCISE: HOW LONG AND HOW OFTEN?	☐	☐	
DAIRY PRODUCT INTAKE/CALCIUM SUPPLEMENTS: QUANTITY	☐	☐	
HEALTH HAZARDS AT HOME OR WORK?	☐	☐	
HAVE YOU BEEN SEXUALLY ABUSED, THREATENED, OR HURT BY ANYONE?	☐	☐	

PERSONAL PROFILE

SEXUAL ORIENTATION: ☐ HETEROSEXUAL ☐ HOMOSEXUAL ☐ BISEXUAL

MARITAL STATUS: ☐ MARRIED ☐ LIVING WITH PARTNER ☐ SINGLE ☐ WIDOWED ☐ DIVORCED

NUMBER OF LIVING CHILDREN:

NUMBER OF PEOPLE IN HOUSEHOLD:

SCHOOL COMPLETED: ☐ HIGH SCHOOL ☐ SOME COLLEGE/AA DEGREE ☐ COLLEGE ☐ GRADUATE DEGREE ☐ OTHER

CURRENT OR MOST RECENT JOB:

TRAVEL OUTSIDE THE U.S.? LOCATION:

PERSONAL PAST HISTORY OF ILLNESSES

MAJOR ILLNESSES	YES (DATE)	NO	NOT SURE	PHYSICIAN'S NOTES
ASTHMA				
PNEUMONIA/LUNG DISEASE				
KIDNEY INFECTIONS/STONES				
TUBERCULOSIS				
SEXUALLY TRANSMITTED DISEASE				
HIV/AIDS				
HEART ATTACK/PROBLEMS				
DIABETES				
HIGH BLOOD PRESSURE				
STROKE				
RHEUMATIC FEVER				
BLOOD CLOTS IN LUNGS OR LEGS				
EATING DISORDERS				
COLLAGEN VASCULAR DISEASE (LUPUS)				
CHICKENPOX				
CANCER				
REFLUX/HIATAL HERNIA/ULCERS				
DEPRESSION/ANXIETY				
ANEMIA				
BLOOD TRANSFUSIONS				
SEIZURES/CONVULSIONS/EPILEPSY				
BOWEL PROBLEMS				
GLAUCOMA				
CATARACTS				
ARTHRITIS/JOINT PAIN/BACK PROBLEMS				
BROKEN BONES				
HEPATITIS/YELLOW JAUNDICE/LIVER DISEASE				
THYROID DISEASE				

American College of Obstetricians and Gynecologists ■ 409 12th Street, SW ■ PO Box 96920 ■ Washington, DC ■ 20090-6920

PATIENT INTAKE HISTORY *(Continued)*

PATIENT NAME:	BIRTH DATE: / /	ID NO.:	DATE: / /

PERSONAL PAST HISTORY OF ILLNESSES *(Continued)*

MAJOR ILLNESSES	YES (DATE)	NO	NOT SURE	PHYSICIAN'S NOTES
GALLBLADDER DISEASE				
HEADACHES				
OTHER				

OPERATIONS/HOSPITALIZATIONS

REASON	DATE	HOSPITAL

INJURIES/ILLNESSES

TYPE	DATE	TYPE	DATE

IMMUNIZATIONS/TEST

	DATE		DATE
TETANUS–DIPHTHERIA BOOSTER		INFLUENZA VACCINE (FLU SHOT)	
HEPATITIS A VACCINE		HEPATITIS B VACCINE	
VARICELLA VACCINE		PNEUMOCOCCAL VACCINE	
MEASLES–MUMPS–RUBELLA (MMR) VACCINE		TUBERCULOSIS (TB) SKIN TEST: RESULT:	

PHYSICIAN'S NOTES:

REVIEW OF SYSTEMS

Please check (x) if any of the following symptoms apply to you now or since adulthood

	NOW	PAST	NOT SURE	PHYSICIAN'S NOTES
1. CONSTITUTIONAL				
WEIGHT LOSS	☐	☐	☐	
WEIGHT GAIN	☐	☐	☐	
FEVER	☐	☐	☐	
FATIGUE	☐	☐	☐	
CHANGE IN HEIGHT	☐	☐	☐	

American College of Obstetricians and Gynecologists ■ 409 12th Street, SW ■ PO Box 96920 ■ Washington, DC ■ 20090-6920

PATIENT INTAKE HISTORY *(Continued)*

PATIENT NAME:	BIRTH DATE: / /	ID NO.:	DATE: / /

REVIEW OF SYSTEMS *(Continued)*

	NOW	PAST	NOT SURE	PHYSICIAN'S NOTES
2. EYES				
DOUBLE VISION	☐	☐	☐	
SPOTS BEFORE EYES	☐	☐	☐	
VISION CHANGES	☐	☐	☐	
GLASSES/CONTACTS	☐	☐	☐	
3. EAR, NOSE, AND THROAT				
EARACHES	☐	☐	☐	
RINGING IN EARS	☐	☐	☐	
HEARING PROBLEMS	☐	☐	☐	
SINUS PROBLEMS	☐	☐	☐	
SORE THROAT	☐	☐	☐	
MOUTH SORES	☐	☐	☐	
DENTAL PROBLEMS	☐	☐	☐	
4. CARDIOVASCULAR				
PAINFUL BREATHING	☐	☐	☐	
CHEST PAIN OR PRESSURE	☐	☐	☐	
DIFFICULTY BREATHING ON EXERTION	☐	☐	☐	
SWELLING OF LEGS	☐	☐	☐	
RAPID OR IRREGULAR HEARTBEAT	☐	☐	☐	
5. RESPIRATORY				
WHEEZING	☐	☐	☐	
SPITTING UP BLOOD	☐	☐	☐	
SHORTNESS OF BREATH	☐	☐	☐	
CHRONIC COUGH	☐	☐	☐	
6. GASTROINTESTINAL				
FREQUENT DIARRHEA	☐	☐	☐	
BLOODY STOOL	☐	☐	☐	
NAUSEA/VOMITING/INDIGESTION	☐	☐	☐	
CONSTIPATION	☐	☐	☐	
INVOLUNTARY LOSS OF GAS OR STOOL	☐	☐	☐	
7. GENITOURINARY				
BLOOD IN URINE	☐	☐	☐	
PAIN WITH URINATION	☐	☐	☐	
STRONG URGENCY TO URINATE	☐	☐	☐	
FREQUENT URINATION	☐	☐	☐	
INCOMPLETE EMPTYING	☐	☐	☐	
INVOLUNTARY/UNINTENDED URINE LOSS	☐	☐	☐	
URINE LOSS WHEN COUGHING OR LIFTING	☐	☐	☐	
ABNORMAL BLEEDING	☐	☐	☐	
PAINFUL PERIODS	☐	☐	☐	
PREMENSTRUAL SYNDROME (PMS)	☐	☐	☐	
PAINFUL INTERCOURSE	☐	☐	☐	
FIBROIDS	☐	☐	☐	
INFERTILITY	☐	☐	☐	
DES EXPOSURE	☐	☐	☐	
ABNORMAL VAGINAL DISCHARGE	☐	☐	☐	
8. MUSCULOSKELETAL				
MUSCLE WEAKNESS	☐	☐	☐	

American College of Obstetricians and Gynecologists ■ 409 12th Street, SW ■ PO Box 96920 ■ Washington, DC ■ 20090-6920

PATIENT INTAKE HISTORY *(Continued)*

PATIENT NAME:	BIRTH DATE: / /	ID NO.:	DATE: / /

REVIEW OF SYSTEMS *(Continued)*

	NOW	PAST	NOT SURE	PHYSICIAN'S NOTES
8. MUSCULOSKELETAL *(Continued)*				
MUSCLE OR JOINT PAIN	☐	☐	☐	
9a. SKIN				
RASH	☐	☐	☐	
SORES	☐	☐	☐	
DRY SKIN	☐	☐	☐	
MOLES	☐	☐	☐	
9b. BREASTS				
PAIN IN BREAST	☐	☐	☐	
NIPPLE DISCHARGE	☐	☐	☐	
LUMPS	☐	☐	☐	
10. NEUROLOGIC				
DIZZINESS	☐	☐	☐	
SEIZURES	☐	☐	☐	
NUMBNESS	☐	☐	☐	
TROUBLE WALKING	☐	☐	☐	
SEVERE MEMORY PROBLEMS	☐	☐	☐	
FREQUENT OR SEVERE HEADACHES	☐	☐	☐	
11. PSYCHIATRIC				
DEPRESSION OR FREQUENT CRYING	☐	☐	☐	
SEVERE ANXIETY	☐	☐	☐	
12. ENDOCRINE				
HAIR LOSS	☐	☐	☐	
HEAT/COLD INTOLERANCE	☐	☐	☐	
ABNORMAL THIRST	☐	☐	☐	
HOT FLASHES	☐	☐	☐	
13. HEMATOLOGIC/LYMPHATIC				
FREQUENT BRUISES	☐	☐	☐	
CUTS DO NOT STOP BLEEDING	☐	☐	☐	
ENLARGED LYMPH NODES (GLANDS)	☐	☐	☐	
14. ALLERGIC/IMMUNOLOGIC				
MEDICATION ALLERGIES	☐	☐	☐	
IF ANY, PLEASE LIST ALLERGY AND TYPE OF REACTION:				
OTHER ALLERGIES	☐	☐	☐	
PLEASE LIST ALLERGY AND TYPE OF REACTION:				

FORM COMPLETED BY: ☐ PATIENT ☐ OFFICE NURSE ☐ PHYSICIAN ☐ OTHER:

SIGNATURE OF PATIENT:

DATE REVIEWED BY PHYSICIAN WITH PATIENT: / /	PHYSICIAN SIGNATURE:
ANNUAL REVIEW OF HISTORY	
DATE REVIEWED: / /	PHYSICIAN SIGNATURE:
DATE REVIEWED: / /	PHYSICIAN SIGNATURE:
DATE REVIEWED: / /	PHYSICIAN SIGNATURE:
DATE REVIEWED: / /	PHYSICIAN SIGNATURE:

American College of Obstetricians and Gynecologists ▪ 409 12th Street, SW ▪ PO Box 96920 ▪ Washington, DC ▪ 20090-6920

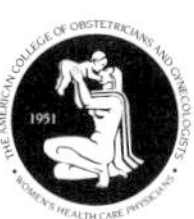

ACOG WOMAN'S HEALTH RECORD

CODING TIPS*

HISTORY

CHIEF COMPLAINT (CC)

REQUIRED FOR ALL VISITS

HISTORY OF PRESENT ILLNESS (HPI)

BRIEF = 1–3 ELEMENTS EXTENDED = 4+ ELEMENTS OR STATUS OF 3+ CHRONIC/INACTIVE CONDITIONS

FACTORS TO BE CONSIDERED INCLUDE:

LOCATION, QUALITY, SEVERITY, DURATION, TIMING, CONTEXT, MODIFYING FACTORS, ASSOCIATED SIGNS AND SYMPTOMS

PAST, FAMILY, AND SOCIAL HISTORY (PFSH)

PERTINENT PFSH = 1 SPECIFIC ITEM FROM EITHER PAST, FAMILY, OR SOCIAL HISTORY

COMPLETE PFSH = NEW PATIENT: 1 SPECIFIC ITEM FROM EACH HISTORY TYPE (PAST, FAMILY, OR SOCIAL HISTORY)
ESTABLISHED PATIENT: 1 SPECIFIC ITEM FROM 2 OF THE 3 HISTORY TYPES (PAST, FAMILY, OR SOCIAL HISTORY)

REVIEW OF SYSTEMS (ROS)

PROBLEM PERTINENT ROS = POSITIVE AND PERTINENT NEGATIVE RESPONSES RELATED TO PROBLEM

EXTENDED ROS = POSITIVE AND PERTINENT NEGATIVE RESPONSES FOR 2–9 SYSTEMS

COMPLETE ROS = POSITIVE AND PERTINENT NEGATIVE RESPONSES FOR AT LEAST 10 SYSTEMS

LEVEL OF HISTORY

(All three elements must be met for a given level of history, eg, brief HPI, problem pertinent ROS, and pertinent PFSH is an Expanded Problem Focused history)

CC	HPI	ROS	PFSH	LEVEL OF HISTORY
REQUIRED	BRIEF (1–3 ELEMENTS)	N/A	N/A	PROBLEM FOCUSED
REQUIRED	BRIEF (1–3 ELEMENTS)	PROBLEM PERTINENT	N/A	EXPANDED PROBLEM FOCUSED
REQUIRED	EXTENDED (4+ ELEMENTS OR STATUS OF 3+ CHRONIC/INACTIVE CONDITIONS)	EXTENDED (2–9 SYSTEMS)	PERTINENT (1 OF 3)	DETAILED
REQUIRED	EXTENDED (4+ ELEMENTS OR STATUS OF 3+ CHRONIC/INACTIVE CONDITIONS)	COMPLETE (10+ SYSTEMS)	COMPLETE (NEW PATIENT: 3 OF 3; ESTABLISHED PATIENT: 2 OF 3)	COMPREHENSIVE

PHYSICAL EXAMINATION

1997 HCFA Guidelines, Female Genitourinary System Examination

The female genitourinary examination template includes 9 organ systems/body areas with 3 shaded boxes and 6 unshaded boxes. The shading only becomes important when a comprehensive examination is performed. For all other levels of examination, the total number of bulleted elements documented in the medical record will determine the level that can be reported.

LEVEL OF EXAMINATION	PERFORM AND DOCUMENT
PROBLEM FOCUSED	1–5 ELEMENTS IDENTIFIED BY A BULLET
EXPANDED PROBLEM FOCUSED	6–11 ELEMENTS IDENTIFIED BY A BULLET
DETAILED	12 OR MORE ELEMENTS IDENTIFIED BY A BULLET
COMPREHENSIVE	PERFORM ALL ELEMENTS IDENTIFIED BY A BULLET DOCUMENT EVERY REQUIRED ELEMENT IN EACH SHADED SECTION AND AT LEAST ONE ELEMENT IN EACH UNSHADED BOX (UNLESS NOTED OTHERWISE)

MEDICAL DECISION MAKING

AMOUNT AND COMPLEXITY OF DATA REVIEWED

MINIMAL/NONE = 1 BOX LIMITED = 2 BOXES MODERATE = 3 BOXES EXTENSIVE = 4+ BOXES

THE FOLLOWING ITEMS (IF CHECKED) COUNT AS TWO BOXES:

- OLD RECORDS REVIEWED AND SUMMARIZED
- HISTORY OBTAINED FROM OTHER SOURCE
- INDEPENDENT REVIEW OF IMAGE/SPECIMEN

CODING TIPS* *(Continued)*

MEDICAL DECISION MAKING *(Continued)*

DIAGNOSES/MANAGEMENT OPTIONS

MINIMAL = MINOR PROBLEM; ESTABLISHED PROBLEM STABLE/IMPROVED

LIMITED = ESTABLISHED PROBLEM, WORSENING

MULTIPLE = NEW PROBLEM, NO ADDITIONAL WORKUP PLANNED

EXTENSIVE = NEW PROBLEM, ADDITIONAL WORKUP PLANNED

RISK OF COMPLICATIONS AND/OR MORBIDITY/MORTALITY FROM DIAGNOSES, DIAGNOSTIC PROCEDURES, AND MANAGEMENT CHOICES:

MINIMAL (EG, COLD, ACHES AND PAINS, OVER-THE-COUNTER MEDICATIONS)

LOW (EG, CYSTITIS, VAGINITIS, PRESCRIPTION RENEWAL, MINOR SURGERY WITHOUT RISK FACTORS)

MODERATE (EG, BREAST MASS, IRREGULAR BLEEDING, HEADACHES, BIOPSY, MINOR SURGERY WITH RISK FACTORS, MAJOR SURGERY WITHOUT RISK FACTORS, NEW PRESCRIPTION)

HIGH (EG, PELVIC PAIN, RECTAL BLEEDING, MULTIPLE COMPLAINTS, MAJOR SURGERY WITH RISK FACTORS, CHEMOTHERAPY, EMERGENCY SURGERY)

2 of the 3 elements must be met or exceeded to qualify for a given type of medical decision making

AMOUNT/COMPLEXITY OF DATA	DIAGNOSES/MANAGEMENT OPTIONS	RISK OF COMPLICATIONS	TYPE OF DECISION MAKING
MINIMAL/NONE	MINIMAL	MINIMAL	STRAIGHTFORWARD
LIMITED	LIMITED	LOW	LOW COMPLEXITY
MODERATE	MULTIPLE	MODERATE	MODERATE COMPLEXITY
EXTENSIVE	EXTENSIVE	HIGH	HIGH COMPLEXITY

CODING SUMMARY

Office or Other Outpatient Services, New Patient

KEY COMPONENTS	99201	99202	99203	99204	99205
HISTORY	PROBLEM FOCUSED	EXPANDED PROBLEM FOCUSED	DETAILED	COMPREHENSIVE	COMPREHENSIVE
EXAMINATION	PROBLEM FOCUSED	EXPANDED PROBLEM FOCUSED	DETAILED	COMPREHENSIVE	COMPREHENSIVE
MEDICAL DECISION MAKING	STRAIGHTFORWARD	STRAIGHTFORWARD	LOW COMPLEXITY	MODERATE COMPLEXITY	HIGH COMPLEXITY
NO. OF KEY COMPONENTS REQUIRED	ALL THREE	ALL THREE	ALL THREE	ALL THREE	ALL THREE
TYPICAL FACE-TO-FACE TIME (MIN)	10	20	30	45	60

Office or Other Outpatient Services, Established Patient

KEY COMPONENTS	99211	99212	99213	99214	99215
HISTORY	N/A	PROBLEM FOCUSED	EXPANDED PROBLEM FOCUSED	DETAILED	COMPREHENSIVE
EXAMINATION	N/A	PROBLEM FOCUSED	EXPANDED PROBLEM FOCUSED	DETAILED	COMPREHENSIVE
MEDICAL DECISION MAKING	N/A	STRAIGHTFORWARD	LOW COMPLEXITY	MODERATE COMPLEXITY	HIGH COMPLEXITY
NO. OF KEY COMPONENTS REQUIRED	N/A	2 OF 3	2 OF 3	2 OF 3	2 OF 3
TYPICAL FACE-TO-FACE TIME (MIN)	5	10	15	25	40

Office or Other Outpatient Consultations, New or Established Patient

KEY COMPONENTS	99241	99242	99243	99244	99245
HISTORY	PROBLEM FOCUSED	EXPANDED PROBLEM FOCUSED	DETAILED	COMPREHENSIVE	COMPREHENSIVE
EXAMINATION	PROBLEM FOCUSED	EXPANDED PROBLEM FOCUSED	DETAILED	COMPREHENSIVE	COMPREHENSIVE
MEDICAL DECISION MAKING	STRAIGHTFORWARD	STRAIGHTFORWARD	LOW COMPLEXITY	MODERATE COMPLEXITY	HIGH COMPLEXITY
NO. OF KEY COMPONENTS REQUIRED	ALL THREE	ALL THREE	ALL THREE	ALL THREE	ALL THREE
TYPICAL FACE-TO-FACE TIME (MIN)	15	30	40	60	80

American College of Obstetricians and Gynecologists ■ 409 12th Street, SW ■ PO Box 96920 ■ Washington, DC ■ 20090-6920

PROBLEM LIST

PATIENT NAME:	BIRTH DATE: / /	ID NO.:

HIGH RISK:	FAMILY HISTORY:
DRUG/LATEX/TRANSFUSION REACTIONS:	**CURRENT MEDICATIONS:**

NO.	ENTRY DATE	PROBLEM/RESOLUTION	ONSET AGE AND DATE	RESOLUTION DATE
1				
2				
3				
4				
5				
6				
7				
8				
9				
10				
11				
12				
13				
14				
15				
16				
17				
18				
19				
20				
21				
22				
23				
24				
25				

American College of Obstetricians and Gynecologists ■ 409 12th Street, SW ■ PO Box 96920 ■ Washington, DC ■ 20090-6920

IMMUNIZATION RECORD*

PATIENT NAME: | BIRTH DATE: / / | ID NO.:

AGE	TETANUS–DIPHTHERIA BOOSTER	INFLUENZA VACCINE	PNEUMOCOCCAL VACCINE	MMR VACCINE	HEPATITIS B VACCINE	FLUORIDE SUPPLEMENTATION	HEPATITIS A VACCINE	VARICELLA VACCINE
13–18	ONCE BETWEEN AGES 11–16	BASED ON RISK	BASED ON RISK	BASED ON RISK	ONE SERIES FOR THOSE NOT PREVIOUSLY IMMUNIZED	BASED ON RISK	BASED ON RISK	BASED ON RISK
19–39	EVERY 10 YEARS	BASED ON RISK	BASED ON RISK	BASED ON RISK	BASED ON RISK		BASED ON RISK	BASED ON RISK
40–64	EVERY 10 YEARS	BASED ON RISK	BASED ON RISK	BASED ON RISK	BASED ON RISK		BASED ON RISK	BASED ON RISK
65 AND OLDER	EVERY 10 YEARS	ANNUALLY	ONCE		BASED ON RISK		BASED ON RISK	BASED ON RISK

DATE								
DATE								
DATE								
DATE								
DATE								
DATE								
DATE								
DATE								
DATE								
DATE								
DATE								
DATE								
DATE								
DATE								
DATE								
DATE								
DATE								
DATE								
DATE								

*For immunizations based on risk refer to the Table of High-Risk Factors.

ROUTINE LABORATORY RECORD

PATIENT NAME: BIRTH DATE: / / ID NO.:

AGE	PAP TEST	CHOLESTEROL TEST*	MAMMOGRAPHY*	FECAL OCCULT BLOOD TEST	SIGMOIDOSCOPY	URINALYSIS	FASTING GLUCOSE TEST*
13–18	YEARLY WHEN SEXUALLY ACTIVE OR BY AGE 18						
19–39	PHYSICIAN AND PATIENT DISCRETION AFTER 3 CONSECUTIVE NORMAL TESTS IF LOW RISK						
40–64	PHYSICIAN AND PATIENT DISCRETION AFTER 3 CONSECUTIVE NORMAL TESTS IF LOW RISK	EVERY 5 YEARS BEGINNING AT AGE 45	EVERY 1–2 YEARS UNTIL AGE 50; YEARLY BEGINNING AT AGE 50	YEARLY OR AS APPROPRIATE BEGINNING AT AGE 50	EVERY 3–5 YEARS AFTER AGE 50		EVERY 3 YEARS AFTER AGE 45
65 AND OLDER	PHYSICIAN AND PATIENT DISCRETION AFTER 3 CONSECUTIVE NORMAL TESTS IF LOW RISK	EVERY 3–5 YEARS BEFORE AGE 75	YEARLY OR AS APPROPRIATE	YEARLY OR AS APPROPRIATE	EVERY 3–5 YEARS	YEARLY OR AS APPROPRIATE	EVERY 3 YEARS

DATE: RESULT:							
DATE: RESULT:							
DATE: RESULT:							
DATE: RESULT:							
DATE: RESULT:							
DATE: RESULT:							
DATE: RESULT:							
DATE: RESULT:							
DATE: RESULT:							

* This test may be appropriate for other patients based on risk (see High-Risk Laboratory Record and Table of High-Risk Factors)

HIGH-RISK LABORATORY RECORD*

PATIENT NAME: BIRTH DATE: / / ID NO.:

	HEMOGLOBIN TEST	CHOLESTEROL TEST	BACTERIURIA TEST	STD TESTING	HIV TEST**	GENETIC TESTING	RUBELLA TITER	TB SKIN TEST	LIPID PROFILE	MAMMOGRAPHY	FASTING GLUCOSE TEST	TSH TEST	COLONOSCOPY	HEPATITIS C VIRUS TEST
DATE: RESULT:														
DATE: RESULT:														
DATE: RESULT:														
DATE: RESULT:														
DATE: RESULT:														
DATE: RESULT														
DATE: RESULT														
DATE: RESULT:														
DATE: RESULT:														
DATE: RESULT														
DATE: RESULT														
DATE: RESULT:														

* See Table of High-Risk Factors.

** Check state requirements before recording results.

HIGH-RISK FACTORS

INTERVENTION	HIGH-RISK FACTOR
BACTERIURIA TESTING	Diabetes mellitus
CHOLESTEROL TESTING	Familial lipid disorders; family history of premature coronary heart disease; history of coronary heart disease
COLONOSCOPY	History of inflammatory bowel disease or colonic polyps; family history of familial polyposis, colorectal cancer, or cancer family syndrome
FASTING GLUCOSE TESTING	Every 3 years for patients who have a first-degree relative with diabetes mellitus; history of gestational diabetes mellitus; are obese or hypertensive; members of high-risk ethnic groups (African American, Hispanic, Native American)
FLUORIDE SUPPLEMENTATION	Live in area with inadequate water fluoridation (<0.7 ppm)
GENETIC TESTING/COUNSELING	Exposure to teratogens; considering pregnancy at age 35 or older; patient, partner, or family member with history of genetic disorder or birth defect; African, Acadian, Eastern European Jewish, Mediterranean, or Southeast Asian ancestry
HEMOGLOBIN LEVEL ASSESSMENT	Caribbean, Latin American, Asian, Mediterranean, or African ancestry; history of excessive menstrual flow
HEPATITIS A VACCINATION	International travelers; illegal drug users; people who work with nonhuman primates; chronic liver disease; clotting-factor disorders; sex partners of bisexual men; measles, mumps, and rubella nonimmune persons; food-service workers; health-care workers; day-care workers
HEPATITIS B VACCINATION	Intravenous drug users and their sexual contacts; recipients of clotting factor concentrates; occupational exposure to blood or blood products; patients and workers in dialysis units; persons with chronic renal or hepatic disease; household or sexual contact with hepatitis B virus carriers; history of sexual activity with multiple partners; history of sexual activity with sexually active homosexual or bisexual men; international travelers; residents and staff of institutions for the developmentally disabled and of correctional institutions
HEPATITIS C VIRUS (HCV) TESTING	History of injecting illegal drugs; recipients of clotting factor concentrates before 1987; chronic (long-term) hemodialysis; persistently abnormal alanine aminotransferase levels; recipient of blood from a donor who later tested positive for HCV infection; recipient of blood or blood-component transfusion or organ transplant before July 1992; occupational percutaneous or mucosal exposure to HCV-positive blood
HUMAN IMMUNODEFICIENCY VIRUS (HIV) TESTING	Seeking treatment for sexually transmitted diseases; drug use by injection; history of prostitution; past or present sexual partner who is HIV positive or bisexual or injects drugs; long-term residence or birth in an area with high prevalence of HIV infection; history of transfusion from 1978 to1985; invasive cervical cancer; pregnancy. Offer to women seeking preconceptional care.
INFLUENZA VACCINATION	Anyone who wishes to reduce the chance of becoming ill with influenza; resident in long-term care facility; chronic cardio-pulmonary disorders; metabolic diseases (eg, diabetes mellitus, hemoglobinopathies, immunosuppression, renal dysfunction); health-care workers; day-care workers; pregnant women who will be in the second or third trimester during the epidemic season. Pregnant women with medical problems should be offered vaccination before the influenza season regardless of stage of pregnancy.
LIPID PROFILE ASSESSMENT	Elevated cholesterol level; history of parent or sibling with blood cholesterol of ≥240 mg/dL; history of sibling, parent, or grandparent with documented premature (<55 years) coronary artery disease; diabetes mellitus; smoking habit
MAMMOGRAPHY	Women who have had breast cancer or who have a first-degree relative (ie, mother, sister, or daughter) or multiple other relatives who have a history of premenopausal breast or breast and ovarian cancer
MEASLES–MUMPS–RUBELLA (MMR) VACCINATION	Adults born in 1957 or later should be offered vaccination (one dose of MMR vaccine) if there is no proof of immunity or documentation of a dose given after first birthday; persons vaccinated from 1963 to 1967 should be offered revaccination (2 doses); health-care workers, students entering college, international travelers, and rubella-negative postpartum patients should be offered a second dose.
PNEUMOCOCCAL VACCINATION	Chronic illness such as cardiovascular disease, pulmonary disease, diabetes mellitus, alcoholism, chronic liver disease, cerebrospinal fluid leaks, functional or anatomic asplenia; exposure to an environment where pneumococcal outbreaks have occurred; immunocompromised patients (from HIV infection, hematologic or solid malignancies, chemotherapy, steroid therapy); pregnant patients with chronic illness. Revaccination after 5 years may be appropriate for certain high-risk groups.
RUBELLA TITER ASSESSMENT	Childbearing age and no evidence of immunity
SEXUALLY TRANSMITTED DISEASE (STD) TESTING	History of multiple sexual partners or a sexual partner with multiple contacts, sexual contact with persons with culture-proven STD, history of repeated episodes of STD, attendance at clinics for STDs; routine screening for chlamydial and gonorrheal infection for all sexually active adolescents and other asymptomatic women at high risk for infection
SKIN EXAMINATION	Increased recreational or occupational exposure to sunlight; family or personal history of skin cancer; clinical evidence of precursor lesions
THYROID-STIMULATING HORMONE (TSH) TESTING	Strong family history of thyroid disease; autoimmune disease (evidence of subclinical hypothyroidism may be related to unfavorable lipid profiles)
TUBERCULOSIS SKIN TESTING	Human immunodeficiency virus (HIV) infection; close contact with persons known or suspected to have tuberculosis; medical risk factors known to increase risk of disease if infected; born in country with high tuberculosis prevalence; medically under served; low income; alcoholism; intravenous drug use; resident of long-term care facility (eg, correctional institutions, mental institutions, nursing homes and facilities); health professional working in high-risk health care facilities
VARICELLA VACCINATION	All susceptible adults and adolescents, including health-care workers; household contacts of immunocompromised individuals; teachers; day-care workers; residents and staff of institutional settings, colleges, prisons, or military installations; international travelers; nonpregnant women of childbearing age

American College of Obstetricians and Gynecologists ■ 409 12th Street, SW ■ PO Box 96920 ■ Washington, DC ■ 20090-6920

APPENDIX H

Guide to Preventive Cardiology for Women*

Coronary heart disease (CHD) is the single leading cause of death and a significant cause of morbidity among American women (1). Risk factors for CHD in women are well documented (2). Compelling data from epidemiological studies and randomized clinical trials show that CHD is largely preventable. Assessment and management of several risk factors for CHD are cost-effective (3). Despite these facts, there are alarming trends in the prevalence and management of risk factors in women (2). Smoking rates are declining less for women than for men. The prevalence of obesity is increasing, and approximately 25% of women report no regular sustained physical activity (4). Approximately 52% of women >45 years old have elevated blood pressure, and approximately 40% of women >55 years old have elevated serum cholesterol (5). The purpose of this statement is to highlight risk factor management strategies that are appropriate for women with a broad range of CHD risk. A more detailed description, including the scientific basis for these recommendations, is available in the 1997 American Heart Association scientific statement "Cardiovascular Disease in Women" (2).

Recently, the Centers for Disease Control and Prevention National Ambulatory Medical Care Survey (6) showed clinicians are missing opportunities to prevent CHD. In this study of 29,273 routine office visits, women were counseled less often than men about exercise, nutrition,

*Endorsed by American Medical Women's Association, American College of Nurse Practitioners, American College of Obstetricians and Gynecologists, and Canadian Cardiovascular Society.

"A Guide to Preventive Cardiology for Women" was approved by the American College of Cardiology Board of Trustees on February 22, 1999, and by the American Heart Association Science Advisory and Coordinating Committee on September 7, 1998.

Source: Mosca L, Grundy SM, Judelson D, King K, Limacher M, Oparil S, et al. Guide to preventive cardiology for women. AHA/ACC Scientific Statement Consensus panel statement. Circulation 1999;99:2480–2484

and weight reduction. In the multicenter Heart and Estrogen/progestin Replacement Study (HERS) (7), only 10% of women enrolled with documented CHD had baseline LDL-cholesterol levels below a National Cholesterol Education Program (NCEP) target of 100 mg/dL. A recent national survey showed that women were significantly less likely than men to enroll in cardiac rehabilitation after an acute myocardial infarction (MI) or bypass surgery (8). This finding is especially important because post-MI patients not enrolled in cardiac rehabilitation are less likely to receive aggressive risk factor management.

Recommendations for the primary and secondary prevention of CHD have been published (9, 10). Although those recommendations apply to women, there are aspects of risk factor management that are unique to women. Pregnancy and the preconception period are optimal times to review a woman's risk factor status and health behaviors to reduce future cardiovascular disease. Pregnant women should be strongly encouraged to discontinue smoking and not to relapse in the postpartum period. Avoidance of excess weight gain during pregnancy may reduce the risk of developing CHD in the future. An emphasis on prevention of CHD in postmenopausal women is particularly important because the incidence of CHD rises with age. The use of estrogen replacement therapy (ERT) to prevent CHD, osteoporosis, and possibly dementia is a difficult health decision for postmenopausal women. The potential benefits of therapy must be weighed against the possible risks, including breast cancer, gallbladder disease, thromboembolic disease, and endometrial cancer, although the last is reduced by concomitant use of a progestin.

The recent findings from HERS (11) have challenged previous observational data regarding the role of hormones in preventing subsequent cardiovascular events. HERS was the first large-scale, randomized, clinical trial in older postmenopausal women with confirmed coronary disease to test the efficacy and safety of hormone replacement therapy on clinical cardiovascular outcome in postmenopausal women. The study population included 2763 women (mean age 66.7 years) with established CHD randomly assigned to 0.625 mg conjugated equine estrogens (CEE) plus 2.5 mg of medroxyprogesterone acetate (MPA) per day or placebo. Participants were monitored for an average of 4.1 years for the main end point of nonfatal MI or CHD death. At study completion, no significant differences existed between groups for any cardiovascular end points.

Surprisingly, after 1 year, HERS showed an increase in cardiovascular events in the treatment arm, but in years 4 and 5, fewer events occurred than in the placebo arm. It has been hypothesized that possible early adverse effects of estrogen in women with CHD may be due to a procoagulant effect that may later be offset by an antiatherogenic benefit. MPA may also have adverse cardiovascular effects and may mitigate some of the beneficial effects of estrogen (2). Although these hypotheses deserve further investigation, the overall null result from HERS does not support initiation of CEE combined with MPA in older postmenopausal women with confirmed coronary disease. For women with CHD already on ERT for ≥1 year, it may be reasonable to continue therapy while awaiting the results of a HERS follow-up study and other ongoing trials of ERT with clinical end points. The results of the HERS trial apply to women with preexisting CHD and may not apply to women free of vascular disease. Furthermore, this study does not take into consideration the other potential benefits of this therapeutic protocol, which are beyond the scope of this statement.

Data are lacking for determining the long-term cardiovascular effects of testosterone administered with ERT. Alternatives to traditional hormone replacement therapy are available, including soy phytoestrogens and selective estrogen receptor modulators (SERMs); however, a recommendation regarding their use for prevention of CHD has not been made at this time because of a lack of sufficient data.

Several other aspects of risk factor management are of heightened importance for women. Diabetes is a powerful risk factor in women, increasing CHD risk 3-fold to 7-fold compared with a 2-fold to 3-fold increase in risk in men (12). This difference may be due to a particularly deleterious effect of diabetes on lipids and blood pressure in women (2, 12). Therefore, recommendations are provided for management of diabetes with an emphasis on controlling concomitant risk factors (13). Low levels of HDL cholesterol are predictive of CHD in women and appear to be a stronger risk factor for women >65 years old than for men >65 (14). Women tend to have higher HDL-cholesterol levels than men, and triglyceride levels may be a significant risk factor in women, especially older women. The current NCEP guidelines are outlined in Table H–1 with a

Table H–1. Guide to Risk Reduction for Women

Lifestyle Factors	Goal(s)	Screening	Recommendations
Cigarette smoking	1. Complete cessation. 2. Avoid passive cigarette smoke.	1. Ask about current smoking status and exposure to others' cigarette smoke as part of routine evaluation. 2. Assess total exposure to cigarette smoke (pack-years) and prior attempts at quitting. 3. Evaluate readiness to stop smoking.	1. At each visit, strongly encourage patient and family to stop smoking. If complete cessation is not achievable, a reduction in intake is beneficial as a step toward cessation. 2. Reinforce nonsmoking status. 3. Provide counseling, nicotine replacement, and other pharmacotherapy as indicated in conjunction with behavioral therapy or a formal cessation program.
Physical activity	1. Accumulate ≥30 min of moderate-intensity physical activity on most, or preferably all, days of the week. 2. Women who have had recent cardiovascular events or procedures should	1. Ask about physical activity (household work as well as occupational and leisure-time physical activity) as part of routine evaluation. 2. In women with symptoms that suggest CVD or in previously	1. Encourage a minimum of 30 min of moderate-intensity dynamic exercise (eg, brisk walking) daily. This may be performed in intermittent or shorter bouts (≥10 min) of activity throughout the day. 2. Women who already meet mini-

Physical activity *(continued)*	participate in cardiac rehabilitation, a physician-guided home exercise program, or a comprehensive secondary prevention program.	sedentary women >50 y old with ≥2 risk factors for CVD, consider a stress test* to establish safety of exercise and to guide the exercise prescription.	mum standards may be encouraged to become more physically active or to include more vigorous activities. 3. Incorporate physical activity in daily activities (eg, using stairs). 4. Muscle strengthening and stretching exercises should be recommended as part of an overall activity program. 5. Recommend medically supervised programs for women who have had a recent MI or revascularization procedure.
Nutrition	1. AHA Step I Diet in healthy women (≤30% fat, 8–10% saturated fat, and <300 mg/d cholesterol). 2. AHA Step II Diet in women with CVD or if a further reduction in cholesterol is needed (≤30% fat, <7%	1. Assess nutritional habits as part of a routine evaluation in all women. 2. Consider formal dietary assessment in women with hyperlipidemia, diabetes, obesity, and hypertension.	1. Encourage a well-balanced and diversified diet that is low in saturated fat and high in fiber. 2. Use skim milk instead of milk with a higher fat content. 3. Diets rich in antioxidant nutrients (eg, vitamin C, E, and beta-

(continued)

Table H–1. Guide to Risk Reduction for Women *(continued)*

Lifestyle Factors	Goal(s)	Screening	Recommendations
Nutrition *(continued)*	saturated fat, and <200 mg/d cholesterol). 3. Limit sodium chloride (salt) intake to 6 g/d. Women with high blood pressure may require further restriction. 4. Total dietary fiber intake of 25–30 g/d from foods. 5. Consume ≥5 servings of fruits and vegetables per day.		carotene) and folate are preferred over nutritional supplements. Note: Daily supplements of 0.4 mg of folic acid are recommended for women of child-bearing age to help prevent neural tube defects. 4. Limit alcohol intake to ≤1 glass of alcohol per day (1 glass=4 oz wine, 12 oz beer, or 1 1/2 oz 80-proof spirits). Pregnant women should abstain from drinking alcohol.
Weight management	1. Achieve and maintain desirable weight. 2. Target BMI (weight in kilograms divided by height in meters squared) between 18.5 and 24.9 kg/m^2 (BMI of 25 kg/m^2=110% of desirable body weight).	Measure patient's weight and height, calculate BMI, and measure waist circumference as part of a periodic evaluation. Note: BMI and waist circumference are used for diagnosis, and measurement of height and weight are used for follow-up.	1. Encourage gradual and sustained weight loss in persons whose weight exceeds the ideal weight for their height. 2. Formal nutritional counseling is encouraged for women with hypertension, hyperlipidemia, or elevated glucose levels associated with overweight.

Weight management *(continued)*	3. Desirable waist circumference <88 cm (<35 inches) in women with a BMI of 25–34.9 kg/m^2.		3. The recommended weight gain during pregnancy is 25–35 lb if the patient's prepregnancy weight is normal. Adjust for multiple gestation and prepregnancy weight (eg, overweight women should gain 15–25 lb, obese women, <15 lb).
Psychosocial factors	1. Positive adaptation to stressful situations. 2. Improved quality of life. 3. Maintain or establish social connections.	1. Assess presence of stressful situations and response to stress as part of a routine evaluation. 2. Evaluate for depression, especially in women with recent cardiovascular events. 3. Assess social support system and evaluate for social isolation.	1. Encourage positive coping mechanisms for stress (eg, substitute physical activity for overeating or excessive smoking in response to stress). 2. Encourage adequate rest and relief for women who are caretakers of others. 3. Consider treatment of depression and anxiety when appropriate. 4. Encourage participation in social activities or volunteer work for socially isolated women.

(continued)

Table H–1. Guide to Risk Reduction for Women *(continued)*

Risk Factors	Goals	Screening	Recommendations
Blood pressure	1. Achieve and maintain blood pressure <140/90 mm Hg and lower if tolerated (optimal <120/80). 2. In pregnant women with hypertension, the goal of treatment is to minimize short term risk of elevated blood pressure in the mother while avoiding therapy that may compromise the well-being of the fetus.	1. Measure blood pressure as part of a routine evaluation. 2. Follow-up is based on initial measurement as follows: SBP, mm Hg — DBP, mm Hg — Follow-up <130 — <85 — Recheck in 2 y 130–139 — 85–89 — Recheck in 1 y 140–159 — 90–99 — Confirm in 2 mo 160–179 — 100–109 — Evaluate in 1 mo ≥180 — ≥110 — Evaluate in 1 wk (Follow-up screening may be modified on the basis of prior history, symptoms, presence of other risk factors, and end organ damage.) 3. In pregnant women with hypertension, evaluate for preeclampsia.	1. Promote the lifestyle behaviors described above (weight control, physical activity, moderation in alcohol intake) and moderate sodium restriction. 2. If blood pressure remains ≥140/90 mm Hg after 3 months of lifestyle modification or if initial level is >160 mm Hg systolic or 100 mm Hg diastolic, then initiate and individualize pharmacotherapy based on the patient's characteristics. 3. In pregnant women with hypertension, reduction of diastolic blood pressure to 90–100 mm Hg is recommended.
Lipids, lipoproteins	Primary goal: Women without CVD <u>Lower risk</u> (<2 risk factors) LDL goal <160 mg/dL (optimal <130 mg/dL)	Women without CVD† Measure nonfasting total and HDL cholesterol and assess nonlipid risk factors. Follow-up is based on the following initial measurements:	1. Promote lifestyle approach in all women (diet, weight management, smoking avoidance, and exercise as described above). Rule out other secondary causes of dyslipidemia.

Lipids, lipoproteins *(continued)*			
	<u>Higher risk</u> (≥2 risk factors) LDL goal <130 mg/dL Women with CVD LDL ≤100 mg/dL Secondary goals: HDL >35 mg/dL Triglycerides <200 mg/dL Note: In women, the optimal level of triglycerides may be lower (≤150 mg/dL) and the HDL higher (≥45 mg/dL).	TC <200, HDL ≥45, follow-up in 5 years; TC <200, HDL <45, follow-up with fasting lipoprotein analysis. TC 200–239, HDL ≥45, and <2 risk factors, follow-up in 1–2 years. TC 200–239, HDL <45 or ≥2 risk factors, follow-up with fasting lipoprotein analysis. TC ≥240, follow-up with fasting lipoprotein analysis. (All cholesterol values in mg/dL.) Women with CVD Fasting lipoprotein analysis (may take 4–6 wk to stabilize after cardiovascular event or bypass surgery).	2. Suggested drug therapy for high LDL levels (defined as [a] ≥220 mg/dL in low-risk, premenopausal women, [b] ≥190 mg/dL in postmenopausal women with <2 risk factors, and [c] ≥160 mg/dL with ≥2 risk factors) is based on triglyceride level as follows: <u>TG <200 mg/dL</u> Statin, Resin, Niacin Note: ERT is an option for postmenopausal women, but treatment should be individualized and considered with other health risks. <u>TG 200–400 mg/dL</u> Statin, Niacin <u>TG >400 mg/dL</u> Consider monotherapy with statin, niacin, fibrate, or a combination of the above.
Diabetes	For patients with diabetes: 1. Maintain blood glucose: preprandial=80–120 mg/dL bedtime=100–140 mg/dL.	1. Monitor glucose and hemoglobin $A1_c$ as part of a routine periodic evaluation in women with diabetes.	1. Encourage adoption of American Diabetes Association Diet (<30% fat, <10% saturated fat, 6–8% polyunsatured fat, cholesterol <300 mg/d).

(continued)

Table H–1. Guide to Risk Reduction for Women *(continued)*

Risk Factors	Goals	Screening	Recommendations
Diabetes *(continued)*			
	2. Maintain Hb $A1_c$ <7%.	2. Screen for diabetes (fasting glucose >125 mg/dL or >200 mg/dL 2 h after 75 g glucose) as part of a periodic examination in women with risk factors for diabetes, such as obesity.	2. A low-calorie diet may be recommended for weight loss.
	3. LDL <130 mg/dL (<100 mg/dL if established CVD). Note: Many authorities believe that LDL should be <100 mg/dL in all patients with diabetes.		3. Encourage regular physical exercise.
			4. Pharmacotherapy with oral agents or insulin should be used when indicated.
	4. Triglycerides <150 mg/dL		
	5. Control blood pressure.		

Pharmacological Interventions	Goal(s)	Screening	Recommendations
Hormone replacement therapy	1. Initiation or continuation of therapy in women for whom the potential benefits may exceed the potential risks of therapy. (Short-term therapy is indicated for treatment of menopausal symptoms.)	1. Review menstrual status of women >40 y old. 2. If menopausal status is unclear, measure FSH level.	1. Counsel all women about the potential benefits and risks of HRT, beginning at age 40 or as requested. 2. Individualize decision based on prior history and risk factors for CVD as well as risks of thromboembolic disease, gallbladder

Hormone replacement therapy *(continued)*			
	2. Minimize risk of adverse side effects through careful patient selection and appropriate choice of therapy.		disease, osteoporosis, breast cancer, and other health risks. 3. Combination therapy with a progestin is usually indicated to prevent endometrial hyperplasia in a woman with an intact uterus and prescribed estrogen. The choice of agent should be made on an individual basis.
Oral contraceptives	1. Minimize risk of adverse cardiovascular effects while preventing pregnancy. 2. Use the lowest effective dose of estrogen/progestin.	Determine contraindications and cardiovascular risk factor status of women who are considering using oral contraceptives.	1. Use of oral contraceptives is relatively contraindicated in women ≥35 y old who smoke. 2. Women with a family history of premature heart disease should have lipid analysis before taking oral contraceptives. 3. Women with significant risk factors for diabetes should have glucose testing before taking oral contraceptives.

(continued)

Table H–1. Guide to Risk Reduction for Women *(continued)*

Pharmacological Interventions	Goal(s)	Screening	Recommendations
Oral contraceptives *(continued)*			
			4. If a woman develops hypertension while using oral contraceptives, she should be advised to stop taking them.
Antiplatelet agents/anticoagulants	Prevention of clinical thrombotic and embolic events in women with established CVD.	1. Determine if contraindications to therapy exist at the time of the initial cardiovascular event.	1. If no contraindications, women with atherosclerotic CVD should use aspirin 80–325 mg/d.
		2. Evaluate ongoing compliance, risk, and side effects as part of a routine follow-up evaluation.	2. Other antiplatelet agents, such as newer thiopyridine derivatives, may be used to prevent vascular events in women who cannot take aspirin
β-blockers	To reduce the reinfarction rate, incidence of sudden death, and overall mortality in women after MI.	1. Determine if contraindications to therapy exist at the time of the initial cardiovascular event. 2. Evaluate ongoing compliance, risk, and side effects as part of a routine follow-up evaluation.	Start within hours of hospitalization in women with an evolving MI without contraindications. If not started acutely, treatment should begin within a few days of the event and continue indefinitely.

ACE inhibitors	To reduce morbidity and mortality among MI survivors and patients with LV dysfunction.	1. Determine if contraindications to therapy exist at the time of the initial cardiovascular event. 2. Evaluate ongoing compliance, risk, and side effects as part of a routine follow-up evaluation	1. Start early during hospitalization for MI unless hypotension or other contraindications exist. Continue indefinitely for all with LV dysfunction (ejection fraction ≤40%) or symptoms of congestive heart failure; otherwise, ACE inhibitors may be stopped at 6 wk. 2. Discontinue ACE inhibitors if a woman becomes pregnant.

CVD indicates cardiovascular disease; BMI, body mass index; SBP, systolic blood pressure; DBP, diastolic blood pressure; TC, total cholesterol; TG, triglycerides; HRT, hormone replacement therapy; and FSH, follicle-stimulating hormone.

*The choice of test modality should be based on the resting ECG, physical ability to exercise, and local expertise and technologies.

†The ACC and AHA recommend cholesterol screening guidelines as outlined by the National Cholesterol Education Panel (measure total and HDL cholesterol at least once every 5 years in all adults ≥20 y old. The consensus panel recognizes that some organizations use other guidelines, such as the US Preventive Services Task Force, which recommends that cholesterol screening in women without risk factors begin at age 45

notation to consider more aggressive targets for HDL cholesterol and triglycerides in women (15). The NCEP also recommends the use of ERT before cholesterol-lowering drugs to reduce LDL cholesterol in postmenopausal women. In this statement, the recommendation has been modified to consider statins a first-line therapy in postmenopausal women on the basis of recent data that suggest women may have at least as much benefit from LDL-cholesterol reduction with statins as men (16).

Recommendations for aggressive risk factor management are based on the future probability of a cardiovascular event. This strategy allows high-risk patients who have not yet had an event to be considered for more intensive treatment (17). It also recognizes that CHD is not a categorical event but rather a continuum of a progressive disease process. As the availability and use of noninvasive tools to detect asymptomatic CHD increase, the line between primary and secondary prevention may become less distinct. Substantial data support aggressive risk factor management in the setting of secondary prevention. However, because first cardiovascular events are often fatal in women, careful consideration should be given to individual risk factor management before onset of clinical CHD in women. The current recommendations are developed from previous guidelines and consensus panel statements along with newer gender-specific data when available (2, 9, 10, 13, 15, 18–23). The recommendations can serve as a guide to risk factor management but cannot replace clinical judgment. As new knowledge is acquired, revised strategies for the prevention of CHD in women should reflect new science.

Acknowledgments

In addition to the American College of Cardiology and the American Heart Association, the following organizations assisted in the development and review of this document: American Medical Women's Association, American College of Nurse Practitioners, and American College of Obstetricians and Gynecologists.

References

1. 1998 heart and stroke facts statistical update. Dallas, Texas: American Heart Association, 1998

2. Mosca L, Manson JE, Sutherland SE, Langer RD, Manolio T, Barrett-Connor E. Cardiovascular disease in women: a statement for healthcare professionals from the American Heart Association. Writing Group. Circulation 1997;96:2468–2482

3. Goldman L, Garber AM, Grover SA, Hlatky MA. 27th Bethesda Conference: matching the intensity of risk factor management with the hazard for coronary disease events. Task Force 6. Cost effectiveness of assessment and management of risk factors. J Am Coll Cardiol 1996;27:1020–1030

4. US Department of Health and Human Services. Physical activity and health: a report of the Surgeon General. Atlanta, Georgia: DHHS, Centers for Disease Control and Prevention, National Center for Chronic Disease Prevention and Health Promotion, 1996

5. National Center for Health Statistics. Health, United States, 1998 with socioeconomic status and health chartbook. Hyattsville, Maryland: NCHS, 1998

6. Missed opportunities in preventive counseling for cardiovascular disease—United States, 1995. MMWR Morb Mortal Wkly Rep 1998;47:91–95

7. Schrott HG, Bittner V, Vittinghoff E, Herrington DM, Hulley S. Adherence to National Cholesterol Education Program treatment goals in postmenopausal women with heart disease. The Heart and Estrogen/Progestin Replacement Study (HERS). The HERS Research Group. JAMA 1997;277:1281–1286

8. Thomas RJ, Miller NH, Lamendola C, Berra K, Hedback B, Durstin JL, et al. National Survey on Gender Differences in Cardiac Rehabilitation Programs. Patient characteristics and enrollment patterns. J Cardiopulm Rehabil 1996;16:402–412

9. Grundy SM, Balady GJ, Criqui MH, Fletcher G, Greenland P, Hiratzka LF, et al. Guide to primary prevention of cardiovascular diseases. A statement for healthcare professionals from the Task Force on Risk Reduction. American Heart Association Science Advisory and Coordinating Committee. Circulation 1997;95:2329–2331

10. Smith SC Jr, Blair SN, Criqui MH, Fletcher GF, Fuster V, Gersh BJ, et al. Preventing heart attack and death in patients with coronary disease. Circulation 1995;92:2–4

11. Hulley S, Grady D, Bush T, Furberg C, Herrington D, Riggs B, et al. Randomized trial of estrogen plus progestin for secondary prevention of coronary heart disease in postmenopausal women. Heart and Estrogen/progestin Replacement Study (HERS) Research Group. JAMA 1998;280:605–613

12. Manson JE, Spelsberg A. Risk modification in the diabetic patient. In: Manson JE, Ridker PM, Gaziano JM, Hennekens CH, eds. Prevention of myocardial infarction. New York: Oxford University Press, 1996:241–273

13. The American Diabetes Association. Clinical practice recommendations 1998. Diabetes Care 1998;21(suppl 1):S23–S32

14. Manolio TA, Pearson TA, Wenger NK, Barrett-Connor E, Payne GH, Harlan WR. Cholesterol and heart disease in older persons and women. Review of an NHLBI workshop. Ann Epidemiol 1992;2:161–176

15. National Cholesterol Education Program. Second Report of the Expert Panel on Detection, Evaluation, and Treatment of High Blood Cholesterol in Adults (Adult Treatment Panel II). Circulation 1994;89:1333–1445

16. Gotto AM Jr. Cholesterol management in theory and practice. Circulation 1997;96:4424–4430

17. Califf RM, Armstrong PW, Carver JR, D'Agostino RB, Strauss WE. 27th Bethesda Conference: matching the intensity of risk factor management with the hazard for coronary disease events. Task Force 5. Stratification of patients into high, medium and low risk subgroups for purposes of risk factor management. J Am Coll Cardiol 1996;27:1007–1019

18. Physical activity and cardiovascular health. NIH Consensus Development Panel on Physical Activity and Cardiovascular Health. JAMA 1996;276:241–246

19. Krauss RM, Deckelbaum RJ, Ernst N, Fisher E, Howard BV, Knopp RH, et al. Dietary guidelines for healthy American adults. A statement for health professionals from the Nutrition Committee, American Heart Association. Circulation 1996;94:1795–1800

20. Gibbons RJ, Balady GJ, Beasley JW, Bricker JT, Duvernoy WF, Froelicher VF, et al. ACC/AHA guidelines for exercise testing: executive summary. A report of the American College of Cardiology/American Heart Association Task Force on Practice Guidelines (Committee on Exercise Testing). Circulation 1997;96:345–354

21. The sixth report of the Joint National Committee on prevention, detection, evaluation, and treatment of high blood pressure [published erratum appears in Arch Intern Med 1998 Mar 23;158(6):573]. Arch Intern Med 1997;157:2413–2446

22. Ryan TJ, Anderson JL, Antman EM, Braniff BA, Brooks NH, Califf RM, et al. ACC/AHA guidelines for the management of patients with acute myocardial infarction: executive summary. A report of the American College of Cardiology/American Heart Association Task Force on Practice Guidelines (Committee on Management of Acute Myocardial Infarction). Circulation 1996;94:2341–2350

23. Clinical guidelines on the identification, evaluation, and treatment of overweight and obesity in adults: the evidence report. Bethesda, Maryland: National Heart, Lung, and Blood Institute, 1998

APPENDIX I

U.S. Organizations Concerned with Gynecology and Women's Health Care

Accreditation Council for Graduate Medical Education
515 North State Street, Suite 2000
Chicago, IL 60610-4322
(312) 464-4920
www.acgme.org/

The Accreditation Council for Graduate Medical Education is responsible for the accreditation of post-MD medical training programs within the United States. Accreditation is accomplished through a peer review process, and is based on established standards and guidelines.

The American Board of Obstetrics and Gynecology
2915 Vine Street, Suite 300
Dallas, TX 75204
(214) 871-1619
www.abog.org/

The American Board of Obstetrics and Gynecology, Inc. examines and certifies almost 2,000 obstetrician–gynecologists and subspecialists in maternal–fetal medicine, reproductive endocrinology, and gynecologic oncology annually. In addition, approximately 2,500 physicians are examined annually for the purpose of recertification.

The American Academy of Family Physicians
11400 Tomahawk Creek Parkway
Leawood, KS 66211-2672
(913) 906-6000
www.aafp.org

The American Academy of Family Physicians is a national, nonprofit medical association representing family physicians, family practice residents, and medical students. The Academy was founded in 1947 to promote and maintain high quality standards for family doctors who are providing continuing comprehensive health care to the public.

The American Association of Gynecologic Laparoscopists
13021 East Florence Avenue
Sante Fe Springs, CA 906704505
(562) 946-8774
www.aagl.com

The American Association of Gynecologic Laparoscopists is a professional association of endoscopic physicians dedicated to promoting the safest, most therapeutic, minimally invasive surgery available in women's health care.

The American Institute of Ultrasound in Medicine, Society of Obstetrical Gynecological Ultrasound
14750 Sweitzer Lane, Suite 100
Laurel, MD 20707-5906
(301) 498-4100
www.aium.org

The American Institute of Ultrasound in Medicine, Society of Obstetrical Gynecological Ultrasound is dedicated to advancing ultrasound in medicine and research with emphasis in education.

The American Medical Association
515 North State Street
Chicago, IL 60610
(312) 464-5000
www.ama-assn.org

The American Medical Association is a voluntary membership organization of physicians, intended to set standards for the practice of medicine and represent the best interests of patients and physicians.

The American Society for Colposcopy and Cervical Pathology
20 West Washington Street, Suite 1
Hagerstown, MD 21740
(301) 733-3640
www.asccp.org

The American Society for Colposcopy and Cervical Pathology serves as the national organization to educate and disseminate information related to the use of colposcopy in the study of the female lower genital tract. The society brings together 3,500 individuals from disciplines including pathology, cytology, cytogenetics, gynecologic oncology, endocrinology, preventive medicine, basic science, and clinical medicine.

American Society for Forensic Obstetricians and Gynecologists
409 12th Street, SW
Washington, DC 20024-2188
(202) 863-1648

American Society for Forensic Obstetricians and Gynecologists uses meetings, education, and exchange of ideas to address an array of medical–legal issues in such areas as medical practice, hospital care, arbitration, and deposition in courts of law.

The American Society for Reproductive Medicine
1209 Montgomery Highway
Birmingham, AL 35216-2809
(205) 978-5000
www.asrm.org

The American Society for Reproductive Medicine is a nonprofit organization devoted to advancing knowledge and expertise in reproductive medicine and biology.

The American Urogynecologic Society
2025 M Street, NW, Suite 800
Washington, DC 20036
(202) 367-1167
www.augs.org

The American Urogynecologic Society was organized to disseminate information regarding the field of urogynecology and pelvic floor reconstruction.

The Association for Hospital Medical Education
The Council on Medical Education Consortia
1200 19th Street, NW, Suite 300
Washington, DC 20036
(202) 857-1196
www.ahme.med.edu

The Association for Hospital Medical Education (AHME) is a national nonprofit professional organization involved in the continuum of medical education. The Council on Medical Education Consortia was established to serve as an information resource on consortia for AHME members and their institutions and to advance AHME's consortium interests in matters of health policy and regulation and medical education accreditation.

The Association of Professors of Gynecology and Obstetrics
409 12th Street, SW
Washington, DC 20024
(202) 863-2507
www.apgo.org

The Association of Professors of Gynecology and Obstetrics promotes excellence in women's health care education. The Association of Professors of Gynecology and Obstetrics considers problems relating to the member departments of gynecology and obstetrics in schools of medicine, advances and improves the study of gynecology and obstetrics, and provides an exchange of information on programs of study, teaching methods, and research activities among gynecologic and obstetric programs.

The Association of Reproductive Health Professionals
2401 Pennsylvania Avenue, NW, Suite 350
Washington, DC 20037-1718
(202) 466-3825
www.arhp.org

The Association of Reproductive Health Professionals is devoted to educating health care professionals and the public on matters regarding human reproduction and health.

Council of University Chairs of Obstetrics and Gynecology
409 12th Street, SW
Washington, DC 20024
(202) 863-1648
www.cucog.org

Council of University Chairs of Obstetrics and Gynecology was established for the charitable and educational purposes of promoting excellence in medical education in the fields of obstetrics and gynecology. Through the unique leadership positions of its 140 members—chairpersons of the department of obstetrics and gynecology—the organization promotes and encourages excellence in medical student, resident, and fellowship training, clinical practice, and basic and clinical research in women's health.

Gynecologic Oncology Group
1600 John F. Kennedy Boulevard, Suite 1020
Philadelphia, PA 19103
800-225-3053 or (215) 854-0770
www.gog.org

Gynecologic Oncology Group is a national organization dedicated to clinical research in the field of gynecologic cancer.

Gynecologic Studies Group
409 12th Street, SW
Washington, DC 20024-2188
(202) 863-1648

Gynecologic Studies Group is an organization of academic institutions dedicated to the development, implementation, analysis, and publication of multicentered trials evaluating nononcologic gynecologic issues.

The Gynecologic Surgery Society
2440 M Street, NW, Suite 801
Washington, DC 20037
(202) 293-5169

The Gynecologic Surgery Society is committed to obstetric and gynecologic surgery and the review and teaching of laser surgery as well as other methods of "cutting edge" technology.

The Infectious Diseases Society for Obstetrics and Gynecology
409 12th Street, SW
Washington, DC 20024-2188
(202) 863-2570

The Infectious Diseases Society for Obstetrics and Gynecology fosters the scientific and clinical study of infectious diseases in obstetrics and gynecology, including bacterial, viral, and parasitic infections, vaginitis and cervicitis, sexually transmitted diseases, urinary tract infections, and post-operative infections.

The Jacobs Institute of Women's Health
409 12th Street, SW
Washington, DC 20024-2188
(202) 863-4990
www.jiwh.org

The Jacobs Institute of Women's Health is a nonprofit organization dedicated to advancing knowledge and practice in the field of women's health. Members of the Jacobs Institute are a multidisciplinary group of health care professionals, researchers, policy makers, and advocates with the common goal of improving the health status of women.

The North American Menopause Society
PO Box 94527
Cleveland, OH 44101-4527
(216) 844-3334
www.menopause.org

The North American Menopause Society is a nonprofit organization dedicated to promoting understanding of menopause and thereby improving the health of women as they approach menopause and beyond.

The North American Society for Pediatric and Adolescent Gynecology
1015 Chestnut Street, Suite 1225
Philadelphia, PA 19107-4302
(215) 955-6331

The North American Society for Pediatric and Adolescent Gynecology is an educational society devoted to bringing programs to health care provider groups who medically manage problems related to pediatric and adolescent gynecologic health.

The North American Society for Psychosocial Obstetrics and Gynecology
409 12th Street, SW
Washington, DC 20024-2188
(202) 863-1646
www.naspog.org

The North American Society for Psychosocial Obstetrics and Gynecology aims to foster scholarly scientific and clinical studies of biopsychosocial aspects of obstetric and gynecologic medicine. The aim is broadly defined to include the psychologic, psychophysiologic, public health, sociocultural, ethical, and other aspects of such functioning and behavior.

Residency Review Committee for Obstetrics–Gynecology
515 North State Street, Suite 2000
Chicago, IL 60610-4322
(312) 464-4683
www.acgme.org/

The Residency Review Committee for Obstetrics–Gynecology, composed of representatives appointed by the American Medical Association Board of Trustees on recommendation of the Council on Medical Education, American Board of Obstetrics and Gynecology, American College of Obstetricians and Gynecologists, and a resident representative, accredits residency programs in the specialty of obstetrics and gynecology.

The Society for Gynecologic Investigation
409 12th Street, SW
Washington, DC 20024-2188
(202) 863-2544
www.socgyninv.org

The Society for Gynecologic Investigation is a scientific organization with members throughout the world. The Society's mission is to promote excellence in reproductive sciences through research, education, and advocacy.

The Society of Gynecologic Oncologists
401 North Michigan Avenue, Suite 24
Chicago, IL 60611
(312) 644-6610
www.sgo.org

The Society of Gynecologic Oncologists is a professional medical organization of board-certified gynecologic oncologists. Its mission is to improve care of gynecologic–oncology patients, advance knowledge, raise standards within the discipline, and encourage research.

The Society of Gynecologic Surgeons
2500 North State Street
Jackson, MS 39216
(601) 984-5314
www.sgsonline.org

The Society of Gynecologic Surgeons' mission is to promote the highest standards for gynecologic surgical care for women in a safe, effective, and ethical manner.

The Society for Maternal–Fetal Medicine
409 12th Street, SW
Washington, DC 20024–2188

The Society for Maternal–Fetal Medicine is dedicated to the promotion and expansion of education in obstetrical perinatology and the exchange of new ideas and research in the field of maternal–fetal medicine.

The Sports Gynecology Society
7 Fullerton Road
Moorestown, NJ 08057
(215) 762-6866

The Sports Gynecology Society's interest is in obstetric and gynecologic care of athletes, research, sports medicine, and exercise advice for women.

INDEX

Note: Page numbers followed by letters *f* and *t* indicate figures and tables, respectively.

A

Abdominal myomectomy, for uterine leiomyomata, 389
Abnormal genital bleeding. *See* Bleeding, abnormal genital
Abortion, 382–385
  and adolescents, 148
  counseling prior to, 383
  obstacles to, 382–383
  patient and professional resources, 384–385
  patient evaluation in, 383–384
  post-procedure care, 384
  spontaneous, 287–290, 364–366
Abstinence, periodic
  deaths associated with, 160*t*
  failure rate of, 158*t*
Abstinence-based sexuality education, 148–149
Abuse, 230–235
  child, 233–234
  domestic violence, 231–233, 283–286
  intimate partner violence, 231–233, 283–286
  of older women, 181–182, 235
  of women with disabilities, 393–394
Accreditation Council for Continuing Medical Education, on conflicts of interest, 26–27
ACE inhibitors
  in preventive cardiology, 465*t*
  in treatment of hypertension, 323*f*
ACOG. *See* American College of Obstetricians and Gynecologists
Acquired immunodeficiency syndrome (AIDS), 319, 372. *See also* Human immunodeficiency virus
Activities of daily living, inability to perform, among older women, 179
Ad hoc committees, 8
ADA. *See* Americans with Disabilities Act
Adenocarcinoma, of endometrium, 343. *See also* Endometrial cancer
Adolescents
  abnormal genital bleeding in, 259
  blood pressure screening for, 207
  confidentiality and, 17–18, 145–147
  consent to services, 17–18
  contraceptive counseling for, 152
  domestic violence and, 231
  eating disorders among, 291, 293–294
  health care of, 145–150
  insurance of, 146
  pregnancy rate of, 147–148
  rape/sexual assault of, 367
  reproductive health care for, 145–146
  sexual activity of, 147–150
  sexual misconduct and, 28–29
  sexuality education for, 148–150
  sexually transmitted diseases of, 147
Advance directives, 185–187

Advanced practice health care clinicians
  certification of, 32, 108–111
  credentialing of, 34
  privileges of, 35
  scope of practice, 35
Adverse outcomes, in quality assessment, 48
Adverse reactions, in ambulatory gynecologic surgery, 251–252
Advisory committees, 9
Aerobic exercise, safety guidelines for, 204
AIDS. *See* Acquired immunodeficiency syndrome
Air transport, in patient transfer, 55
Alcohol abuse, 375–381
  behavior modification for, 267
  and depression, 281
  of health care professionals, 21–24
  patient and professional resources for, 267, 380–381
  and rape/sexual assault, 367
  screening questionnaires for, 377–378
  treatment for, 380
Allergic reactions
  to latex, 252, 336–338
  postoperative, 252
  preoperative assessment of, 250
Alternative therapies, in pain management, 356–357
Alzheimer's disease, 178–179
  hormone replacement therapy and, 315
AMA. *See* American Medical Association
Ambulatory care facilities
  facilities and equipment management in, 81–82
  governance of, 11
  health care services in, 118
  patient flow in, 112
  staffing requirements for, 105
  surgery in, 241–243
Ambulatory gynecologic surgery, 240–254
  adverse reactions to, 251–252
  in ambulatory facilities, 241–243
  anesthesia in, 244–247
Ambulatory gynecologic surgery *(continued)*
  common procedures, 240
  discharge plans, 252–254
  intraoperative care, 250–251
  length of stay after, 252–254
  in offices, 243
  patient preparation for, 249–250
  patient selection, 241–243
  perioperative considerations, 247–254
  postoperative care, 250–251
  preoperative evaluation, 247–249
  recovery period after, 252–254
  site selection, 241–243
Amenorrhea, 201, 297
American Board of Obstetrics and Gynecology, 106
American College of Nurse–Midwives, 108
American College of Obstetricians and Gynecologists (ACOG)
  Code of Professional Ethics of, 14, 74, 397–404
  Committee on Ethics of, 29–30
  operational mission statement of, 433
  quality assessment screening tools of, 40–41
  screening recommendations of, *see* Primary and preventive care
  on sexual misconduct, 29–30
  statement of Scope of Practice of Obstetrics and Gynecology, 433
  on universal coverage, 119
  vision statement of, 433
  Voluntary Review of Quality Care program of, 41
  woman's health record, 434–452
American College of Surgeons, surgical facilities classification of, 83
American Medical Association (AMA)
  on conflicts of interest, 26–27
  Council on Ethical and Judicial Affairs of, 29–30
  and Medicare, 137
  on patients' bill of rights, 66–69
  on sexual harassment, 28
  on sexual misconduct, 29–30

American Nurses Association, 108
American Society for Reproductive Medicine
endometriosis classification of, 299–302, 300*f*–301*f*
on infertility services, 331–333
Americans with Disabilities Act (ADA), 50, 428–432. *See also* Women with disabilities
and auxiliary aids, 431
definitions in, 429
employment obligations in, 429
persons protected by, 428
on physician discrimination, 430–431
and public accommodations, 430
and reasonable accommodation, 429–430
resources, 431–432
Title III of, 394
Analgesia, 97
Analgesic ladder, 356
Anaphylactic reaction, following immunizations, 326–327
Ancillary services, 95–98
Androgen therapy, for sexual dysfunction, 229, 371
Anesthesia, 97
in ambulatory care facilities, 242–243
in ambulatory gynecologic surgery, 244–247
conscious intravenous sedation, 246–247
general, 97
local, 97, 244–246
recovery period and, 252–254
Anorexia nervosa, 291
complications of, 295
diagnostic criteria for, 292
Antibiotic prophylaxis, 249
Anticardiolipin antibodies, and recurrent pregnancy loss, 364–365
Anticoagulants, in preventive cardiology, 464*t*
Antiplatelet agents, in preventive cardiology, 464*t*
Appointments
management of patients, 112–113
of medical staff, 31–34
Arousal, lack of, 229
ART. *See* Assisted reproductive technologies
ASCUS test results, 261. *See also* Cervical cytology
Assisted reproductive technologies (ART). *See also* Infertility
ethics and, 62
genetics and, 310
outcomes for, 334*t*
Association of Women's Health, Obstetrics, and Neonatal Nurses, staffing guidelines of, 105
Asthma, occupational, 337
Autoclaving, in sterilization, 87
Autonomy
as ethical principle, 63
and honesty, 65–66
and informed consent, 65

B

Bacterial vaginosis, 224
Bacteriuria screening for, risk factors for, 122*t*, 126, 128, 130, 132
Barium enema. *See* Double contrast barium enema
Battered women. *See* Domestic violence
Behavior modification, 266–268
Beneficence
as ethical principle, 63–64
and honesty, 65–66
β-blockers
in preventive cardiology, 464*t*
in treatment of hypertension, 323*f*
Billing
avoiding fraud, 27–28, 50, 61
and liability, 61
management of, 111–112
Binge-eating disorder, 291
Biotin intake, 202*t*
Bipolar disorder, 281
Bladder prolapse, 360

Bleeding
abnormal genital, 257–261
in adolescents, 259
causes of, 258
classification of, 258–259
differential diagnosis of, 258
evaluation of, 260
health care impact of, 257–259
patient and professional resources, 260–261
treatment for, 259–260
uterine, 257–260
Blood pressure
classification of, 207*t*
measurement of, 207–208, 322
in preventive cardiology, 460*t*
Bloodborne pathogens, exposure to
communication of hazards to employees, 415–416
disinfection and sterilization procedures for, 92
engineering and work practice controls, 50–51, 408–409
exposure control plan, 50–51, 406–407
housekeeping and, 411–412
and isolation precautions, 92–93
mandatory universal precautions, 407–408
Occupational Safety and Health Administration regulations on, 50–51, 405–417
personal protective equipment, 50–51, 409–411
postexposure evaluation and follow-up, 50–51, 413–414
record-keeping of, 50–51, 416–417
BMI. *See* Body mass index
Body mass index (BMI), 194–195, 195*t*
Bone densitometry, 350–353
Bone loss, postmenopausal, 201. *See also* Osteoporosis
Bowel habits, among aging women, 180
Bowel preparation, preoperative, 249
BRCA1 mutation, 345
Breast cancer, 216–217, 339–341. *See also* Mammography
hormone replacement therapy and, 174–175, 315–316
prevention of, 129, 131, 133, 176, 340
relative location of lesions, 139*f*
tamoxifen and, 176
Breast Cancer Risk Assessment Tool, 340
Breast disorders, 269–271
diagnosis of, 269
evaluation of, 269–270
fibrocystic, 269
patient and professional resources, 271
Breast examination, 138–139
Bulimia nervosa, 291
complications of, 295
diagnostic criteria for, 292–293
Bupropion, for depression, 280

C

CAGE Questionnaire, 377–378
Calcium intake/supplementation, 172, 199, 202*t*
Calendar method of contraception, failure rate of, 158*t*
Cancer, 214–218, 214*t*, 339–350
breast, 174, 216–217, 315–316, 339–341
cervical, 140–141, 261–265, 341–342
colon, 218
colorectal, screening for, risk factors for, 122*t*, 126–128, 130, 132
endometrial, 174, 217, 259, 315, 343–345
lung, 215
of older women, 180–181
ovarian, 174, 217, 345–346
pain management for, 356
patient and professional resources, 349–350
risk factors for, 214–217
screening for, 214–218
vulvar, 346–347
Cancer Rights Act of 1998, 341

Candidal vaginitis, 224–225
Cardiology, preventive, 453–468, 456*t*–465*t*
Cardiovascular disease (CVD), 201–210
cholesterol and, 209–210, 272–273
hormone replacement therapy and, 173–175, 315
hypertension and, 206–208
among older women, 180
prevention of, 453–468, 456*t*–465*t*
in postmenopausal women, 314–315
risk factors, 201
evaluation of, 126, 128, 130–132
modifiable, 205–206
nonmodifiable, 205
CDC. *See* Centers for Disease Control and Prevention
Centers for Disease Control and Prevention (CDC)
Hospital Infection Control Practices Advisory Committee of, 92–93
on immunizations, 327
on infection control, 86
on sexually transmitted diseases, 372–373
vaccination guidelines of, 51
Centers for Medicare and Medicaid Services. *See* Health Care Financing Administration
Central nervous system, effects of hormone replacement therapy on, 315
Cerebrovascular disease, cholesterol and, 209–210
Certificate for Provider-Performed Microscopy Procedure, 419–421
Certificates of Waiver, 418–419
Certification
from foreign countries, 32
of nurse practitioners, 108–109
of physician assistants, 109–110
of physicians, 32, 106–107
and recertification, 37–38
subspecialty, 107
Certified nurse–midwives, 34, 108. *See also* Advanced practice health care clinicians
Cervical atresia, and endometriosis, 299
Cervical cancer, 261–265, 341–342, risk factors for, 140–141
Cervical cap
contraindications and side effects of, 156*t*
failure rate of, 158*t*
Cervical cytology, 140–143
abnormal, 261–265
evaluation of, 261–265
health care impact of, 261
patient and professional resources, 265
new techniques for, 143
Cervical intraepithelial neoplasia, risk factors for, 140–141
Chaperons, 18–19
CHD. *See* Coronary heart disease
Chemical dependency, of health care professionals, 21–24
Child abuse, 233–234
Childproofing, of reception areas, 80
Children, sexual misconduct and, 28–29. *See also* Adolescents; Pediatric gynecology; Pediatric patients
Chlamydia, 220, 372
Chlamydia trachomatis, 220
Chloroprocaine, as local anesthetic, 245
Cholelithiasis, hormone replacement therapy and, 174
Cholesterol, 209–211, 272–274
and cardiovascular disease, 209–210, 272–273, 455, 466
high, treatment for, 273
patient and professional resources, 273–274
and preventive cardiology, 454, 460*t*–461*t*, 466
screening for, risk factors for, 122*t*, 126, 128, 130, 132, 209–211, 272–273
Choline intake, 202*t*
Chronic pelvic pain. *See* Pelvic pain, chronic
Cigarette smoking. *See* Smoking
Circumcision, female. *See* Female circumcision/female genital mutilation

Cleaning
  in infection control, 86–87
  as standard precaution, 93
CLIA. *See* Clinical Laboratory Improvement Amendments of 1988
Clinical indicators, in quality assessment, 40
Clinical Laboratory Improvement Amendments of 1988, 51–53, 418–421
  Certificate for Provider-Performed Microscopy Procedure, 419–421
  Certificates, 52–53
  Certificates of Waiver, 418–419
Clinical Nurse Specialists, 108
Coagulation disorders, and uterine bleeding, 257–258
Code of Professional Ethics of the American College of Obstetricians and Gynecologists, 14, 74, 397–404
Codes of ethics, 14
Coding. *See* Billing
Cognitive changes, in aging women, 178–179
Collaborative practice, 35
Colon cancer, 218
Colonoscopy, 130, 132
Colorectal cancer, screening for, risk factors for, 122*t*, 126–128, 130, 132
Committee on Ethics, of American College of Obstetricians and Gynecologists, on sexual misconduct, 29–30
Committees
  ad hoc, 8
  advisory, 9
  of Department of Obstetrics and Gynecology, 7–9
  executive, 9
  standing, 8
Communicable diseases, of health care professionals, 24–25
Communication
  and confidentiality, 15
  and end-of-life considerations, 184
  of hazards, to employees, 415–416
  and informed consent, 65
  management of, 101–104
  and medical history interviews, 135
  with older women patients, 177
  in quality assessment, 47–48
  with women with disabilities, 391–392
Compliance
  with government regulations, 50–57
  monitoring of, 103
Complications, medical, in quality assessment, 48
Comprehensive Accreditation Manual for Ambulatory Care, 136
Comprehensive Accreditation Manual for Hospitals, 136
Compulsive eating. *See* Binge-eating disorder
Condoms
  contraindications and side effects of, 156*t*
  deaths associated with, 160*t*
  failure rate of, 158*t*
  and latex allergy, 336–337
Conferences, of Department of Obstetrics and Gynecology, educational, 9–10
Confidentiality, 15–18
  and adolescents, 17–18, 145–147
  and domestic violence, 285
  as ethical concept, 66
  of medical records, 100
  of peer review, 43
  and private area for discussions, 82
  staff reminders of, 11
  technology and, 101–102
  violation of, 16
Conflicts of interest, 25–27
Conscious intravenous sedation, 97, 246–247
  emergency backup for, 247
  selection of agents, 246–247

Consent. *See also* Informed consent
adolescent clients and, 17–18
parental, 17
in pediatric gynecology, 359
Consultations, and referrals, 20, 59–61. *See also* Referrals
Continuing competence evaluations, 37–38
Continuous quality improvement (CQI), 40–49. *See also* Quality assessment
collection and analysis of data in, 42–43
and corrective actions, 43–46
interdepartmental, 44–45
in offices, 46–49
program leadership, 40
trending in, 41
Contraceptive counseling, 152–153, 383
Contraceptives
characteristics of, 157*t*
choice of method, 152
contraindications and side effects of, 154*t*–156*t*
deaths associated with, 160*t*
emergency, 160–162, 161*t*
failure of, 158*t*–159*t*, 162
in family planning, 150–162
periodic reassessment of, 153–160
prescription of, 151
Coronary heart disease (CHD). *See also* Cardiovascular disease
cholesterol and, 272–274
with oral contraceptive use, 151–152
in postmenopausal women, 314–315
and preventive cardiology, 453–468
risk reduction for, 456*t*–465*t*
Corrective actions, failure of, 43–46
Council on Ethical and Judicial Affairs, of American Medical Association, on sexual misconduct, 29–30
Counseling
in family planning, 152–153
during menopause, 171–172
in periodic assessments, 126–133
in preconceptional care, 166–169
preoperative, 249–250
for sexually transmitted diseases, 226
CQI. *See* Continuous quality improvement
Credentials
evaluation of, 31–38
special, 36–37
Crisis intervention, 277–278
Criteria sets. *See* American College of Obstetricians and Gynecologists, quality assessment screening tools of
Critical items, disinfection and sterilization of, 87–90, 88*t*–89*t*
Cultural competency, and patient communication, 103–104, 170–171
Cultural knowledge, 73
CVD. *See* Cardiovascular disease
Cystic lesions, of breast, 139

D

Data
collection and analysis of, in quality assessment, 42–43
operating room tracking of, 113
DCBE. *See* Double contrast barium enema
Decision making, ethical, 71–75
and institutional ethics committees, 72–74
and institutional responsibility, 74–75
Decontamination, and occupational exposure to bloodborne pathogens, 411–412
Delirium, among older women, 179
Dementia
among older women, 178–179
hormone replacement therapy and, 315
Department chair/head, 4–7
and granting of privileges, 34
responsibilities of, 5–6
Department of Obstetrics and Gynecology
committees of, 7–9
conferences of, 9–10
department chair/head of, 4–7
education programs of, 10
functions of, 3
goal of, 4

Department of Obstetrics and Gynecology (*continued*)
 governance of, 3–11
 meetings of, 9–10
 officers of, 4–7
 organization of, 4
 outreach programs of, 10–11
 responsibilities of, 4
 staff fund of, 7
Depression, 235–236, 279–282
 diagnosis of, 235–236, 279–280
 differential diagnosis of, 235–236, 281
 patient and professional resources, 282
 and premenstrual syndrome, 362
 recurrence of, 279–280
 referral options for, 281
 treatment for, 279–280
Diabetes mellitus, 210–213
 and coronary heart disease, 455, 461*t*–462*t*
 diagnosis of, 211–213
 nutrition and, 213
 preconceptional counseling and, 168
 testing for, 122*t*, 126, 128, 130, 132, 210–213
 types of, 213
Diagnostic imaging services. *See* Radiology services
Diaphragm (contraceptive)
 contraindications and side effects of, 156*t*
 deaths associated with, 160*t*
 failure rate of, 158*t*
 and latex allergy, 336–337
Diazepam, in conscious intravenous sedation, 246
Dietary reference intakes, 202*t*–203*t*
Digital rectal examination, 130, 132
Disabilities
 Americans with Disabilities Act, 428–432
 World Health Organization definition of, 391
 women with, 391–395
Discharge plans, 97–98, 252–254
Disciplinary actions, for impaired clinicians, 22
Disease detection and prevention, 192–239
Disease transmission, and infection control, 86–94
Disinfection, in infection control, 87–92, 88*t*–89*t*
Do-Not-Resuscitate orders, 184–185
Documentation
 of corrective actions, 44
 of institutional review board activities, 71
 of occupational exposure of bloodborne pathogens, 416–417
Domestic violence, 231–233, 283–286
 clinician responsibilities in addressing, 284
 patient and professional resources, 285–286
 and women with disabilities, 393–394
Double contrast barium enema, 130, 132
Doxycycline, in antibiotic prophylaxis, 249
Drug(s). *See* Medication(s)
Drug abuse, 375–381
 behavior modification for, 266–268
 and depression, 281
 of health care professionals, 21–24
 patient and professional resources for, 267–268, 380–381
 and rape/sexual assault, 367
 treatment for, 380
Dry heat, in sterilization, 87
Dual employment, 32–34
Dual-energy X-ray absorptiometry (DXA), in bone density assessment, 351, 353
Due process, of corrective actions, 44
DXA. *See* Dual-energy X-ray absorptiometry
Dying patients, end-of-life considerations, 183–189
Dyspareunia, 229

E

Eating disorders, 291–296
 behavior modification for, 266–268
 complications of, 295
 diagnosis of, 294

Eating disorders *(continued)*
patient and professional resources, 295–296
screening for, 291–294
treatment of, 294
ECC. *See* Endocervical curettage
Ectopic pregnancy, 287–290
diagnosis of, 288–289
patient and professional resources, 289–290
treatment for, 288–289
Education programs, of Department of Obstetrics and Gynecology, 10–11
Educational conferences, 9–10
Elderly, abuse and neglect of, 235. *See also* Older women
Emancipated minors, 17
Emergency contraception, 160–162, 161*t*
Emergency equipment/supplies, maintenance of, 80
Emergency medical conditions
determination of, 423
of pregnant women, 423–424
Emergency plans, 79–81
Emotional problems, and sexual dysfunction, 230
Employee training, on occupational exposure risks, 415–416
Employment, dual, 33–34
End-of-life considerations, 183–189
ethics and, 62
legal rights, 185–187
pain management, 189
terminal care, 187–189
Endocervical brush, 141–142
Endocervical curettage (ECC), 261
Endocrine disorders, 297–298
Endometrial ablation, for anovulatory uterine bleeding, 259–260
Endometrial assessment, for abnormal uterine bleeding, 176, 259
Endometrial biopsy, 343–344
Endometrial cancer, 217, 259, 343–345
hormone replacement therapy and, 174–175, 315
screening for, 343
Endometrial hyperplasia, hormone replacement therapy and, 315
Endometriosis, 299–305
and chronic pelvic pain, 274
classification of, 299–302, 300f–301*f*
pain management of, 302–303
patient and professional resources, 304–305
referrals for, 304
surgical therapy for, 303–304
Endoscopic equipment, disinfection of, 90–91
Environmental engineer, and facilities planning, 80
Environmental factors, in preconceptional care, 166
Epinephrine, and local anesthetics, 245
Equipment
in ambulatory settings, 81–82
disinfection and sterilization of, 87–92, 88*t*–89*t*
general requirements for, 79–85
in inpatient facilities, 84–85
maintenance of, 80–81
in offices, 81–82
in quality assessment, 48
in surgical facilities, 82–84
Estrogen replacement therapy. *See also* Hormone replacement therapy
and endometriosis, 304
after hysterectomy, 304
preventive aspects of, 454–455, 466
Ethical concepts, 64–66
Ethical principles, 63–64
Ethics, 62–75
and billing fraud, 27–28, 61
codes of, 14
and conflicts of interest, 25–27
and decision making, 71–75

Ethics *(continued)*
  definition of, 62–63
  and patient protection, 66–71
  and sexual harassment, 28
Ethics committees, institutional. *See* Institutional ethics committees
Evaluations, for continuing competence, 37–38
Examination rooms, 82
Executive committees, 9
Exercise, 200–201
  in preventive cardiology, 456*t*–457*t*
  safety guidelines for, 204–205
  among women with disabilities, 393
Expert witnesses, 20–21
Exposure Control Plan, for occupational exposure to bloodborne pathogens, 50–51, 407–408
External peer review, as corrective action, 45
Eye protection
  for occupational exposure to bloodborne pathogens, 410–411
  as standard precaution, 93

F

Face protection
  for occupational exposure to bloodborne pathogens, 410–411
  as standard precaution, 93
Facilities
  ambulatory care
    facilities and equipment management in, 81–82
    governance of, 11
    health care services in, 118
    patient flow in, 112
    staffing requirements for, 105
    surgery in, 241–243
  emergency plans, 79–81
  general requirements for, 79–85
  inpatient, 84–85
  in offices, 81–82
Facilities *(continued)*
  medical equipment, 80–81
  surgical, 82–84, 105
Falls, among older women, 179–180
Family history
  of genetic disorders, 310
  in medical history, 138
Family planning, 150–162
  contraceptive failure and, 162
  counseling in, 152–153
  emergency contraception in, 160–162, 161*t*
  initial evaluation in, 150–152
  periodic reassessment in, 153–160
Fasting glucose testing, 122*t*, 126, 128, 130, 132, 211–213
Fat intake, 197
FC/FGM. *See* Female circumcision/female genital mutilation
FDA. *See* U.S. Food and Drug Administration
Fecal occult blood testing, 130, 132
Fellows, privileges of, 33
Female circumcision/female genital mutilation (FC/FGM), 305–309
  awareness of, 307–308
  classification of, 306
  professional resources on, 308–309
Female condom, contraindications and side effects of, 156*t*
Female sterilization, 153, 159*t*
Fentanyl citrate, in conscious intravenous sedation, 246
Fetal surgery, ethics and, 62
Fiber intake, 197
Fibroids. *See* Uterine leiomyomata
Financial records, of patients, 101
Fitness, 193–201
  evaluation of, 126, 128, 130, 132
  exercise, 200–201
  nutrition, 196–200
  weight for height, 193–195, 194*t*
Fluid management, intraoperative, 251
Fluoride intake/supplementation, 122*t*, 126, 202*t*

Folate intake, 202*t*
Folic acid intake/supplementation, 165–166, 199
Follow-up services, 97–98
Food Guide Pyramid, 197, 198*f*
Foreign bodies, and vaginitis, in pediatric gynecology, 358–359
Fractures
  among older women, 180
  osteoporosis-related, 350
Functional assessment, of older women patients, 177–180

G

Gamete donors, genetic screening and, 310
Gardnerella vaginitis, 224
Gas bead sterilizers, 87
Gate theory, of pain management, 356–357
Gender disparity, in end-of-life considerations, 187
General anesthesia, 97
Generic drug names, and conflicts of interest, 26–27
Genetic testing/counseling, 126, 128, 131, 310–311
  for breast–ovarian cancer, 340, 345–346
  preconceptional, 168
  risk factors for, 122*t*
Genetics, 309–311
  and assisted reproductive techniques, 310
  conditions with genetic risk factors, 309–310
  counseling and testing, 310–311
  patient and professional resources, 311
Genital bleeding. *See* Bleeding, abnormal genital
Genital herpes, 222–223, 372
Genital mutilation, female. *See* Female circumcision/female genital mutilation
Geriatrics. *See* Older women
Germicides, for sterilization, 90–91
Gestational trophoblastic disease (GTD), 347–348
Gloves
  latex, 336
  for occupational exposure to bloodborne pathogens, 410
  as standard precaution, 93
Goggles, for occupational exposure to bloodborne pathogens, 93, 410
Gonadotropin-releasing hormone (GnRH) agonist, for endometriosis, 302
Gonorrhea, 219–220, 372
Governance, 3–12
  of ambulatory surgical facilities, 11
  of Department of Obstetrics and Gynecology, 3–11
  and granting of privileges, 34–37
  of offices, 11–12
  and quality assessment, 8
Government regulations, compliance with, 50–57
Gowns
  for occupational exposure to bloodborne pathogens, 410
  as standard precaution, 93
GTD. *See* Gestational trophoblastic disease
Gynecologic surgery, ambulatory. *See* Ambulatory gynecologic surgery
Gynecologic ultrasonography, 312–314

H

Haemophilus vaginitis, 224
Hand-washing, as standard precaution, 93, 408
HAV. *See* Hepatitis A virus
HBV. *See* Hepatitis B virus
hCG. *See* Human chorionic gonadotropin
HCV. *See* Hepatitis C virus
HDL cholesterol. *See* High-density lipoprotein cholesterol
Health Care Financing Administration, 52, 136–137

Health care industry, and conflicts of interest, 26
Health care power of attorney, 186–187
Health care professionals
  associations representing, 106, 469–477
  communicable diseases of, 24–25
  communication of hazards to, 415–416
  continuing competence evaluations of, 37–38
  hepatitis B vaccination for, 412–413
  impaired, 21–24
  referrals to and from, 19–20
  troubled, 24
  types of, 105–111
  violence against, 81
Health Care Quality Improvement Act of 1986, 43
Health Insurance Portability and Accountability Act of 1996, 50
Hearing disorders, among older women, 179
Heart and Estrogen/Progestin Replacement Study (HERS), 173, 454–455, 466
Heart disease. *See* Cardiovascular disease, and Coronary heart disease
Heart rate, during exercise, 200–201
Height, weight proper for, 193–195, 194*t*
Hemoglobin level assessment, risk factors for, 122*t*, 126, 128, 130, 132
Hepatitis A virus (HAV), vaccination for, 122*t*, 127, 129, 131, 133
Hepatitis B virus (HBV), 225
  among adolescents, 147
  and health care professionals, 24–25
  vaccination, 127, 129, 131, 133
    CDC guidelines for, 51
    for health care workers, 412–413
    risk factors for, 123*t*
Hepatitis C virus (HCV)
  and health care professionals, 24–25
  risk factors for, 123*t*
  testing for, 126, 128, 130, 132
Herpes simplex virus (HSV), 222–223, 372
HERS. *See* Heart and Estrogen/Progestin Replacement Study
Heterocyclic agents, for depression, 280
High blood pressure. *See* Hypertension
High-density lipoprotein (HDL) cholesterol, 209–210, 455, 466
Hip, fracture of, 180, 350
History. *See* Medical history
HIV. *See* Human immunodeficiency virus
Home, terminal care in, 187–189
Honesty, as ethical concept, 65–66
Hormone replacement therapy (HRT), 172–176, 314–318
  and breast cancer, 174–176, 315–316
  and cardiovascular disease, 172–175
  concerns about, 174–175
  contraindications to, 175
  endometrial assessment during, 176
  and endometrial cancer, 174–175, 344
  during menopause, 172–176
  and ovarian cancer, 174
  patient and professional resources, 317–318
  preventive aspects of, 172–174, 314–315, 454–455, 466
  in preventive cardiology, 454–455, 462*t*–463*t*, 466
  treatment regimens of, 175–176
  and uterine leiomyomata, 389
Hospice, terminal care in, 187–189
Hospital
  in patient transfer, 54, 422–427
  terminal care in, 187–189
Hospital Accreditation Standards, of Joint Commission on Accreditation of Healthcare Organizations, 68
Hospital Infection Control Practices Advisory Committee, of the Centers for Disease Control and Prevention, 92–93
Hospitalists, 108
Housekeeping, and occupational exposure to bloodborne pathogens, 411–412

HPV. *See* Human papillomavirus
HRT. *See* Hormone replacement therapy
HSIL test results, 263–264. *See also* Cervical cytology
HSV. *See* Herpes simplex virus
Human chorionic gonadotropin (hCG), and ectopic pregnancy, 288–289
Human immunodeficiency virus (HIV), 225, 319–321, 372
  confidentiality and testing, 15–16
  exposure to, 51
  health care professionals with, 24–25, 319
  knowledge of, 320
  patient and professional resources, 320–321
  precautions for health care workers, 92–93, 319
  testing for, 123*t*, 126, 128, 130, 132, 225, 319
Human papillomavirus (HPV), 223–224
  among adolescents, 147
  and cervical cancer, 215, 223, 341
  testing for, 143, 224
Human resources, 13–30
  personnel, 13–14
  and professional behavior, 14–30
Hydatidiform moles, 347–348
Hyperglycemia, in diabetes mellitus, 210–213
Hypersensitivity reactions, following immunizations, 326–327. *See also* Allergic reactions
Hypertension, 206–208, 321–324
  classification of, 207–208
  hormone replacement therapy and, 174
  management of, 322
  patient and professional resources, 324
  risk groups for, 321
  treatment algorithm for, 323*f*
Hysterectomy
  for cervical cancer, 264
  for chronic pelvic pain, 274
  for endometriosis, 303–304
  for uterine leiomyomata, 388

I

Immunizations, 325–329
  ACOG recommendations for, 325–326. *See also* Primary and preventive care
  contraindications to, 326–327
  for health care professionals, 24
  hypersensitivity reactions following, 326–327
  patient and professional resources, 328–329
Impaired clinicians, 21–24
Inappropriate conduct, of health care professionals, 21–24
Incontinence, 179–180, 360, 386–387
Industry, guidelines for relationships with, 26–27
Infection(s)
  and cancer, 215
  of older women, 181
Infection control, 86–94, 405–417. *See also* Bloodborne pathogens
  cleaning in, 86–87
  disinfection in, 87–92, 88*t*–89*t*
  isolation precautions, 92–93
  sterilization in, 87–92, 88*t*–89*t*
Infertility, 330–335
  counseling for, 330
  patient and professional resources, 331, 335
  and uterine leiomyomata, 389
Influenza vaccination, 127, 129, 131, 133, and risk factors for, 123*t*
Information management, 99–104
  and informed consent, 104
  medical records, 99–101
  and patient communication, 101–104
Informed consent
  as ethical concept, 65
  and female sterilization, 153
  inability to provide, 65
  and information management, 104
  and institutional ethics committees, 73–74
  and institutional review boards, 70–71

Inpatient facilities
  equipment of, 84–85
  organization of, 84–85
Institutional ethics committees, 72–74
  education of, 73
  functions of, 72
  and informed consent, 73–74
  membership in, 72–73
  and quality assessment, 74
Institutional responsibility, in ethical decision making, 74–75
Institutional review board (IRB)
  documentation of activities, 71
  and informed consent, 70–71
  and patient protection, 69–71
  and research programs, 10–11, 69, 71
  selection of members, 69–70
Insurance
  of adolescents, 18, 146
  and billing/collections, 111–112
  and conflicts of interest, 26
  coverage, 119
  and practice coverage, 113–114
  and referrals, 19–20
  universal coverage, 119
Interhospital patient transfer, 53–56, 422–427
Interns, and credentials evaluation, 32
Interviews, in medical history, 135–136
Intimate partner violence, 231–233, 283–286
Intraoperative care, 250–251
Intrauterine device (IUD)
  contraindications and side effects of, 155*t*
  deaths associated with, 160*t*
  failure rate of, 158*t*
Iodine intake, 203*t*
IRB. *See* Institutional review board
Iron intake, 203*t*
Isolation precautions, 92–93
IUD. *See* Intrauterine device

J

JCAHO. *See* Joint Commission on Accreditation of Healthcare Organizations
Job descriptions, 13, 35
Joint Commission on Accreditation of Healthcare Organizations (JCAHO)
  on continuous quality improvement, 45
  on facilities/equipment requirements, 80
  Hospital Accreditation Standards of, 68
  on medical history, 136
  on pain management, 356
  on patients' bill of rights, 66–69
  on privileges, 35
  on quality assessment, 40
Justice, as ethical principle, 64

K

Kortokoff sounds, in blood pressure measurement, 207–208

L

Laboratory tests, 96
  government regulation of, 51–53, 418–421
  office tracking system for, 103
  patient notification of, 103
  preoperative, 248–249
Laparotomy, patient positioning during, 250–251
Latex allergy, 252, 336–338
Laundry, contaminated, and occupational exposure to bloodborne pathogens, 412
LDL cholesterol. *See* Low-density lipoprotein cholesterol
LEEP. *See* Loop electrosurgical excision procedure

Legal issues
and end-of-life considerations, 185–187
expert witnesses, 20–21
impaired clinicians, 21–24
Leiomyomata, uterine, 388–390
Length of stay, after ambulatory gynecologic surgery, 252–254
Lesbian health, 169–171
Levonorgestrel subdermal implants
contraindications and side effects of, 154*t*
failure rate of, 158*t*
Liability, 57–61
and billing, 61
and practice coverage, 59–61
and referrals, 59–61
and risk reduction, 57–59
Lidocaine, as local anesthetic, 245
Linens, standard precautions with, 93
Lipid testing, 126, 128, 130, 132. *See also* Cholesterol
blood samples for, 209–211
risk factors for, 124*t*
Lipids, in preventive cardiology, 460*t*–461*t*
Lipoproteins, in preventive cardiology, 460*t*–461*t*
Living will, 185–187
Local anesthesia, 97, 244–246
emergency backup for, 245–246
selection of, 245
Loop electrosurgical excision procedure (LEEP), for squamous intraepithelial lesions, 263. *See also* Cervical cytology
Low-density lipoprotein (LDL) cholesterol, 209–210, 272–273
LSIL test results, 262–263. *See also* Cervical cytology
Lung cancer, 215
Lupus anticoagulant, and recurrent pregnancy loss, 364–365
Luteal phase defect, and recurrent pregnancy loss, 365

M

Magnesium intake, 202*t*
Male sterilization, failure rate of, 153, 159*t*
Malpractice suits, statute of limitations on, 101
Mammography, 128, 130, 132, 139, 217, 339
U.S. Food and Drug Administration regulations on, 50, 56–57, 82
risk factors for, 124*t*
Mammography Quality Standards Act, 56–57
Mammography Quality Standards Reauthorization Act, 57
Managed care
and conflicts of interest, 26–27
and practice coverage, 113–114
and referrals, 19–20
on timing of office visits, 121
Mandatory universal precautions, and occupational exposure to bloodborne pathogens, 407–408
MAOIs. *See* Monoamine oxidase inhibitors
Marijuana, 375
Masks
for occupational exposure to bloodborne pathogens, 410
as standard precaution, 93
Mastectomy, 341
Maternal age, preconceptional counseling and, 168–169
Mature minor, 17–18
Measles–mumps–rubella (MMR) vaccination, 124*t*, 127, 129, 131
Medicaid records
and end-of-life considerations, 185
retention of, 101
Medical equipment. *See* Equipment
Medical history
chief complaint in, 137
content of, 136–138
history of present illness in, 138

Medical history *(continued)*
past, family, and social history in, 138
in periodic assessments, 126, 128, 130, 132
in preconceptional care, 164
review of systems in, 138
in women's health examination, 135–138
woman's health record, 434–452
Medical office. *See* Offices
Medical practice, closing of, and patient referrals, 60–61
Medical procedures, patenting of, 27
Medical Products Reporting Program (MedWatch), of U.S. Food and Drug Administration, 95
Medical records
confidentiality of, 15–18, 100
information in, 99–100
management of, 99–101
in quality assessment, 47
requests for, 100–101
retention of, 101
woman's health record, 434–452
Medical staff appointments, 31–34
Medical tests, results of
confidentiality of, 15–16
office tracking systems for, 103
patient notification of, 103
Medicare
billing, 61
documentation, 136–137
and end-of-life considerations, 185
retention of records, 101
Medication(s)
dispensation of, 95
in preconceptional care, 164–165
names of, and conflicts of interest, 26–27
in quality assessment, 48
secure management of, 114
use by older women, 182–183
Medroxyprogesterone acetate
for endometriosis, 303
injectable
contraindications and side effects of, 154*t*
failure rate of, 158*t*
MedWatch, 95
Meetings, of Department of Obstetrics and Gynecology, 9–12
Memory, of older women patients, 177
Menopause, 171–176
confirmation of, 153
counseling during, 171–172
and hormone replacement therapy, 172–176, 314–318
symptoms of, 171
and vaginal lubrication, 229–230
Menorrhagia, 259
Meperidine, in conscious intravenous sedation, 246
Metabolism, of older women, 181
Methotrexate, for ectopic pregnancy, 288
Metronidazole, for trichomonas, 221
Metrorrhagia, 258
Midazolam, in conscious intravenous sedation, 246
Minors, rights of, 17–18
Minutes, of department meetings, 9
MMR vaccination. *See* Measles–mumps–rubella vaccination
Mobiluncus vaginitis, 224
Molar pregnancy, 347–348
Monoamine oxidase inhibitors (MAOIs), for depression, 280
Mood disorders, depression, 279–282
Moonlighting, 32–34
Morphine, in conscious intravenous sedation, 246
Mortality and morbidity, leading causes of, 134
ages 13–18, 127
ages 19–39, 129
ages 40–64, 131
ages 65 and older, 133
Mouthpieces, as standard precaution, 93

Müllerian fusion defects, and endometriosis, 299
Myomas. *See* Uterine leiomyomata
Myomectomy, abdominal, for uterine leiomyomata, 389

N

National Cholesterol Education Program Expert Panel on Detection, Evaluation, and Treatment of High Blood Cholesterol in Adults, 209, 272
National Heart, Lung, and Blood Institute
  body mass index classifications of, 195, 195*t*
  Sixth Report of the Joint National Committee on Prevention, Detection, Evaluation, and Treatment of High Blood Pressure, 207
  on waist circumference, 197
National Osteoporosis Foundation, on bone density measurements, 352
National Practitioner Data Bank (NPDB), 23
  contact information for, 33
  and credentials evaluation, 32, 38
Needlestick Safety and Prevention Act of 2000, 51, 406
Neglect, of elderly, 235
Neisseria gonorrhoeae, 219–220
Neoplasms, 339–350. *See also* Cancer
Neural tube defects
  risk of, 166, 199
  folic acid supplementation for prevention of, 166, 199
Niacin intake, 202*t*
Noncompliance
  behavior modification for, 266–268
  monitoring of, 103
Noncritical items, disinfection and sterilization of, 88*t*–89*t*, 91–92
Nonmaleficence, as ethical principle, 63–64
Nonsteroidal antiinflammatory drugs, in pain management, 356
NPDB. *See* National Practitioner Data Bank
Nurse practitioners, 34, 108–109. *See also* Advanced practice health care clinicians
Nurses' Health Study, 173
Nutrition
  and diabetes mellitus, 213
  dietary reference intakes, 202*t*–203*t*
  and fitness, 196–200
  history, 196
  of older women, 181
  and preconceptional care, 165–166
  in preventive cardiology, 457*t*–458*t*
  Recommended Dietary Allowances, 202*t*–203*t*
  among women with disabilities, 393

O

Observation of practitioner, as corrective action, 45–46
Obstetric and gynecologic privileges, 35
Obstetrician–gynecologists, 106–107
Occupational Safety and Health Administration (OSHA)
  on infection control, 86
  Occupational Exposure to Bloodborne Pathogens Standard of, 50–51, 405–417
Occupational Safety and Health Administration Compliance Consultation, 84
Office manager, 14
Office tracking systems, 103
Office visits, timing of, 121
Officers, of Department of Obstetrics and Gynecology, 4–7
Offices
  ambulatory gynecologic surgery in, 243
  facilities and equipment management in, 81–82
  governance of, 11–12

Offices *(continued)*
- human resource needs in, 14
- patient flow in, 112
- quality assessment in, 46–49
- risk management in, 49
- staffing requirements for, 105

Older women, 176–183
- cognitive changes in, 178–179
- common medical conditions of, 180–181
- communication with, 177
- functional assessment of, 177–180
- intraoperative management of, 251
- medication use by, 182–183
- psychosocial concerns of, 181–182

Oophorectomy
- for endometriosis, 304
- for ovarian cancer, 346

Operating room data tracking, 113

Opioids, in pain management, 356

Oral contraceptives
- for anovulatory uterine bleeding, 259
- combined
  - contraindications and side effects of, 154*t*
  - failure rate of, 158*t*
- deaths associated with, 160*t*
- as emergency contraception, 160–162, 161*t*
- for endometriosis, 302–303
- evaluation for, 151–152
- in preventive cardiology, 463*t*–464*t*
- progestin-only
  - contraindications and side effects of, 154*t*
  - failure rate of, 158*t*
- risks with, 151–152

Oral glucose tolerance test, 211–213

Organizations of gynecology and women's health care, resource list of, 469–477

Orgasm, lack of, 229

OSHA. *See* Occupational Safety and Health Administration

Osteoporosis, 350–353
- evaluation of, 352
- menopause and, 171–172
- among older women, 180
- patient and professional resources, 353
- postmenopausal, 314–315, 350
- treatment for, 352

Outreach surgeons, privileges of, 37

Ovarian cancer, 174, 217, 345–346

Ovulation method, failure rate of, 158*t*

P

Pain management, 354–357
- assessment in, 354–356
- at end-of-life, 189
- for endometriosis, 302–303
- gate theory of, 356–357
- principles of, 355

Palliative care, at end-of-life, 184–185

Pantothenic acid intake, 202*t*

Pap tests, 142, in periodic assessments, 126, 128, 130, 132. *See also* Cervical cytology

Parental consent, 17

PAs. *See* Physician assistants

Patenting, of medical procedures, 27

Paternalism, 64

Pathology services, 96, 251

Patient communication
- barriers to, 103–104
- management of, 101–104
- in quality assessment, 47

Patient flow
- management of, 112–113
- in quality assessment, 47

Patient history. *See* Medical history

Patient information. *See* Medical records

Patient notification, of test results, 103

Patient positioning
- in pediatric gynecology, 358
- during pelvic examination, 139–143
- during surgery, 250–251

Patient preparation, for ambulatory gynecologic surgery, 249–250
Patient protection, 66–71
  and institutional review boards, 69–71
  and patients' bill of rights, 66–69
Patient relations, in quality assessment, 47
Patient screening, federal requirements for, 53–56, 422–427
Patient Self-Determination Act of 1990, 185
Patient transfer
  air transport, 55
  education about, 56
  federal requirements for 53–56, 422–427
  procedures for, 425
  refuse to consent to, 425–426
Patients' bill of rights, 66–69
Pediatric gynecology, 358–359
Pediatric patients, 144. *See also* Adolescents; Children
Peer review
  confidentiality of, 43
  external, as corrective action, 45
Pelvic examination, 139–143, 312–314, in periodic assessments, 126, 128, 130, 132
Pelvic floor dysfunction, 360–361
Pelvic inflammatory disease (PID), 220–221
Pelvic mass, evaluation of, 346
Pelvic organ prolapse, 360
Pelvic pain, chronic, 274–276
  conditions associated with, 275
  diagnosis of, 274, 276
  and endometriosis, 302
  evaluation of, 274, 276
  patient and professional resources, 276
  treatment for, 274, 276
Penicillin, in vaccines, 327
Periodic abstinence, 158*t*, 160*t*
Periodic assessment
  ages 13–18, 126–127
  ages 19–39, 128–129
  ages 40–64, 130–131
  ages 65 and older, 132–133
Perioperative considerations, in ambulatory gynecologic surgery, 247–254
Personal protective equipment, for occupational exposure to bloodborne pathogens, 93, 409–411
Personnel management, 13–14, 48. *See also* Human resources
Pharmacy services, 95
Phenylketonuria, preconceptional counseling and, 168
Phosphorus intake, 202*t*
Physical examination, 138–143, in periodic assessments, 126, 128, 130, 132
Physician assistants (PAs), 34, 109–110. *See also* Advanced practice health care clinicians
Physicians. *See* Health care professionals
PID. *See* Pelvic inflammatory disease
PMS. *See* Premenstrual syndrome
Pneumococcal vaccination, 127, 129, 131, 133, risk factors for, 124*t*
Polypharmacy, among older women patients, 182–183
Postexposure evaluation, in infection control, 320, 413–414
Postoperative care, 250–251
Postovulation method, failure rate of, 158*t*
Postpartum depression, 169
Power of attorney, 186–187
Practice coverage, 59–61, 113–114
Practice management, 105–115
  billing and collections, 111–112
  medication security, 114
  patient flow, 112–113
  practice coverage, 113–114
  staffing, 105–111
Practitioner–patient relationship, termination of, 103
Preanesthetic assessment, 97
Preconceptional care, 163–169
  counseling in, 166–169
  history in, 163–166
    of environmental factors, 166
    medical, 164

Preconceptional care, history in *(continued)*
of medication and substance abuse, 164–165
reproductive, 165
nutrition in, 165–166
physical assessment in, 166
Pregnancy
among adolescents, 147–148
and domestic violence, 232, 283
early complications of, 287–290
ectopic, 287–290
emergency medical conditions in, 423–424
termination of, 382–385
unintended, 153
Pregnancy loss. *See also* Spontaneous abortion
causes of, 364–365
patient and professional resources, 366
recurrent, 364–366
testing of, 365*t*
Premenstrual syndrome (PMS), 362–363
Preoperative evaluation, 247–249
Primary and preventive care, 118, 121–144, 192–193
periodic assessment in
ages 13–18, 126–127
ages 19–39, 128–129
ages 40–64, 130–131
ages 65 and older, 132–133
risk factor indications in, 122*t*–125*t*
women's health examination in, 134–143
Privileges
added skills or qualifications, 36–37
in ambulatory surgical facilities, 11
blanket approval for, 35
delineation of, 34–37
granting of, 31–38
obstetric and gynecologic, 35
of outreach surgeons, 37
provisional status of, 36
reduction of, 38, 46
renewal of, 37–38
restriction of, 38, 46
Privileges *(continued)*
revocation of, 38, 46
special, 36–37
temporary, 36
termination of, 38, 46
voluntary surrender/restriction of, 38
Proctoring, as corrective action, 45
Professional behavior, 14–30
and billing fraud, 27–28
and chaperons, 18–19
and communicable diseases, 24–25
and confidentiality, 15–18
and conflicts of interest, 25–27
and ethical conduct, 14
and expert witnesses, 20–21
and impaired clinicians, 21–24
and referrals, 19–20
and sexual harassment, 28
and sexual misconduct, 28–30
Progestins
and breast cancer, 316
cyclic, for anovulatory uterine bleeding, 259
Protective clothing, for occupational exposure to bloodborne pathogens, 93, 410–411
Provider-Performed Microscopy Procedure, certificate for, 419–421
Provisional status, 36
Psychiatric disorders, and premenstrual syndrome, 362. *See also* Depression
Psychological factors, in preventive cardiology, 459*t*
Psychosocial issues
abuse, 230–235
depression, 235–236
evaluation of, 126, 128, 130, 132
with older women, 181–182
sexuality, 227–230
substance abuse, 237
in women's health care, 226–237
Psychotherapy, for depression, 280
Public accommodations, in Americans with Disabilities Act, 430

Q

Quality assessment, 40–49
  collection and analysis of data in, 42–43
  and continuing competency evaluations, 38
  and corrective actions, 43–46
  and institutional ethics committees, 74
  institutional governance and, 8
  meetings concerning, 9
  in offices, 46–49
  screening tools, 40–41
Quality indicators, gynecologic, 42

R

RADAR Model, of domestic violence assessment, 233
Radiation, exposure to, 81
Radiology services, 96, 103
Rape, 367–370
  legal issues with, 368–369
  patient and professional resources, 369–370
  screening for, 367–368
Reasonable accommodation, in Americans with Disabilities Act, 429–430
Reception areas, 80–82
Recertification, 37–38
Recommended Dietary Allowances, 202*t*–203*t*
Record-keeping. *See* Documentation
Recovery period, after ambulatory gynecologic surgery, 252–254
Rectovaginal examination, 130, 132, 140
Recurrent pregnancy loss, 364–366
Referrals, 19–20
  with closing of medical practice, 60–61
  and liability, 59–61
  physician self-interest and, 11
  reluctant, 60
Refuse to consent to transfer, 425–426
Refuse to consent to treatment, 104, 424–425
Regional block anesthesia, 97
Registered nurse first assistants, 110–111
Registered nurses (RNs), 107–108
Remedial education, as corrective action, 44–45
Reporting
  of domestic violence, 285
  of rape/sexual assault, 368
  of test results, 15–16
Reproductive awareness, 150
Reproductive health care, for adolescents, 145–146
Reproductive history, 165
Reproductive years, women's health care during, 150–169
Research programs
  and institutional review boards, 69, 71
  patient protection in, 66
  at teaching hospitals, 10–11
Residency Review Committee for Obstetrics–Gynecology, 10
Residents
  and credentials evaluation, 32
  and dual employment (moonlighting), 32–33
  privileges of, 33
Restrooms, in offices, 82
Resuscitation devices, in ambulatory surgery facilities, 246–247
Riboflavin intake, 202*t*
Risk factors
  in adolescents, 146–147
  in primary and preventive care, screening, 122*t*–125*t*, 126–133
Risk management, 57–61
  clinical care issues in, 58–59
  elements of, 57–58
  in offices, 49
RNs. *See* Registered nurses
Rubella titer assessment, 126, 128, risk factors for, 124*t*

S

Safety, in health care settings, 81
Scheduling, management of, 112–113
Scope of practice
  ambulatory women's health care services, 117–119
  obstetrics and gynecology, 433
Screening. *See* Primary and preventive care
Sedation, conscious intravenous, 246–247
Selective estrogen receptor modulators (SERMs)
  for breast cancer prevention, 176, 316
  in hormone replacement therapy, 176
  for osteoporosis, 176, 316
Selective serotonin reuptake inhibitors (SSRIs), for depression, 280
Selenium intake, 203*t*
Self-assessment inventory for patients, 192
Semicritical items, disinfection and sterilization of, 88*t*–89*t*, 90–91
SERMs. *See* Selective estrogen receptor modulators
Sex discrimination, 28
Sexual abuse, 234
Sexual activity, among adolescents, 147–150
Sexual assault, 367–370
  legal issues with, 368–369
  patient and professional resources, 369–370
  screening for, 367–368
Sexual assault assessment kit, 368
Sexual desire, 228
Sexual dysfunction, 227–230
  patient and professional resources, 371–372
  treatment of, 370–371
Sexual function, 227–230
Sexual harassment, 12, 28
Sexual history, 227
Sexual misconduct, 28–30
Sexual orientation, 22. *See also* Lesbian health
Sexual response pattern, 370
Sexuality, 227–230, evaluation of, 126, 128, 130, 132
Sexuality education, 148–150
Sexually transmitted diseases (STDs), 218–225, 372–374
  of adolescents, 147
  counseling for, 226
  evaluation of, 219–225
  among lesbians, 169–170
  partner treatment and, 373
  patient and professional resources, 373–374
  prevention of, 219
  risk factors for, 124*t*, 218–219
  testing for, 126, 128, 130, 132
Sharp instruments, standard precautions with, 93, 408
Sharps injury log, 417
Sigmoidoscopy, flexible, 130, 132
Sixth Report of the Joint National Committee on Prevention, Detection, Evaluation, and Treatment of High Blood Pressure, 207
Skin examination, 126, 128, 130, 132, risk factors for, 125*t*
Skin preparation, preoperative, 250
Smoking, 375–381
  behavior modification for, 267
  and coronary heart disease, 456*t*
  and lung cancer, 215
  patient and professional resources for, 267–268, 380–381
  treatment for, 379
Sodium intake, 197
Sonography, in breast examination, 139
Special credentials and privileges, 36–37
Spermicides
  contraindications and side effects of, 156*t*
  deaths associated with, 160*t*
  failure rate of, 158*t*
Spinal anesthesia, 97
Spontaneous abortion, 287–290
  diagnosis of, 288–289
  patient and professional resources, 289–290

Spontaneous abortion *(continued)*
recurrent, 364–366
treatment for, 289
SSRIs. *See* Selective serotonin reuptake inhibitors
Staffing, 105–111
Standard precautions, for infection control, 92–93, 407–408
Standing committees, 8
State medical societies, on impaired clinicians, 22–23
STDs. *See* Sexually transmitted diseases
Sterilization, in infection control, 87–92, 88*t*–89*t*
Sterilization (contraceptive)
failure rate of, 159*t*
female, 153
Strengthening exercises, safety guidelines for, 205
Stretching exercises, safety guidelines for, 205
Subspecialties, 107
Substance abuse, 164–165, 237, 375–381, *See also* Alcohol abuse; Drug abuse
Suicide
adolescents and, 147, 281
depression and, 236, 279, 281
domestic violence victims and, 285
Supporting services, 95–98
Surgeons, outreach, privileges of, 36–37
Surgery
ambulatory gynecologic (*See* Ambulatory gynecologic surgery)
in medical records, 100
privileges, 34–37
Surgical assistants, 110–111
Surgical facilities
ambulatory
facilities and equipment management in, 81–82
governance of, 11
staffing requirements for, 105, 110–111
American College of Surgeons classification of, 83
Surgical facilities *(continued)*
equipment of, 82–84
organization of, 82–84
physical design of, 83–84
Surgical instruments
critical items, 87–90, 88*t*–89*t*
disinfection and sterilization of, 87–92, 88*t*–89*t*
noncritical items, 88*t*–89*t*, 91–92
semicritical items, 88*t*–89*t*, 90–91
Symptothermal method, failure rate of, 158*t*
Syphilis, 221, 372

T

Tamoxifen
for breast cancer prevention, 176, 217, 340
and endometrial cancer, 344
Target heart rate, 201
Teaching hospitals, research programs of, 10–11
Technology, and patient communication, 101–102
Teen pregnancy, 147–148
Telemedicine, 102
Telephone communications
protocols for, 102
in quality assessment, 47–48
Temporary privileges, 36
Teratogens, sources of information on, 167
Terminal care, 187–189
Termination of pregnancy, 382–385. *See also* Abortion
Test(s). *See also* Laboratory tests; Medical tests
in Clinical Laboratory Improvement Amendments, 52
results of
confidentiality of, 15–16
patient notification of, 103
Testimony, from expert witnesses, 20–21
Tetanus–diptheria booster immunization, 127, 129, 131, 133

Thermometers, disinfection of, 91
Thiamin intake, 202*t*
Third party, and confidentiality, 66
Thromboembolic disease, hormone replacement therapy and, 174
Thromboprophylaxis, 250
Thyroid disorders, 298
Thyroid-stimulating hormone testing, 125*t*, 128, 130, 132
Tobacco use, 215, 375–381. *See also* Smoking
Toxicology screenings, for substance abuse, 379
Transfer, of patients. *See* Patient transfer
Transport team, in patient transfer, 55
Trazodone, for depression, 280
Treatment programs, for impaired clinicians, 22
Trending, in continuous quality improvement, 41
Trichomonas vaginalis, 221
Tricyclic agents, for depression, 280
Troubled clinicians, 24
Tubal sterilization, 153
Tuberculosis skin testing, 126, 128, 130, 132, risk factors for, 125*t*

U

Ultrasonography, 96, gynecologic, 312–314
Universal precautions, 92–93, 407–408
Urinalysis, 132
Urinary incontinence, 179–180, 360, 386–387
U.S. Department of Agriculture
  Food Guide Pyramid of, 197, 198*f*
  height/weight chart of, 193, 194*t*
U.S. Food and Drug Administration (FDA)
  and institutional review boards, 69
  Mammography Quality Standards Act of, 50, 56–57
  Medical Products Reporting Program (MedWatch) of, 95
U.S. Preventive Services Task Force
  on bone density measurements, 351–352
  on cholesterol screenings, 209
Uterine leiomyomata, 388–390
  imaging techniques for, 389
  patient and professional resources, 389–390
  treatment for, 389

V

Vaccinations, 51, 325–329. *See also* Immunizations; Primary and preventive care
Vaginal atresia, and endometriosis, 299
Vaginal lubrication, lack of, 229–230
Vaginismus, 229
Vaginitis
  candidal, 224–225
  Gardnerella, 224
  Haemophilus, 224
  Mobiluncus, 224
  in pediatric gynecology, 358–359
Vaginosis, bacterial, 224
Varicella vaccination, 125*t*, 127, 129, 131, 133
Vasectomy, 153
Vasovagal reactions, 252
Venous thromboembolism, prevention of, 250
Violence. *See also* Abuse
  domestic, 283–286
  against health care professionals, 81
Visual disorders, among older women, 179
Vitamin A intake, 202*t*
Vitamin B_6 intake, 202*t*
Vitamin B_{12} intake, 202*t*
Vitamin C intake, 203*t*
Vitamin D intake, 202*t*
Vitamin E intake, 203*t*
Vitamin K intake, 203*t*
Voluntary Review of Quality Care, of American College of Obstetricians and Gynecologists, 41
Vulvar cancer, 346–347

W

Waist circumference, as risk indicator, 197
Waived tests, in Clinical Laboratory Improvement Amendments, 52
Warning labels/signs, and occupational exposure risk, 415
Weight, proper for height, 193–195, 194*t*
Weight management, in preventive cardiology, 458*t*–459*t*
Wellness programs, 267
White coat hypertension, 208
Withdrawal method of contraception, failure rate of, 158*t*
Woman's Health Record, of ACOG, 434–452
Women with disabilities, 391–395
  abuse of, 393–394
  Americans with Disabilities Act, 428–432
  communication with, 391–392
  physician understanding of disability, 393
  professional resources, 394–395
Women's health care
  during adolescence, 145–150
  ambulatory services, 118
  continuum of, 144–191
  and lesbian health, 169–171
  during menopause, 171–176
  for older women, 176–183
  organizations, 106, 469–477
  psychosocial issues in, 226–237
  during reproductive years, 150–169
  for women with disabilities, 391–394
Women's health examination, 134–143
  breast examination, 138–139
  general examination, 138
  medical history in, 135–138
  pelvic examination, 139–143
Women's Health Initiative, 173
Work practice controls, for occupational exposure to bloodborne pathogens, 407–408
World Health Organization
  classification of female circumcision/female genital mutilation, 306
  definition of disability, 391

Y

Yeast infections, 224–225

Z

Zinc intake, 203*t*